Dear Reader

said that th

To Ronald with very best wishes from Myles
hoping that it might stimulate your interest
in Medical History further

Myles

The Dawn
of Drug Safety

Myles D B Stephens

The discovery, reporting and management of adverse drug reactions prior to and including the Thalidomide disaster

The farther backward you can look, the farther forward you are likely to see ~ *Winston Churchill*

Historical knowledge is indispensable for those who want to build a better world ~ *Ludwig von Mises*

If you would understand anything, observe its beginning and its development ~ *Aristotle*

Published by
George Mann Publications
Easton, Winchester,
Hampshire SO21 1ES
+44(0)1962 779944

A CIP catalogue record for this book
is available from the British Library

ISBN 9780956087485

George Mann Publications

Contents

Part 3. Regulatory Responses to Adverse Drug Reactions

The drugs being marketed prior to 1960 and subsequently removed/restricted from the market:

Amidopyrine	Mercury
Antimony	Mercury Amide Hcl
Arsenic Sodium	Methapyrilene
Aspirin (paediatric)	Nialamide
Bismuth	Oxomemazine
Buformin	Oxyphenbutazone
Bunamiodyl	Oxyphenisatin
Carisoprodol	Phenacetin
Chloral hydrate	Phenformin
Chloramphenicol	Phenobarbitone
Chloroform	Phenolphthalein
Cincophen	Phenylbutazone
Clioquinol	Piperazine
Coralgin	Pyrithyldione
Cuproxane	Stalinon
Dantron	Sulfamethoxydiazine
Datura	Sulfamethoxypyridazine
Diamthazole	Sulfathiazole
Diethylstilboestrol	Tetracycline (paediatric)
Dihydrostreptomycin	Thalidomide
Dinitrophenol	Thenalidine
Dipyrone	Thiomersal
Ethchlorvynol	Thorotrast
Glutethimide	Triparanol
Iproniazid	Urethane

Preface

This book is not a history book. It investigates how adverse drug reactions were discovered, what information was given and how it was given. The progress of regulations to control the safety of drugs is followed until the Thalidomide disaster. Thalidomide was such a watershed that the whole approach to drug safety changed. The literature published over such a long period is vast and I have only reviewed a small amount of it, but I hope that it is sufficiently representative that it has not missed too much. In order to link the chronologically listed pharmacovigilance events in time I have also included some important medical events. It has been necessary to include the sources inspected, but which yielded no information, so that the reader can draw their own conclusions as to whether the sources are sufficiently representative as to support the conclusions that I draw. Six marker drugs have been chosen to follow and perhaps I should have chosen a different set, but they do seem representative of the pharmacopoeias over time. The terminology of the various adverse events described has changed with the passing of time to such an extent that it is difficult to group them for analysis. The analyses are in a tabular format, which I hope is not too daunting for the reader.

There is a strong bias towards the English language publications and a bias towards French, Italian and German literature in that order. Publications in other languages have not been accessed due to language difficulties and, therefore, only secondary English language sources have been used. For the benefit of those whose second language is English much of the spelling has been changed to modern British spelling.

My main sources have been: the Wellcome Library, the Royal Society of Medicine library , the British Medical Association library, Medline, Embase, PubMed Central, Medicina Antiqua, Bulletin de Médecine Ancienne, US National Library of Medicine, the Internet Library of Early Journals and, of course, Wikipedia and Google. I am also indebted to the great scholarship of Professor Mann's 'Modern Drug Use' an enquiry on historical principles, and Dr Sneader's 'Drug Discovery', both superb books.

This book is based on published works and as such may give a biased impression as to what was really happening in the world. Adverse drug reactions occurring to those in remote areas of developed countries or in undeveloped countries had little chance of being reported. An account of rural general practice in Essex, UK, in the nineteen thirties revealed that the doctors prepared and dispensed their own drugs including 'Vinum Ferri' for their richer patients; this was made by putting a pound of nails into a Winchester jar and filling it with cooking sherry. The mixture was shaken every day for 3-4 weeks and then allowed to settle. It was prescribed for anaemia (Barber, 1974). No doubt a similar lag occurred in other ages and countries.

Acknowledgements

My task would have been impossible without the help of the Wellcome Library. Both the Royal Society of Medicine library and the BMA library have been essential for my research. I am also grateful to the following individuals:

Dr Jeffrey Aronson for his general advice and specific suggestions for the Introduction and Chapter 1.

Dr Patrick Waller for his advice and suggestions on part 3.

Dr Abdul Kaadan for help with the translation of Kitab a-Munjih al-fibb.

David JB Stephens for help with German and French translations.

Dr Mike Hadoke for translation of the German papers on Aspirin and for his review of the book

Dr Nikolai Serikoff for help with the Arabic papers at the Welcome Library

Mr Will Percival for Latin translations

Dr You-Ping Zhu of Groningen University for information on Adverse Drug Reactions in Traditional Chinese Medicine

Sir John Crofton for help with the toxicity of streptomycin

Mr George Mann for his advice and superb crafting of the book from my rough manuscript.

Illustrations

I am very grateful for permission to use the following images and graphs:

Wellcome Collection Library, London for the images of arsenic adverse effects, mercury adverse effects, Morison's Pills, the doctors dispensatory, antimoine, opium poppy, Hyoscyamus niger and black hellebore.

Scribid Library for *World average income per person* and *Global population growth* from Alasdair Laurie's book *Proving Jesus*.

The American Medical Association for the Phenacetin warning leaflet.

I am very grateful to Lee W. Gilbert of Manly NSW, Australia, for permission to use his photograph of 'Dawn, Tasman Sea' for the cover of this book.

Introduction

Abroad definition of pharmacovigilance is *'the watchfulness in guarding against danger from drugs or providing for drug safety'* (Abenheim et al, 1999). There are many different definitions, some place emphasis on post-marketing activities while others cover both pre and post marketing activities (Stephens, 2004). The definition given by the WHO in 1969 was: *'pharmacovigilance: one means by pharmacovigilance the notification, the registration and the systematic evaluation of the adverse reactions to medicines delivered with or without a prescription'*; this was the earliest reference to 'pharmacovigilance' that I have found (WHO, 1969). The information on these reactions can be obtained, either by voluntary notifications by general practitioners or from hospitals and centres previously designated (spontaneous pharmacovigilance), or by the application of epidemiological techniques allowing the systematic collection of information from certain sources: hospitals, representative samples of the medical profession, etc. (intensive pharmacovigilance).

The pharmacovigilance cycle starts with the patient, who after taking a drug and then having an adverse event reports it to a health professional who reports it to a national authority (or pharmaceutical company) which investigates it, establishes the full facts, and assesses them before passing it to the WHO monitoring centre. If this new adverse event supports other data to suggest an adverse drug reaction (ADR) then this is a signal[1]. This signal is then followed up and if on the balance of probabilities it is considered an ADR then it is likely to be published and communicated to all those who prescribe drugs, enabling them to use the information for the benefit of future patients. Unless the cycle is completed pharmacovigilance has failed.

---

[1] signal = anything that suggests that action should be taken is a signal, but a more formal definition is 'information that arises from one or multiple sources (including observations and experiments), which suggests a new potentially causal association, or a new aspect of a known association, between an intervention and an event or set of related events, either adverse or beneficial, which would command regulatory, societal or clinical attention, and is judged to be of sufficient' (Hauben & Aronson, 2009).

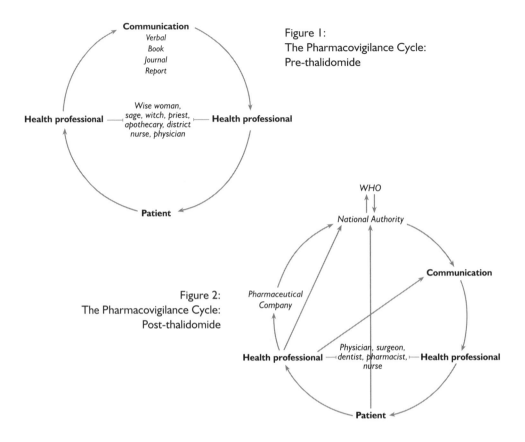

Communication
Verbal
Book
Journal
Report

Wise woman, sage, witch, priest, apothecary, district nurse, physician

Health professional — **Health professional**

Patient

Figure 1:
The Pharmacovigilance Cycle:
Pre-thalidomide

WHO

National Authority

Communication

Pharmaceutical Company

Figure 2:
The Pharmacovigilance Cycle:
Post-thalidomide

Physician, surgeon, dentist, pharmacist, nurse

Health professional — **Health professional**

Patient

The Pharmacovigilance Cycle

In the beginning the diameter of the cycle was small–involving only parent or grandparent to child or family, but as tribes developed the diameter would have increased to cover the whole tribe and a learned elder/philosopher/ priest would have entered the cycle as a pseudo 'health professional'. When the tribes united into a nation and a central government was formed another authoritative figure would have taken control and issued edicts concerning the production and use of herbs and other materials used as medicines (Figure 1). The method of communication changed from oral in the first instance to the written word and then finally to the printed word. The method used would have influenced the form of the message and comprehension of the recipient. Only the literate would have been able to understand the message and so another person, again a health professional, would have had to interpret the message for the masses. The means of communication were:

13,000–25,000 BC Cave paintings, limited by the presence of suitable caves and the availability of pigments.

3200 BC Small clay tablets were used by Assyrians, Sumerians and the Babylonians (from Mesopotamia) (Bottered, 2000), which was between the Tigris and the Euphrates – present-day Iraq). Cuneiform characters were engraved on the tablets using a stylus. Later the tablets were left to dry or even fired in a kiln.

3000 BC Papyrus is an early form of paper produced from the pith of the papyrus plant, *Cyperus papyrus*, a wetland sedge that was once abundant in the Nile Delta of Egypt. Papyrus is first known to have been used in ancient Egypt and was produced as early as 3000 BC, but it was also widely used throughout the Mediterranean region, as well as inland parts of Europe and south-west Asia.

c1200 BC In China, documents were written on bone or bamboo, making them heavy and awkward to transport. The earliest examples of Chinese writing date to the late Shang period.

868 BC Wood block printing by Tong dynasty.

301 BC Parchment was first mentioned. Parchment is a thin material made from calf skin, sheep skin or goat skin. Parchment is not tanned, but stretched, scraped, and dried under tension, creating a stiff white, yellowish or translucent animal skin. The finer quality parchment was called vellum.

973 AD First Chinese Herbal printed.

c1000 AD Paper was introduced by the Arabs.

1040 AD Invention of movable type in China.

1452 AD Printing was invented by Johann Guttenberg. It was a further 100 years before the number of medical books started to soar.

1476 AD William Caxton set up his printing press in London.

The communications described here fall into different categories:

a) Poetry, in which the aim is solely to entertain rather than to be helpful to patients; here the information is stated as common knowledge.

b) Aphorisms, many of which are succinct statements whose frequent aim is to appear witty; others are statements of principles. There is a very strong publication bias in favour of decrying drugs.

c) Sources of true helpful advice addressed to prescribers. Many of these are herbal recipe books, dispensatories or pharmacopoeias describe drugs/herbs and the methods for preparing them for use; but frequently without giving the indications for use or their adverse effects. The flood of publications after the widespread introduction of printing contained a lot of dross, which had accumulated over the centuries, as well as the helpful publications (Ring, 1972).

d) Scientific papers giving details of individual cases, which often contain the first reports of new ADRs.

Bayes'[2] theorem can be applied in Pharmacovigilance as:

Prior probability of adverse reactions + Human experience = Posterior probability of adverse reactions

The prior probability consists of the total information known about the drug before its first use in humans. Historically, the early evidence of toxicity would have been its effect on animals. Since the early users were aware of the potential toxicity of herbs/mineral they are likely to have to have been more alive to that possibility when the new herb was similar in any way to a known toxic herb/mineral.

Ideal knowledge of an adverse drug reaction

The information on an adverse drug reaction that should be available in order to give the maximum help to the prescriber is:

- ✧ The manifestation (clinical or laboratory) both subjective and objective
- ✧ Graded both for severity and seriousness
- ✧ Frequency or incidence, both absolute and relative to similar drugs with confidence intervals
- ✧ Mechanism of action
- ✧ Causality
- ✧ Predisposing factors
- ✧ Treatment and its effect
- ✧ Reversibility or sequelae

Although this is achievable, it is very rare that even with a modern drug and with all the modern facilities for investigation, those responsible bother to attain it. Using these criteria we shall see how little we know about the 'well known' reactions to our six marker drugs.

To illustrate the process of pharmacovigilance over the centuries six 'marker' drugs have been followed in this book:

---

[2] Bayes = Thomas Bayes (1702 – 1761) was an English clergyman who proposed a theory of probabilities; his work was published posthumously in 1774.

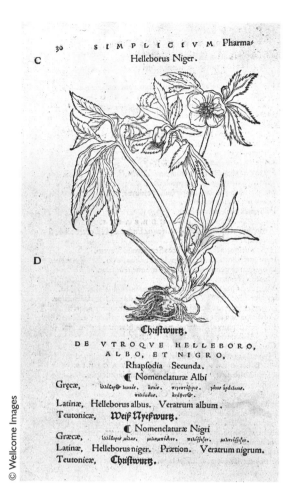

I. Hellebore

There are two types of hellebore: Helleborus (buttercup family) with 20 species and Veratrum (lily family, Liliaceae), with 45 species.

(i) Black Hellebore (*Helleborus niger*, Christmas Rose, *Helleborus officinalis*)

Dating from 585 BC and in frequent use as a purgative but with serious type A reactions. It contains the glycosides: helleborin, $C_{36}H_{42}O_6$ a potent narcotic, helleborein, $C_3H_{44}O_{15}$, helleboresin, $C_3OH_{38}O_4$, and helleboretin, $C_{14}H_{20}O_3$, hellebrin, $C_{36}H_{52}O_{15}$, a digitalic narcotic. Used for purging and as an abortifacient and emmenagogue. Its action is due to enhanced sodium ion conductivity, which activates the Bezold-Jarish reflex[3] causing slowing of the heart rate and lowering of the blood pressure.

The high amounts of ranunculin or protoanemonin in the leaves, stems and flowers of *H. niger* are responsible for dermatitis, which can follow exposure to bruised root material, leaves, stems and flowers. The cardiac glycosides present are responsible for toxic digitalis-like effects: bradycardia, prolonged P-R interval, idioventricular rhythm, bundle-branch block, ventricular fibrillation, slow, irregular pulse and asystole. These are thought to be more with the other species of the hellebores rather than with *H. niger*.

(ii) Any of various plants of the genus *Veratrum,* especially *V. viride* of North America, having large leaves and greenish flowers and yielding a toxic alkaloid used medicinally. The name was given to a number of toxic plants, whose precise identification still causes confusion.

---

[3] Bezold-Jarish reflex = when the cardiac sensory receptors are stimulated by stretch or drugs there is increased parasympathetic activity and inhibition of sympathetic activity promoting reflex bradycardia, vasodilatation and hypotension and at the same time modulating renin release and vasopressor secretion (Mark, 1983)

(a) White Hellebore, now known as *Veratrum album*

The latter plant is highly toxic, containing Veratrine, protoveratrine A and B, and the teratogen cyclopamine and jervine. Used as an emetic. A European plant.

Veratrum is irritating and ingestion can result in a burning sensation in the upper abdominal area followed by salivation, vomiting, purging, sneezing, gastric erosion, hypotension, and bradycardia. There have been several poisonings reported in humans with the different species. Although the latter plant is highly toxic, it is believed to be the 'hellebore' used by Hippocrates as a purgative. Some maintain that *V viride* and a*lbum* are identical. Reveratrol was isolated in 1940 from the roots of white hellebore.

(b) Green hellebore or Veratrum viride or American hellebore.

Not too dissimilar from *Veratrum album*, but with slightly different constituents. It causes sneezing, watery eyes, excess saliva, vomiting, diarrhoea, a burning sensation in the mouth and throat, and inability to swallow. These symptoms are followed by a tingling sensation, dizziness, possible blindness, paralysis of the arms and legs, mild seizures, slowed heartbeat, irregular heartbeat, and low blood pressure. Death occurs when the drug stops either the heart or the lungs. (Jaffe et al, 1990 ; Peterson, 1905). It was still used in 1952 for hypertension as Veriloid or Sabidilla (SED 1952).

2. Henbane (*Hyoscyamus niger, Jusquiame noire, L. Solanacées***)**

Used from about 3500 BC. Other herbs with similar actions include *Datura stramonium,* (jimson weed, angel's trumpet, thorn apple), *Atropa belladonna* (deadly nightshade), *Mandragora*

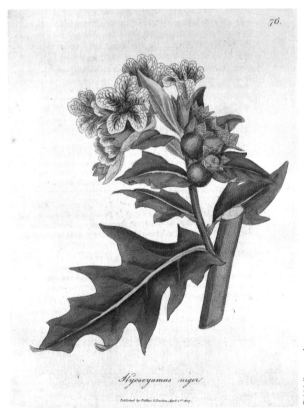

76.

Hyoscyamus niger

Published by Phillips & Jordan, April 1st 1809.

officinarum (mandrake). These plants contain the tropane alkaloids: atropine, scopolamine (hyoscine), and hyoscyamine. Henbane contains not less than 0.05% hyoscyamine and also hyoscine and atropine. Used as an hypnotic and anodyne. There are 15 species of annuals, biennials, and perennials in this genus, which is distributed through Western Europe, northern Africa, and central and south-western Asia. H. niger is found in base sandy soil, near the sea. Its use faded as it its component alkaloids were identified and manufactured. One of these alkaloids, scopolamine, was used until recent years with a form of morphia, colloquially known as 'Om & Scop,' (Omnopon + scopolamine) as an anaesthetic premedication. Used in 1694 for madness, melena, asthma, difficulty in breathing, epilepsy, and as a purge and as a diuretic.

3. Mercury

Included because of its use from at least 1500 BC and its resurgence as a treatment for syphilis in the 1500s AD until now when it is finally disappearing. Tomb (nr 1) of the ancient cemetery of Costebelle, attributed to the 4th century AD, contained the skeleton of a pregnant female and that of her fœtus in the pelvic cavity. This was aged seven months, was almost complete and showed an exceptional example of bony lesions suggestive of infection. Its pathology suggested the likelihood of early congenital syphilis. This case raises the question of the theory of the importation of venereal disease into Europe, about a 1,000 years later, by the crews of Christopher Columbus in 1493 AD. The fœtus of Costebelle is not an isolated example: other osteo-archaeological findings make a case for the existence of a treponeme (venereal or non venereal) in Europe before 1493 (Palfi et al, 1995).

The end of the use of thiomersal (*O*-(ethylmercurithio) benzoic acid), which contains 50% mercury by weight and is metabolized into ethyl mercury and thiosalicylate, as a preservative in vaccines is imminent. The different inorganic forms of mercury are: mercuric iodide HgI_2, mercuric oxide HgO, corrosive sublimate (mercuric chloride $HgCl_2$), calomel (mercurous chloride $HgCl$) and the pure metal Hg (Quicksilver). Its various forms have differing adverse effects. The crude ore is cinnabar, which contains mercuric sulphide, HgS. Mercury's principal use was in syphilis, but it was also used in gout, cancer, palsy, asthma, obstructions of the liver and gall bladder, leprosy and women's disorders (Harris, 1734).

4. Opium, *Papaver somniferum*

Opium is included because its use spans 4200 BC to the present day and its adverse effects are well known. It consists of many alkaloids including: morphine < 23%, papaverine < 11% (peripheral action depressing plain muscle), codeine < 1% (only 1/20 as much narcotic action as morphia but ¼ its action on cough and respiratory centre), thebaine 1%, narcotine < 10% (excitant action on the respiratory centre) and noscapine <8% each with its own actions and adverse effects.

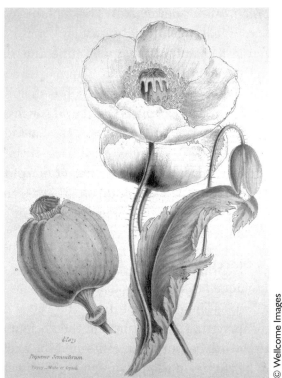

5. Aspirin Acetylsalicylic acid

This is one of the earliest synthetic drugs, 1899, and yet is still a major drug today. Its beneficial and adverse effects have only slowly become fully known. Its precursors were the active principles isolated from several common salicylate-containing herbs:

- ✧ *Betula lenta* (sweet birch)
- ✧ *Betula pendula* (white birch)
- ✧ *Filipendula ulmariaor* or *Spiraea ulmaria* (meadowsweet). The name *Spiraea* was incorporated into the trade name of acetylsalicylic acid by Bayer–Aspirin.
- ✧ *Gaultheria procumbens* (wintergreen)
- ✧ *Populus balsamifera* (balsam poplar)
- ✧ *Populus nigra* (black poplar)
- ✧ *Populus candicans* (balm of Gilead)
- ✧ *Salix alba* (white willow)
- ✧ *Viburnum prunifolium* (black haw)

The resulting drugs, obtained from these herbs, were:

- ✧ Salicin $C_{13}H_{18}O_7$. Used for acute rheumatism, typhus, typhoid, cerebrospinal fever (i.e. meningitis), scarlet fever, diphtheria and pneumonia.
- ✧ Salol (phenyl salicylate) $C_{13}H_{10}O_3$. Used as an antipyretic and for: duodenal catarrh, catarrh of the bile ducts, catarrhal jaundice,

gonorrhoea, infective diarrhoea and typhus.

✧ Sodium salicylate $NaC_7H_5O_3$. Used for acute and chronic rheumatism, headaches, phlegmasia[4] alba, osteoarthritis, gout and back pain,

✧ Methyl salicylate $CH_3C_7H_5O_3$. Used as ointment but it is absorbed and therefore also has systemic effects.

✧ Salicylic acid $C_7H_5O_3$. Used for acute rheumatism, typhus, typhoid, cerebro-spinal fever, scarlet fever, diphtheria, pneumonia, dyspepsia, worms, aphthae, thrush, lumbago, neuralgia, diabetes and hectic fever.

✧ Acetylsalicylic acid $C_9H_8O_4$. Aspirin, whose uses are too many to number.

All of these salicylates were in the 1914 British Pharmacopoeia.

6. Streptomycin

Molecular Formula: $C_{21}H_{39}N_7O_{12}$

Description: an antimicrobial organic base produced by the growth of certain strains of the Actinomycete *Streptomyces griseus*, or by any other means. Discovered in January 1944 by Schatz, Bugie and Waksman and used for many different types of infection. Its place here is justified by its use for tuberculosis in the first randomised controlled clinical trial in 1946 when the first supplies of streptomycin became available in the UK. It had been available in limited amounts for studies in the USA since its discovery. Each of the literature sources has been searched for references to these marker drugs.

Discussion

The axiom that there is no such thing as a safe drug means that if a substance has any active principle that influences the body then it is called a drug and that active principle may, if given in the wrong dose, cause an adverse event or if the person is allergic to it they may suffer an allergic drug reaction. The official definition of a drug: *Any substance or mixture of substances destined for administration to man for use in the diagnosis, treatment, investigation or prevention of disease or for the modification of physiological function'.* Safety can only be discussed in the context of the balance between the chance that it will do good and the chance that it will do harm—the so-called risk/benefit ratio. The choice of drug to be used must depend on the balance of the cost/benefit ratio of one drug compared with the cost/benefit ratio of all the other treatments that might benefit the patient.

---

[4] Phlegmasia = phlegmasia alba = inflammation of the femoral vein causing a white swollen leg

Part 1. Chronicles of Drug Safety

The verbatim descriptions of the adverse events associated with herbs and drugs, in chronological order, with special reference to the six marker herbs and drugs. All these are put into context with the important contemporary medical events, and the relevant laws and regulations.

Chapter 1: Pre-biblical Era: Inserts: Alchemy.

Chapter 2: Biblical Era – 1200 AD: Inserts: Adulteration of drugs, and Medical Philosophies.

Chapter 3: 1200 to 1500 AD: Inserts: The Age of Herbals and Dispensatories, Apothecaries.

Chapter 4: 16th Century: Inserts: Dose, Dichotomy

Chapter 5: 17th Century: Inserts: Journals, Tracts and Monographs.

Chapter 6: 18th Century: Inserts: Terminology, and Self-experiments.

Chapter 7: 19th Century: Inserts: Secret remedies, Placebo, Disease nomenclature, Adverse Reaction Committees, Interactions, and Health Insurance schemes.

Chapter 8: 20th Century: Inserts: Type B allergic reactions, Poison, Demise of drugs, Persistence of drugs, Panaceas, The strength of the evidence that an adverse event was caused by a drug, Books on the side-effects of drugs, and Regulations and laws.

Chapter 1. Pre-biblical period

From the beginning of time until ~~untit~~ 30 AD. Alchemy was born out of superstition and magic.

One can only conjecture that animals and primitive man could distinguish, by trial and error, between plants and berries that were edible and those that were poisonous, and by an extension of this that they knew that some were beneficial when they were ill and that whether the plant or berry was beneficial or produced adverse effects depended on the amount they took. Some modern research supports this hypothesis.

An African chimpanzee that was ill because of a parasitic intestinal infection with the nematode worm, *Oesophagostomum stephanostomum*, chewed the pith of *Vernonia amygdalina*, with recovery in 24 hours. The pith of *V. amygdalina* was found to contain vernonioside B1 and vernoniol B1, which had antiparasitic activity. Chimpanzees avoid the leaves, which contain the highly toxic compound vernodalin. (Huffman, 2001) For several African ethnic groups, a concoction made from *V. amygdalina* is used for treating for malarial fever, schistosomiasis, amoebic dysentery, several other intestinal parasites and stomach aches (Huffman, 2001). In two cases, recorded in detail, recovery from such symptoms was evident 20-24 hours after the individuals chewed the bitter pith. In one of these cases, the eggs per gram (EPG) of faeces of an *Oe. stephanostomum* infection could be measured; it fell from 130 to 15 in 20 hours (Huffman, 2001).

Most domestic or wild ungulates[5] that graze on rangelands with poisonous plants do not succumb to these plants. Animals can cope with poisonous plants, using both behavioural and physiological adaptations. Behavioural mechanisms converge on postingestive feedback and aversive conditioning, as animals learn which plants cause illness. Physiological mechanisms centre on detoxifying plant compounds in the gut by rumen microbes or in the liver through enzymatic reactions that allow toxins to be excreted. Domestic livestock are more often made ill or killed by toxic plants than are wild ungulates, probably because wild animals have more developed avoidance or detoxifying capabilities than do livestock (James, 1999).

---

[5] ungulates = hoofed mammals

Stone Age – Middle Palaeolithic (180,000 - 22,000 BC)

80,000–60,000 BC

Evidence of the use of herbal remedies goes back some 60,000 years to the Shanidar burial site at the foothills of the Zagros Mountains in north-eastern Iraq, where the remains of a Neanderthal man were uncovered in 1960 by Ralph Solecki (Solecki, 1975). Here there were what appeared to be ordinary human bones 60-80,000 years old and plant remains surrounded the dead man. Study of the plants suggested that the plants *may* have been chosen for their specific medicinal properties. Yarrow, Cornflower, Bachelor's Button, St. Barnaby's Thistle, Ragwort or Groundsel, Grape Hyacinth, Joint Pine or Woody Horsetail and Hollyhock were represented in the pollen samples, Achillea-type, Centaurea solstitialis, Senecio-type, Muscari-type, Ephedra altissima, and Althea-type, all of which have medicinal properties. There was also evidence of alcohol use, seeds belonging to the psfraisis plant, used in pits and fermented to produce a primitive alcoholic drink, were found in abundance next to the burial site (Lietava, 1992; Sommer, 1999).

25,000–13,000 BC

Medicinal plants were depicted at Lascaux, France, where the rock paintings in the caves have been radiocarbon dated to 13,000–25,000 BC. The Well Scene probably shows a shaman[6] in a trance state induced by psychedelic substances.

Stone Age – Neolithic Age (7,000 BC)

7000–5000 BC In the rock cave paintings in the Tassili-n-Ajjer Mountains in southern Algeria, dated 7000-5000 BC, there are images of dancers with fists full of mushrooms and have mushrooms sprouting from their bodies (McKenna, 1992; Lewin, 1991; Samorini, 2001). These two examples show the early use of psychoactive mushrooms, probably a mushroom from the Psilocybe genus, which contains high dosages of psilocybin, which induces vivid psychedelic experiences.

---

[6] shaman = person having access to the world of good and evil spirits

5000 BC Dried peyote buttons (from the Mexican cactus, *L ophophora williamsii*, which contains mescaline), subsequently found in Shumla Cave, Texas, provide evidence of peyote use.

A number of Linearbandkeramik[7] sites in the Rhineland and Swiss Neolithic lake villages dated to 5000-4500 BC have yielded samples of opium poppy seeds (*Papaver somniferum*) (Merlin, 1984).

4200 BC Alcohol was used, as shown by illustrations of the process of fermentation on pottery from Mesopotamia made around 4200 BC.

Archaeological samples of henbane have been found at the Bronze Age site of Feudvar in Serbia (Sherratt, 1995) and at a Neolithic ritual site at Balfarg in Fife, Scotland (Barclay and Russel-White, 1993).

Siddha medicine, which flourished in Southern India and dates back to almost 5000 BC, is a form of medical treatment using substances of all possible origins in a way that balances the possible harmful effect of each substance. This form of medicine was professed and practised by Siddha who wrote their recipes on palm leaves for the use of future generations. Siddha medicine was developed by outstanding Dravidians (ancient Tamils), locally called Cittars. Preparations are made mainly out of the parts of the plants and trees such as leaves, bark, stem, root, but also include mineral and some animal substances. This form of medicine is still well known today in South India, and is a form of Ayurveda. The use of metals like gold, silver and iron powders in some preparations is a special feature of Siddha medicine, which claims it can detoxify metals to enable them to be used for stubborn diseases. This claim is especially relevant in the case of mercury which is relatively often used in the system; this means that medicine containing purified mercury should only be received from a highly qualified practitioner of the art. Fruits such as the lemon and leaves of certain plants were frequently prescribed because of their medicinal properties, such as Margosa leaves for smallpox.

c4200 BC Evidence for opium found at Cueva de los Murcialagos (Spain) ('Bat Cave') has been radiocarbon dated to c4200 BC. A large

---

[7] Linearbandkeramik = first true farming communities in Central Europe. c5400-4900 BC

number of burials were accompanied by globular bags of esparto grass containing a variety of items including large numbers of opium poppy capsules. This suggested that the seeds had a symbolic significance beyond their use as a food source, and that this symbolism was particularly appropriate as an accompaniment for the dead (Sherratt, 1991).

4000 BC Further examples of rock art from Siberia, dating to c4000 BC, show spirits or shamans with mushrooms on their heads. These are likely to be the species Amanita muscaria, which was used extensively by Tungus Reindeer shamans to induce trances.

Sumerian[8] ideograms, dated to 4,000 BC, show the poppy as a plant of joy – probably the first record of human opium consumption (Scott, 1969).

3500 BC Sumerian pre-cuneiform script, mentioning the opium poppy (*Papaver somniferum*), has been discovered on tablets dating to around 3500 BC–5000 BC. These tablets were found at Nippur, a spiritual centre of the Sumerians located south of Baghdad, and described the cultivation of the opium poppy, including the collection of poppy juice in the early morning, with the subsequent production of opium. They also mention henbane (*Hyoscyamus sp*). The Assyrians[9] and the Egyptians were aware of the analgesic effects of a decoction of myrtle or willow leaves for joint pains.

3350 and 3100 BC

The Iceman was discovered on September 19, 1991 on Tisenjoch Glacier in Northern Italy. On two strips of hide, attached to his clothing, the Iceman carried spherical forms made of birch fungus. And microbiologists have identified them as the fruit of the birch fungus, *Piptoporus betulinus*, which is common in cold environments. If the fungus is ingested, it can bring on short bouts of diarrhoea because the fungus contains compounds that are both purgative and antimicrobial, as well as antimetazoan (Capasso, 1998). An autopsy showed that in the man's colon there were eggs of a parasitic whipworm, *Trichuris trichiura*. This infestation causes diarrhoea and acute stomach pains.

---

[8] Sumerians = relating to the early and non-Semitic elements in the civilisation of ancient Babylon.
[9] Assyrians = inhabitant of Assyria, region on the upper Tigris in North Mesopotamia.

3000 BC The discovery was made in late 1849 of the Royal Palace of King Sennacharib[10] (705–681 BC), which contained thousands of clay tablets and fragments containing texts of all kinds (royal inscriptions, chronicles, mythological and religious texts, contracts, royal grants and decrees, royal letters, assorted administrative documents, etc.) from the 7th century BC. The oldest clay tablets go back to 3000 BC.

c2500 BC *Pen Tsao* – a pharmacopoeia, or book containing an official list of medicines, was compiled under the direction of Emperor Shen-nung of China about 2500 BC. It describes the use of 365 medicinal plants, including opium (*Papaver somniferum*), ephedra (Ma huang, *Ephedra sinica/vulgaris/equisetina*), hemp, and chaulmoogra. It took approximately 2,000 years before the work of Shen Nung and his followers was documented in a book called *Shen Nung Pen Ts'ao Ching* [elsewhere it is called *Shen Nong Ben Cao Jing* or *Pen-Ching* or *Shenong Herbal*] by Ts'ao Hung-Ching (451–536 AD) and published in c500 AD. It contained the oldest known therapeutic description of *Cannabis sativa*. Henbane: *'forces one to walk madly and see demons.'* Shen-nung was reputed to have tasted all kinds of herbs and encountered seventy kinds of toxic substances in a single day, but he was a semi-mythical legend (Baohua & Xingjun, 2002).

Bronze Age (2,300–600 BC)

2000 BC At an archaeological site, Gonur South, in the Margiana district of Turkestan in the Kara-kum desert old bowls dating back to between the first and second millennium BC have been found with traces of cannabis, ephdra and opium, which are believed to be the constituents of Soma, a hallucinogenic potion.

Around 2,000 BC, people began to settle on the Japanese islands and engage in farming. They left behind unique earthenware with braid-like patterns on them. This period is generally called the Joumon era, (Joumon means braid). When archaeologists excavated the remains of residences dating to this period, they discovered the bark of Kihada *(Phellondron amurense Rupr.)*. It is the oldest herbal drug discovered in Japan.

---

[10] Sennacharib = ruler of Assyria

Archaeological samples of henbane have been found at the Bronze Age site of Feudvar in Serbia (Sherratt, 1995).

1760 BC The code of laws promulgated by Hammurabi, King of Babylon, 1792-1750 BC. These are inscribed on a stone monument, which was discovered at Susa, Iran.

§ 215. If a doctor has treated a gentleman for a severe wound with a bronze lancet and has cured the man, or has opened an abscess of the eye for a gentleman with the bronze lancet and has cured the eye of the gentleman, he shall take ten shekels of silver.

§ 218. If the doctor has treated a gentleman for a severe wound with a lancet of bronze and has caused the gentleman to die, or has opened an abscess of the eye for a gentleman with the bronze lancet and has caused the loss of the gentleman's eye, one shall cut off his hands.

§ 219. If a doctor has treated the severe wound of a slave of a poor man with a bronze lancet and has caused his death, he shall render slave for slave (Gutenberg project).

It is to be noted that there is no mention of drugs in these laws, solely surgery, but there remains the possibility that there was a similar set of laws concerning medicines. These stringent laws must have dissuaded surgeons from operating on cases with a poor prognosis in a similar way to the present situation where operative mortality lists might dissuade junior surgeons from operating on cases with a poor prognosis.

1600–1500 BC Mercury was shown to be present in the tombs of the 18th/19th dynasty of Egypt (Almkvist, 1932).

1550 BC The Ebers[11] Papyrus is a collection of 829 prescriptions, mentioning 700 drugs in just 135 pages. Compounded medications during this time period included gargles, snuffs, inhalations, suppositories, fumigations, enemas, poultices, decoctions, infusions, pills, troches, lotions, ointments and plasters. Beer, milk, wine and honey were popular vehicles for drugs while honey and wax were used as binding agents. Salts

---

[11] Ebers = George Ebers, 1837 – 1898, was a German Egyptologist who discovered the papyrus at Luxor (Thebes) Egypt.

of minerals of lead, iron, copper, antimony and mercury were used. Amongst the herbs mentioned are: hyoscyamus (henbane), opium and colchicum. (Mann, 1986). However, there is no mention of adverse drug effects (Ebers, 1937).

The use of the poppy during the Minoan age was more widespread as is shown by further archaeological discoveries in other parts of the island. Thus, in a grave at Pachyammos in the district of Hierapetra, opium was found in a jar of the Late Minoan III period (1300–1250 BC).

1400 BC Melampus, soothsayer and physician, used black hellebore for madness (Pliny, 77).

Iron Age (1200 BC – 400 AD)

1134 BC Podalirius is thought to have been the first person to practise blood-letting when he treated Princess Syrna for concussion (Halls Dalle, 1927).

1100 BC *Nicotiana tabacum* has been demonstrated definitively by study of mummies and desiccated corpses dating from at least 1100 BC.

The Druids, the Gallo-Celtics, used the leaves of gui, mistletoe, as a drink, which protected one from everything and made women fertile.

950 BC Homer's Odyssey IV
−750 BC

    Such useful medicines, only borne in grace
    Of what was good, would Helen ever have.
    And this juice to her Polydamna gave
    The wife of Thoon, all Ægyptian born,
    Whose rich earth herbs of medicine do adorn
    In great abundance. Many healthful are,
    And many baneful. Every man is there
    A good physician out of Nature's grace,
    For all the nation sprung of Paeon's race.

He is thought to have used the snowdrop, *Galanthus nivalis* (Moly), as an antidote for datura poisoning and as such would be the oldest recorded use of an anticholinesterase to reverse anticholinergic intoxication (Plaitakis & Duvoison, 1983).

1065–771 BC Wu Shi Er Bing Fang [Prescriptions for fifty-two diseases] lists 283 known prescriptions and 247 drugs, but contains no apparent reference to adverse effects. It was discovered in 1973 during the excavation of Ma Wang Dui tomb at Changsha, Hunan province of China (Leung, 1990).

1000 BC-800 AD

Ayurvedic[12] medicine flourished in Northern India during the time of Buddha (around 520 BC), and in this period the Ayurvedic practitioners were commonly using mercuric-sulphur combination-based medicines. They used also drugs of vegetable origin (fruits, leaves, bark, and roots), drugs of animal origin, and minerals such as gold, copper and iron. In the '*Caraka Samhita*' which is believed to have arisen around 400–200 BC, 2000 such drugs are included. A few such ancient drugs are still in use in modern medicine in their refined form, the well-known examples being quinine from cinchona bark, reserpine from rauwolfia and bromhexine from *Adathoda vascica*. Ayurveda's popularity declined between the 10th and 12th centuries. *http://ncbi.nlm.nih.gov/books/bv.fcgi?rid=hstat1.section.95686. Accessed* 23rd August 2009).

A study published in the Journal of the American Medical Association found significant amounts of toxic heavy metals such as lead, mercury and arsenic in 20% of Ayurvedic preparations that had been made in South Asia for sale in America. If taken according to the manufacturers' instructions, this 20% of remedies could have resulted in heavy metal intakes above published regulatory standards. Similar studies have been performed in India, and have confirmed these results. In response to the study, some practitioners of Ayurveda claimed that heavy metals are integral to some formulations and have been used for centuries. '*There is no point in doing trials as they have been used safely and have mention in our ancient texts.*' Chemical analysis of some modern antiarthritic medicines from Ayurveda has led to a finding that synthetic anti-inflammatory drugs like phenylbutazone, indomethacin and/or corticosteroids have been added (Saper et al., 2004).

---

[12] Ayurvedic = ayur = life, veda = knowledge.

Start of Roman Age

c600 BC King Assurbanipal of Sumeria, Assyria (668–626 BC) ordered the compilation of the first known materia medica, containing 250 herbal drugs. Examination of clay tablets in his library identified 120 mineral drugs and 250 vegetable drugs including asafoetida, calamus, cannabis, castor, crocus, galbanum, glycyrrhiza, *hellebore*, mandragora, mentha, myrrh, *opium*, pine turpentine, styrax[13], and thyme.

585 BC During the Siege of Kirrha (Greece), hellebore was reportedly used by the Greek besiegers to poison the city's water supply. The defenders were subsequently so weakened by diarrhoea that they were unable to defend the city from assault.

430 BC Empedocles (490–440 BC) from Agrigentum in Sicily wrote of the four 'roots or elements', which were water (cold and wet), air (hot and wet), fire (hot and dry) and earth (cold and dry). When combined in different ways, these succeed in producing all the varieties of vegetable and animal species on earth (Stathakou et al., 2007). These four elements became linked with the four humours. One of his comments was *'Refrain entirely from laurel leaves'*.

429–347 BC During the time of Plato the physicians of Greece were prohibited under penalty of death, from prescribing mercury.

410 BC Euripides *The Bacchae*

> *For a most cruel insanity*
> *Has warped your mind*
> *While drugs may well have*
> *Caused it, they can bring no cure.*

400 BC–700 AD

Papyrus was used in Egypt from late fourth century BC until the middle of the seventh century.

4th Century BC An inscription at the Acropolis dating from the 4th century BC commemorated that Evanor, the physician, had been chosen as inspector of drugs (Goldberg, 1986). (Uncorroborated).

400 BC Hellebore root extracts were used to induce vomiting without

---

[13] Styrax = genus of many species of large shrubs and small trees (*Styracus.*)

Greek physicians realizing that the root contains substances so irritating and poisonous that the patient quickly got rid of any ingested, although many died from the treatment. Mention was found on Sumerian clay tablets.

384 BC Aristotle (384–322 BC) Experimentation and observation were the cornerstones of Aristotle's science. He affirmed the precedence of facts over theory by declaring that if newly discovered facts contradicted a previously held theory, the theory had to be modified or discarded to accommodate them. In Aristotle, we can see the origins of modern science and the scientific method (http://www.greekmedicine.net/whos_who/ Aristotle.html).

370 BC Hippocrates (c460–370 BC) advocated an underlying theory of disease based on the four humours (blood, yellow bile, black bile and phlegm) and the four elements (earth, fire, water, air) with their pairs of associated qualities (wet and dry, hot and cold). Imbalances of one element led to an increase in the production of its associated humour, causing disease (Cahill, 2005). Belief in the 'humours' lasted into the early 20th century, and the humours were responsible for the practices of bloodletting, emesis and purging, which tormented patients over the centuries.

Hippocrates first reported adverse reactions to cow's milk around 370 BC. It is often quoted that Hippocrates said '*Primum non nocere*'. This is unsubstantiated and similarly Galen and Ambrose Paré have been cleared of responsibility. (Smith, 2005) However, it is the opinion of many scholars that Hippocrates did, in fact, originate the phrase, but did so in his *Epidemics,* Book. I, Section. XI. One translation reads: '*Declare the past, diagnose the present, foretell the future; practice these acts. As to diseases, make a habit of two things — to help, or at least to do no harm'.* Although this is an exhortation or command it should be interpreted as a hope. Whether the translation is accurate and it really means ' make a habit...to do no harm' is questionable. There must have always been a balanced judgement as to whether any action might cause harm or benefit. 'Cutting off of a doctor's hands' if he caused the patient to die only happened, one hopes, if the doctor was negligent. Now, of course, '*We must operate on sensible risk/benefit principles'* (Shelton, 2000). Hippocrates recommended chewing willow leaves for analgesia in childbirth. He was familiar with blood-letting.

Hippocrate's aphorisms:

> *'In acute diseases employ drugs very seldom and only at the beginning. Even then, never prescribe until you have made a thorough examination of the patient.'*

> *'Drugs may be administered to pregnant women from the fourth to the seventh month of gestation.'* (Chadwick & Mann, 1950).

> *'Leave your drugs in the chemist's pot if you can heal the patient with food.'*

> 37. *'Purgative medicines agree ill with persons in good health.'*

> 16. Hellebore (alias Christmas Rose, *Veratum niger* or *Helleborus niger*) *'is dangerous to persons whose flesh is sound, for it induces convulsion. ... Convulsions following the administration of hellebore are fatal.'* (The rhizome contains helleborin, and hellebrigenin. Helleborin is a potent narcotic with a burning acrid taste, while hellebrin is listed as a digitalic, narcotic and said to possess anticarcinomic characteristics. In its role as a digitalic it also can function as a purgative. It is a cardiac glycosides). Hippocrates was among those who used hellebore *'It was in such wide use that the old physicians used the medicine in similar cases that it produced the proverb* 'to need Hellebore' means that *'you have lost your senses.'* (Le Clerc, 1702).

354 BC *The Economist* by Xenophon[14] *'None whatever, unless we are prepared to admit that hyoscyamus, as they call it, is wealth, a poison the property of which is to drive those who take it mad.'* *'A dose of henbane, ' "hogs'-bean," so called.'* Diosc. 4. 69; 6. 15; Plut. 'Demetr'. xx. (Clough, v. 114).

320 BC Theophrastus of Eresos (372–286 BC), a Greek philosopher who had been a pupil of Aristotle and Plato, wrote *'De Historia Plantarum'* [About the history of plants] consisting of nine books, one of which is called *'Saps and medicines'*. Its full title:

---

[14] Xenophon = Exophanes, a Greek philosopher from Colophon

'De historia plantarum libri decem, græce & latine. In quibus textum græcum variis lectionibus, emendationibus, hiulcorum, supplementis: latinam gazæ versionem nova interpretatione ad margines: totum opus absolutissimis cum notis, tum De Causis Plantarums'. [Ten books about the history of plants, in Greek and in Latin. The Greek version has various readings, amendments, gaps and additions: the Latin version of the treasure house is with new interpretations in the margins: the whole work not only with very many notes but also Concerning the Causes of plants] Part of this work is devoted to plant lore and the medicinal uses of plants, making it the earliest complete extant herbal and pharmacopoeia as well. Contains 500 plants. He was aquainted with tolerance *'The virtues of all drugs become weaker to those who are accustomed to them, and in some cases become entirely ineffective. Thus some eat enough hellebore to consume whole bundles and yet suffer no hurt'.*

265 BC *Huang Di Nei Jing Su Wen* (The Yellow Emperor's Classic of Medicine). Although the *Huang Di Nei Jing* book's authorship is attributed to the Yellow Emperor, it was actually written by several authors over a long period of time. Differing opinions date the book between 800 BC and 200 BC. It is a compendium of medical theory and practice attributed to the Yellow Emperor who is thought to have lived around 4700 BC or to be a mythical character whose age and royal status would provide credence to a contemporary work (Hong, 2004). It is in the form of a dialogue between the master and a student. Translation by Mao Shing Ni, Publisher Shambuala, 1995.

This book is divided into two sections. The first is *Suwen* (The book of plain questions). The second part, called the *Lingshu* (The Vital Axis), was written sometime in the second century BC with revisions taking place up to the Han Dynasty (206 BC-25 AD). The three themes that run through the book are the theory of Taoism, Yin and Yang, and the five elements. *'There are toxic herbs and non-toxic ones. When greatly poisonous herbs are used to treat a disease the treatment should be stopped when this disease is recovered 60%. When commonly poisonous herbs are used the treatment should be stopped when this disease is recovered 70%.'* (xiaopg@public.bta.net.cn.). There is no mention of adverse effects.

c197–130 BC Nicander of Colophon[15] wrote *Alexipharmaca* (A poem in 630 hexameters), which deals with plant and animal poisons and their cures. He lists animal, vegetable, and mineral poisons, including aconite, white lead, hemlock, and opium, together with their symptoms and specific remedies. He describes poisons in general, and analyses 19 specific poisons (8 animal and 11 vegetable).

Poppy: '*Those who drink the juice of the poppy which carries its seed in the head suffer as follows: learn further that when men drink the tears of the poppy, whose seed are in the head, they fall fast asleep; for their extremities are chilled; their eye do not open but are bound quite motionless by their eyelids. With the exhaustion an odorous sweat bathes all the body, turns the cheeks pale, and causes the lips to swell; the bonds of the jaw are relaxed, and through the throat the laboured breath passes faint and chill. And often either the livid nail or wrinkled nostril is a harbinger of death; sometimes too the sunken eyes.*'

Henbane: '*Let no man fill his belly with Henbane, as men often do in error, or as children who, having lately put aside their swaddling clothes and head-bindings, and their perilous crawling on all fours, and walking now upright with no anxious nurse at hand, chew its sprays of baleful flowers through witlessness, since they are just bringing to light the incisor teeth in their jaws, at which time itching assails their swollen gums.*'

120–63 BC Mithridates VI, King of Pontus[16], had concocted by his physician Zopyrus an antidote to any possible poison, 'Mithridatium', which the king is said to have taken daily in gradually increasing doses and thereby developed multivariant tolerance such that, when later he was captured and imprisoned and tried to commit suicide, he was immune to the action of the poison (Hayes, 2001). It seems strange that having concocted an antidote and used it prophylactically that he should contemplate using a poison; it shows little faith in his own antidote. The king had tested it in 'clinical trials' on convicted criminals and slaves. It contained costmary, sweet flag, hypericum, gum, sagapenum, acacia juice, Illyrian iris, cardamom, anise, Gallic nard, gentian root and dried rose-leaves, poppy-tears, parsley, casia, saxifrage, darnel, long pepper, storax, castoreum, frankincense, hypocistis juice, myrrh, opopanax, malabathrum leaves, flower of round rush, turpentine-

---

[15] Colophon = ancient Greek city..
[16] Pontus = region on the south coast of the Black Sea

resin, galbanum, Cretan carrot seeds, nard, opobalsam, shepherd's purse, rhubarb root, saffron, ginger, cinnamon. These are pounded and taken up in honey (http://en.wikipedia.org/wiki/ Mithridate. Accessed 29th June 2009).

Andromachus the elder (c60 AD), physician to Emperor Nero, added squill, viper flesh and opium content, and called his preparation 'Theriaca Andromachi'.

When Mithridatium was used against poisoning, a piece the size of an almond was given in wine. In other affections an amount corresponding in size to an Egyptian bean is sufficient. The ingredients changed over the years: Celsus used 36 ingredients; Pliny said 54, Andromachus 64, Servilius Damocrates 48, and Galen 77 (Nutton, 1995). The different formulas and ingredients for 'Mithridatium' led to different names being given for them. Galen said that 'Mithridatium' had 41 ingredients and that another version, now called 'Galene', had 55 constituents. 'Galene' subsequently was called 'Theriaca' and this term finally became 'Venetian Treacle' (Griffin 2004), the word 'treacle' being a derivative of 'Theriaca'. It was also used for malaria and gradually became a universal panacea. The use of this medication continued until the 1780s. Heberden was loud in its denunciation: *As many people busy themselves with the practice of Physick who are unqualified to know what they are doing it may be advisable, for the sake of such as fall into their hands, to discountence a medicine which upon tradition of its sovereign virtue, or as a sudorific is often applied at random and, by means of the opium, does much mischief. The prescribed lies too much at the mercy of the person who gives the ingredients whether what he gives for an ordinary dose shall not contain dangerous or fatal quantity of opium and indeed it is hardly to be expected in such a multiplication of ingredients, that the usual dose will contain a just proportion of all of them'.* (Heberden, 1745).

A.E. Housman refers to it in *'A Shropshire Lad'* saying that the king was poisoned with arsenic and strychnine, which makes it strange as Mithridatium did not contain these poisons and would not have given any protection (presumably there was some poetic licence).

There was a king reigned in the East:
There, when kings will sit to feast,

They get their fill before they think
With poisoned meat and poisoned drink.
He gathered all that sprang to birth
From the many-venomed earth;
First a little, thence to more,
He sampled all her killing store;
And easy, smiling, seasoned sound,
Sate the king when healths went round.
They put arsenic in his meat
And stared aghast to watch him eat;
They poured strychnine in his cup
And shook to see him drink it up:
They shook, they stared as white's their shirt:
Them it was their poison hurt.
I tell the tale that I heard told.
Mithridates, he died old.

90–30 BC Diodorus Siculus, a Greek historian wrote '*Bibliotheca Historica*' a multi-volume history:

> '*Now during that day the army was disheartened, terrified as it was at both the strange happening and the great number of the unfortunates; but on the next day at about the same hour all came to themselves, gradually recovered their senses, and rose up from the ground, and their physical state was like that of men recovered after a dose of a drug.*'

49 BC Titus Lucretius Carus wrote the poem *De Rerum Natura* [On The nature of things] that includes the following lines:

> I will unfold, or wherefore what to some
> Is foul and bitter, yet the same to others
> Can seem delectable to eat,–why here
> So great the distance and the difference is
> That what is food to one to some becomes
> Fierce poison, as a certain snake there is
> Which, touched by a spittle of a man, will waste
> And end itself by gnawing up its coil.
> Again, *fierce poison is the hellebore*
> To us, but puts the fat on goats and quails.
> That thou mayst know by what devices this

Is brought about, in chief thou must recall
What we have said before, that seeds are kept
Commixed in things in divers modes...

(The Internet Classic Archives)

One is tempted to believe that the first passage suggests a personal idiosyncrasy, but it may refer to either a dose problem where tolerance has developed or the large differences in dose necessary for some drugs *'It may therefore be assumed that in a group of 100 persons there will be at least a fourfold difference between the doses required to produce equal effects upon the most susceptible and least susceptible individuals.'* (Wilson & Schild, 1952). The second passage is the first recording of the bane of toxicology in that the actions of drugs in animals do not necessarily foretell their action in man.

43–17 BC Ovid's *'Metamorphoses'*,
'Or perhaps the juice of some herb caused it?'
Ovid, Tristia (II.296) *'Eripit interdum, modo dat medicina salutem, quaeque iuuet, monstrat, quaeque sit herba nocens.'*

[Sometimes it rescues, but medicine gives health, it shows that always it may help, or always it may be a harmful plant].

'Medicine sometimes snatches away health, sometimes gives it.'

'Medicine sometimes grants health, sometimes destroys it, showing which plants are helpful, which do harm.'

42 BC *'Some remedies are worse than the disease.'* in *'Sententiae'* [Opinions] by Publilius Syrus.

29 BC Aegrescitque medendo [And people fall ill from being cured]
Vergil, Aeneid 12:46.

23 BC Horace. The poems of Horace consisting of odes, satyres, and epistles. Rendered in English verse by several persons. 1666

He was highly melancholy;
For this a lusty dose of *Hellebore*
He took, which did him to himself restore;
But being cur'd, he cry'd, and said, Alas!
Such an unhappy remedy ne'ere was;
For now by this unfortunate occasion,
I've lost the pleasure of imagination.

Alchemy

From the Arabic *al-kimiya*, al 'the' + *kimiya* 'transmutation'.

The term refers to the transmutation of inferior metals to gold or silver via the philosopher's stone, to the search for a universal panacea and the search for immortality. The substances most used were mercury and sulphur. The use of other metals in transmutation led to their use in medicine and accounts for the early detection of their side-effects. In addition to the physical research there was also an occult philosophy which seemed to involve the transmutation of 'man' into a superior being. Occult in this context meaning hidden from a logical mind. Some date its origin as early as 2000 BC, but the first acknowledged alchemist was Geber alias Abou Moussah Djafar al Sofi alias Abu Musa Jabir ibn Hayyan in the 8th century.

Summary

There is evidence that the medicinal use of herbs predated 50,000 BC but written evidence of their use was probably first recorded in about 3,500 BC. The reference to henbane in *Pen Tsao,* which was compiled by Emperor Shen-nung in about 2,500 BC, is the first reference that I have found of an adverse effect of a drug/herb, but since this work was not published until c 500 AD it cannot be considered reliable, especially as Emperor Shen-nung may have been a mythological figure. The statement that he tasted 70 toxic substances a day is obviously wrong; it was unlikely that there were 70 toxic substances available; it would have been impossible to take 70 substances a day unless he took many of them simultaneously, and there would have been insufficient time to assess their action. Homer's comment in 'The Odyssey' in 950 BC that many herbs are healthful and many baneful is more reliable. Thenceforth we start seeing reports of the adverse effect of individual herbs; firstly with hellebore in 585 BC and 400 BC and then with the specific problems concerning convulsions with hellebore from Hippocrates in 370 BC. Xenophon refers to henbane in *'The Economist'* in 354 BC as driving people mad. The adverse effects of poppy are first found in Nicander's *Alexipharmacas* in 197–130 BC and are given in some detail. By the beginning of the Christian era it was well known that herbs can be poisonous and that hellebore can cause diarrhoea, vomiting and convulsions. The main effects of the poppy were known and it was also known that henbane could cause madness. 'Known' means that there was written evidence, but it is likely that much more was known but not recorded. From Titus Lucretius Carus in 47 BC we learn that animals and humans may react differently and that there is individual variation in response to herbs with humans. The dating of a report gives us no information as to when the event reported took place and that is especially relevant during this early period.

Chapter 2. Biblical period to 1200 AD

From the time of Christ (30 AD) until 1200 AD covering the Roman age and the beginning of the Dark Ages, the Early Middle Ages and the start of the High Middle Ages.

30 AD Aulus Cornelius Celsus (25 BC–?37 AD) says in his book '*De Medicina*' [Concerning medicine]... '*A great deal has also been recorded concerning the powers of medicaments, as in the works of Zeno[17] or of Andreas[18] or of Apollonius[19], surnamed Mys. On the other hand, Asclepiades[20] dispensed with the use of these for the most part, not without reason; and 'since nearly all medicaments harm the stomach and contain bad juices, he transferred his treatment rather to the management of the actual diet'.*

Book 2, 12. '*Some endeavour to induce sleep by draught of pepper or hyoscyamus*'. He also stated that a boiled vinegar extract of willow leaves could be employed for the relief of pain (Rainsford, 2004). It appeared in print in 1478 soon after the introduction of the printing press. Although a Roman he used a few Greek words directly and also latinised other Greek words as well as translating Greek words into Latin (Wulff, 2004). He mentions white hellebore for an emetic and the black hellebore as a purgative. Opium/henbane: '*If... patients are wakeful, some endeavour to induce sleep by draughts of decoction of poppy or hyoscyamus.*' He used henbane for spastic or soft tissue pains, as a poultice for joints, leaves in an eye salve, the juice for earache and the root for toothache (Mann, 1984).

47 AD Scribonius Largus, (c1–50 AD) court physician to the Roman emperor Claudius, who came to Britain in AD 43, wrote '*De Compositiones Medicamentorum*' [Concerning the composition

---

[17] Zeno = Greek philospopher c490 BC–430 BC
[18] Andreas= physician to Ptolemy IV, died 217 BC
[19] Apollonius = physician c30 BC–c30 AD
[20] Asclepiades = Greek physician 124 BC–c40 BC who reduced the use of drugs, venesection and purgatives, preferring diet and water

of medicaments] describing 306 ingredients. The word 'anodyne' meaning able to relieve pain, is first found here. He recommended an inhalation of burned henbane seeds to drive out the 'tooth-worms', which caused decay. He was said by Lewin to be familiar with opium induced mental confusion, vertigo and headache (Lewin, 1883). In his account of opium he says *'The drug causes heaviness of the head, coldness and lividity of the limbs, and cold sweats. In addition, it causes difficulty of breathing, dullness of the mind and loss of consciousness'.* (Prioreschi, 1996).

77 AD Pliny the Elder, Gaius Plinius Secundus (23–79 AD) in *'Historia naturalis'* [Natural history].

Poppy: *'This juice is possessed not only of certain soporific qualities, but, if taken in too large quantities, is productive of sleep unto death even: the name given to it is 'opium.'*

Black Hellebore: according to Pliny, was used as a purgative in mania by Melampus, a soothsayer and physician, 1,400 years before Christ. He gave the uses of black hellebore as:*' paralysis, insanity, dropsy (provided there is no fever), chronic gout, joint disease, and it has the effect of carrying off the bilious secretions and morbid humours by stool. If given in any considerable quantity in combination with a sweet substance it is highly dangerous'.*

White Hellebore: It was used for: *'epilepsy, white elephantiasis, leprosy, tetanus, vertigo, melancholy, insanity, delirium, palsy, gout, dropsy, incipient tympanitis, stomach affections, cynic spasms, sciatica, quartan fevers, which defy other treatments, chronic coughs, flatulency, and other griping in the bowels.*

It is universally recommended not to give hellebore to aged people or children, to persons of a soft and effeminate habit of body or mind, or a delicate or tender constitution. … also it is not recommended in cases where the viscera are ulcerated or tumified, and more particularly when the patient is afflicted with spitting of blood, or with maladies of the side of the fauces'. He also gives advice on when to use hellebore. *'In order to secure a beneficial result, due precautions must be taken not to administer hellebore in cloudy weather, for if given at such a time, it is sure to be productive of excruciating agonies'.*

<u>Hyoscyamus</u>: *'known also as the Apollinaris, Henbane or Altercum. The root is sometimes made use of; but the employment of this plant in any way for medical purposes is, in my opinion, highly dangerous. For it is a fact well ascertained, that the leaves even will exercise a deleterious effect upon the mind, if more than four are taken at a time; though the ancients were of opinion that the leaves act as a febrifuge, taken in wine'... 'they have all of them, the effect of producing vertigo and insanity'. 'An oil (I say) is made of the seed thereof, which if it be taken into ears, is enough to trouble the brain.'* (*Naturalis Historiæ* translated by Philemon Holland 1601).

<u>Quicksilver</u>: *'It acts as a poison upon everything, and pierces vessels even, making its way through them by the agency of its malignant property.'* He also said *'The dung of wood-pigeon is particularly good taken internally as an antidote to quicksilver'.* (Bostock & Riley, 1855).

He used poplar bark infusions for pain in sciatica (Rainsford, 1984).

<u>Willow:</u> He also recommended a paste made from the ash of willow bark for removing corns and callosities (local application of salicylic acid is still used for warts). He goes on to say that *'the bark and leaves, boiled in wine , form a decoction that is remarkably useful as a fomentation for affections of the sinews'.*

Also he said *'Marvellous efficacy of human experiment, which has not left even the dregs of substance and the fouled refuse untested in such numerous ways'* (medicinal). There seems to have been no substance animal, vegetable or mineral that has not been used as a drug at some time.

He also criticised doctors: '*...but of all these facts the doctors, if they will permit me to say so, are ignorant—they are governed by names; so detached they are from the process of making up drugs, which used to be the special business of the medical profession. Nowadays whenever they come on books of prescriptions, wanting to make up some medicines out of them, which means to make trial of the ingredients in the prescriptions at the expense of their unhappy patients, they rely on the fashionable druggists' shops, which spoil everything with fraudulent adulterations, and for a long time they have been buying plasters and eye-salves ready-*

made; and thus is deteriorated rubbish of commodities and the fraud of the druggists' trade put on show'. (Book XXXIV.25).

78 AD Pedanius Dioscorides (c 40–90 AD) wrote *'De Materia Medica Libri Quinque'* [Concerning medical materials. Five books]:

> Book I   contains aromatics, oils, ointments and trees.
> Book II   lists living creatures, milk and dairy products, cereals and sharp herbs.
> Book III   describes roots, juices and herbs.
> Book IV   herbs and roots;
> Book V   vines and wines and metallic ores.

This text contains 950 curative substances, of which 600 are plant products and the rest are of animal or mineral origin (Ackerknecht, 1973). Each entry includes a drawing, a description of the plant, an account of its medicinal qualities and method of preparation, and warnings about undesirable effects.

Hellebore: *'White hellebore helps melancholy, the falling sickness, madness, gout, etc., but not to be taken of old men, youths, such as are weaklings, nice, or effeminate, troubled with headache, high-coloured, or fear strangling,'* saith Dioscorides. The pods and seeds: *'These both cause delirium and sleep and are scarcely usable.'*

Thorn Apple (*Datura strammonium*): *'The root being drank with the quantity of a dragm, has the power to effect not unpleasant fantasies. But 2 dragms being drunk, make one beside himself for three days and 4 being drank kill him. But the remedy of this is Melicrate (honey water), much being drank, and vomited up again.'*

Opium (*Papaver somniferum*): *'Taken as a drink too often it hurts, making men lethargic and it kills.'* Noted 'pruritus opii' (Dioscorides, 1516).

Mercury: *'Taken as a drink it eats through the internal organs by its weight.'*

Willow: Dioscorides suggested: *'The leaves [of the willow] being beaten small and drank with a little pepper and wine do help such as are troubled with the Iliac Passion [colic]... The decoction of the leaves and bark is an excellent fomentation[21] for the Gout ...'*

Colchicum: He also mentioned the poisonous properties of

---

[21] fomentation = a piece of cloth wrung out of boiling water or solution and placed on the disease site = poultice

colchicum (*Colchicum autumnale*) and he believed that an excessive use of coriander (*Coriandrum sativum*) affected the brain (Cilliers and Retief, 2000).

Henbane: '*Presently he filled a cresset[22] with firewood, on which he strewed powdered henbane, and lighting it, went round about the tent with it till the smoke entered the nostrils of the guards, and they all fell asleep, drowned by the drug.*' (History of Gharib and his Brother Ajib, Vol. VII, p. 7).

Nightshade; '*a drachm of the extract from the root when dissolved in water produces fleeting images that please the sense but if the dose be doubled it can cause immediate death.*' (Dioscorides P, c100 AD).

c150 AD Claudius Galen (c129–c199 [?131–201 AD]). Galen says that those substances which are assimilated are called foods and that all others are called drugs. The latter he breaks down to four classes:

'*There is one kind that remain as they are when taken, and transform and overpower the body, in the same manner that the body does foods; these drugs are of course deleterious and destructive to the animal's nature. The other kind takes the cause of its change from the body itself, then undergoes putrefaction and destruction, and in that process causes putrefaction and destruction to the body also. These too are clearly deleterious. In addition to these, a third kind heats the body reciprocally but does not harm; and a fourth both acts and is acted upon, so that they are gradually completely assimilated. This last kind, therefore, falls into the category of both drugs and foods.*'

He also says '*There are four faculties of the body as a whole: that which attracts familiar substances, that which retains these, that which transforms substances and that which expels alien substances. These faculties are those that belong to the entire substances of each of the bodies, which substance, as we have seen, is composed of a mixture of hot, cold, dry, and wet.*' (Singer, 1997). This philosophy of the four humours has no logical basis and when it affects the drawing of conclusions from the observation of medical events it may lead to false conclusions.

---

[22] cresset = fire basket

However, when the observer just reports his observation then we have a valuable statement. Examples follow:

'*All those who drink of this remedy recover in a short time, except those whom it does not help, who die. Therefore, it is obvious that it fails only in incurable cases*'. In '*Facultatum simplicium mediamentorum*' [Of the abundance of simple remedies] Galen saith *the seed (of poppy) is dangerous to be used inwardly.*'

<u>Hellebore</u> '*In subjects who have taken hellebore the pulse just before the vomiting, while they are undergoing compression, is broad, sparse, fairly faint, and fairly slow; as they are vomiting and retching it is uneven and irregular, as they recover it is regular, but still uneven, though less so than before; when they are close to the normal state it is even, larger than before and more vigorous.*' (Singer, 2002). This is from a chapter on the pulse showing that he paid a lot of attention to the minutiae.

Of <u>Jusquiame (henbane)</u> he said '*the jusquiame, which has the black berry, provokes sleep, and troubles the understanding. The one, which has the rather red berry, has almost the same properties as the other. However and one and the other are dangerous and venomous.*'

He used willow leaves for skin conditions (Brock, 1916). Galen also mentions interactions '*All such (cooling) drugs, then, when taken in small amounts and in conjunction with substances which are able to counteract the extreme nature of their cooling effect, may sometimes be of value to our bodies.*'

He developed the practice of using herbs in complex mixtures, which became known as 'Galenicals'. After Galen there was a period when experimentation ceased (Mann, 1984). His influence persisted until the 19th century.

150–250 AD Acharya Nagarjuna lived in India some time during the period 150–250 AD: he was a great alchemist and was later known as the "Father of Indian Chemistry". He was the first to use metal oxides, black sulphide of mercury (Kajjali) and other mercury preparations in medicine (Lamotte, 1966).

230 AD Hua T'o employed anaesthesia during surgical procedures. It was probably *Cannabis indica* mixed with wine or fumes of aconite, datura and hyoscyamus (Atkin 1995).

220 AD The first Chinese Herbal classic, '*Shen Nong Ben Cao*[23] *Jing*' [Classic of herbal medicine] was published, which divided 365 herbs into three categories according to their toxicity: These were reported in '*The Yellow Emperor's Classic of Medicine*' as a dialogue between Huang Di, who asks '*Can you tell me about the three grades of herbs that were recorded in the Shen Nong Ben Cao?*' and Qi Bo replies '*In ancient times the art of herbology was practised by categorizing all herbs into three classifications:*

The first category of herbs was called superior or immortal foods because of their lack of side effects and strengthening qualities (e.g. ginseng). These were often incorporated into one's diet and were used as preventative measures.

The second category of herbs was called medium or medicinal and were used to rectifying imbalances in the human body. These were used until the patient recovered from their illness and then withdrawn.

The third category of herbs was called inferior or radical herbs (e.g. croton) (*Croton tiglium*) which helps to relax the bowels, relieve oedema (swelling) or eliminate', *so named because they are strong in action and not without side effects; sometimes they are toxic. Therefore these were used often in small amounts and once the desired action took place they were discontinued immediately.*' (Maoshing Ni, 1995).

The concept of 'side-effects' is not recognised as such in Chinese medicine. The toxic effects of certain medicinals are recognized according to degree, and if it is necessary to use a 'toxic' substance medicinally, it will be prepared in a special manner or combined with other medicinals to reduce or eliminate toxicity if possible (Rosenberg, 1997). The difference between 'side-effects' and 'toxic effects' in this context is rather obscure. None of the books I have looked at have any specific adverse effects mentioned.

The Chinese meaning of 'toxic' should not be equated with the western connotation. 'What are recorded as toxic drugs only apply to those that have been found over time to be consistently toxic, though in different degrees, when used in the traditional manner. There are countless others that ordinarlily are not toxic

---

[23] Ben Cao = essential herb

but may be toxic if used outside of tradition' (Leung, 2001) www.phyto-tech.com/lchn/2001-0102.html (accessed 16th November 2009). I have not been able to find out how a herb is classified as 'toxic'. The many anomalies baffle me, e.g. arsenic disulfide–non-toxic, honeycomb–toxic. The '*Shen Nong Ben Cao*' has a phrase '*Take mercury over a long period, you will become a celestial being of immortality*'.

'*Toxicity can be reduced by proper processing, or by adding another herb to counter the toxicity.*' (Zhu, 2002). This reference to interactions is further explained by Paul Unschuld as 7 categories:

> xiāng xū, '*one helps the other*' means the mutual enhancement of similar effects of different drugs when administered together. This is also called 'mutual reinforcement'.
>
> xiāng shǐ, '*one endows the other*' means the mutual enhancement of different actions of different drugs when administered together. This is also termed 'assistance'.
>
> xiāang wèi, '*one fears the other*' the reduction of undesired effects of a drug by another drug with which it is administered. This is also called 'restraint', e.g. mercury restrains arsenic.
>
> xiāng shā, '*one kills the other*'. the elimination of undesired effects of a drug through another drug with which it is administered. This is also called 'neutralization'.
>
> xiāng wù, '*one hates the other*'. means the mutual reduction of desired effects of different drugs when administered together. This is also called 'counteraction'.
>
> xiāang fān, '*one clashes with the other*'. means producing undesired new effects through simultaneous administration of different drugs that are not produced when the drugs are administered individually. This is also called 'incompatibility', e.g. Radix *Veratri nigri* incompatible with Radix Ginseng, *Codopsis pilosulae*, Scrophulariae, *Salviae miltiorrhizae*, *Paeoniae alba* and also *Herba asari*.
>
> dān xíng, '*one goes alone*'. means administering a single drug without being influenced by other drugs administered simultaneously (Unschuld, 1998; Liu Yanchi, 1988).

While its attributed author is Shen Nong, no one knows for sure who wrote it. The book lists a total of 365 Chinese medicines from which 252 were of plant origin, 67 from animals, and 46 from minerals. Each medicine was divided into one of three categories. The superior category included 120 medicines. The second category included average medicines of which 120 were listed. The third category included 125 inferior medicines that were considered to be toxic with side effects It is difficult to follow the names of the herbals as they all seem to have several alternative names that look and/or sound alike, but may have additional words in the title and the English translations vary considerably. In the Pharmacopoeia of the People's Republic of China dated 2000 *Hyoscyamus niger* (Henbane) is labelled 'very toxic' and *Papaver somniferum* (opium) as 'toxic' (Zhu, 2002).

1st quarter of the 2nd century AD

'The Lord hath created medicines out of the earth; and he that is wise will not abhor them. Was not the water made sweet with wood that the virtue thereof might be known? And he hath given men skill, that he might be honoured in his marvellous works. With such doth he heal [men] and taketh away their pains. Of such doth the apothecary make a confection; and of his work there is no end; and from him is peace over all the earth....' The King James Bible, Apocrypha, Ecclesiasticus (38:4).

Early 4th century AD

The start of Western Monasteries. These monasteries were built as accommodation for travellers and gradually gave some medical care with herbs, e.g. Cluny in France had a large hospice in 1000-1050, which became a hospital. Hospices were under the Church whilst hospitals were controlled by physicians. Church hospices were frequently closed by the church since disease was God's punishment and curing it went against this principle. However since hospitals were now under the physicians' control they remained open. The first hospital was probably the one founded in Bagdad by Jibra'il ibn Bakhtishu c805. The Hotel Dieu in Paris opened in the 9th century and by the 15th century had 279 beds. From the point of view of adverse drug reactions this was the first time that a lot of sick patients were brought together under the care of physicians and they had many more patients than those purely in private practice. They had, therefore, better opportunites to study disease and adverse reactions leading, in due course, to the writing of case series.

452–536 AD Tao Hong-Jing wrote *'Ben Cao Jing Ji Zhu'* [Collection of commentaries on the divine husbandman's classic of materia medica] based on *'Shen Nung Pen Ts'ao Ching'*. He divided the herbs into categories and qualities then added 365 new herbs to his materia medica bringing the total number of herbs in this book to 730. In the *Shen nong Ben cao Jing, Ma huang*[24] is described this way: *'Bitter and warm; it is non-toxic, treating mainly wind, stroke, cold damage, headache, and warm malaria. It effuses the exterior through sweating, eliminates evil heat qi, suppresses cough and counterflow of qi, eliminates cold and heat, and breaks concretions and hardness, accumulations and gatherings.'*

454–473 AD *'Xiao Pin Fang'* written by Chen Yan Zhi. He discusses when to use higher doses or lower doses, e.g. *'In mild illnesses, or the early stages of an illness (in patients with normal strength), the amount of physical strength consumed by the illness is small. Therefore, the patient still has enough strength to endure the adverse effects of the medication and the dose can be increased.'* He was familiar with drug tolerance, e.g ephedrine. He says that the adverse effects of purgatives are that *'they exhaust the vital essence of life and reduce physical strength.'* He states that 'pulse palpation' is important for prognosis (Mayanagi, 1987).

476 AD End of Roman Age with the fall of Rome and start of the Dark Ages or Early Middle Ages.

480 AD Several works survive from Anglo-Saxon medicine in England, among them a 9th–10th century translation of *'Herbarium Apuleius'* the author was unknown and he is referred to as 'Pseudo-Apuleius (c480). It was one of the most copied herbal manuscripts, available in English. This work contains recipes and uses of 131 herbs, including *Papaver somniferum* (opium), *Herba symphoniaca* (henbane) and *Herba solatrim* (deadly nightshade); and is therefore more a prescription book than a

---

[24] *Ma huang* = from Ephedra sinica and contains ephedrine, an α and ß agonist and works mainly by releasing noradrenaline from the nerve endings (Cupp, 200)

herbal. The stylised diagrams of plants are very crude and there is no mention of any adverse events (Prioreschi, 2001) (see 1483 AD).

The Dark Ages from the 5th to the 8th centuries. They formed part of the Early Middle Ages.

5th Century AD The Irish used foxglove for weekly bed fever[25].

659 AD A physician named Su Jing, along with approximately 20 other of his compatriots wrote the '*Xin Xiu Ben Cao*' [Newly revised materia medica] (this may be the same as '*Hsin-hsiu Pen-ts'ao*' by Su Ching or '*Tang Ben Cao*' [Tang herbal], which was the first official pharmacopoeia in China and in the world (Wang, 1987). The pharmacopeia describes 850 drugs. It became a standard textbook in Japan in 787 AD.

In the seventh century the Japanese government sent physicians to China to study Chinese medicine. In 702 AD the Japanese government issued an Imperial Order to copy the medical educational system of the Chinese Tang Dynasty and set up a specialty of acupuncture and moxibustion (counter-irritation produced by igniting a cone or cylinder of moxa[26] placed on the skin). No apparent references to adverse effects. The Japanese developed their own system called 'Kanpo or Kampo Medicine' which means 'The Han method' referring to the herbal system in China during the Han Dynasty. In 753 AD a Chinese Buddhist priest, Jian Zhen, arrived in Japan and set up a school. In 1649 a Dutchman, Caspar Schomberger, brought western medicine to Japan.

6th–7th Century AD

Vagbhatta (Ayurvedic[27] physician) recommends internal use of mercury for therapeutic ends.

777–857 AD Yuhanna Ibn Masawaih Damasqui (Mesue Major), a Nestorian[28] physician, wrote '*Daghal al-'ain*' [Disorder of the eye] he also wrote '*Sumum wa Tiriaq*' [Poisons and antidotes] '*Ioanne Mesue*

---

[25] weekly bed fever = this was probably relapsing fever caused by *Spirillum obermeieri*, sometimes called famine fever or seven-day fever because of its association with destitution and periodicity of one week fever, one week recovering and then relapsing. I have found no other reference to this use of foxglove
[26] moxa = an Indian moss used for gout
[27] ayurevedic = a traditional Hindu system of medicine based on the idea of balance in bodily systems and emphasizing diet, herbal treatment and yogic breathing
[28] Nestorian = follower of Nestorius (c. 386–c. 451) became Archbishop of Constantinople

says that one needs to throw out the White Hellebore because it is poisonous and provokes the body.' He was said to have used charred mercury for external use on itchy skin (Abramowitz, 1934).

8th Century AD

The first acknowledged alchemist was Geber alias Abou Moussah Djafar al Sofi alias Abu Musa Jabir ibn Hayyan in the 8th century. He wrote on sulphur, mercury, arsenic, gold, silver, lead, tin, copper, iron, and magnesium (Waite, 1970). The discovery of sulphuric acid (H_2SO_4), nitric acid (HNO_3) and hydrochloric acid (HCl) has also been attributed to him. He wrote *'Kitab Assomoum wa Dafu Madariha'* [Poisons and their antidotes], in which he described poisons by their traits and natural origins, modes of action, dosages, methods of administration and choice of drugs. He also identified the target organ of each poison (Saad et al., 2006).

800 AD The monks of the Benedictine monastery at Monte Cassino in southern Italy used a mixture of opium, henbane, mulberry juice, lettuce, hemlock, mandragora and ivy, which had been soaked up by dry mushrooms and allowed to dry. It was called *Spongia somnifera,* [Sleep-bringing sponge] and they were softened and then were tamped into the nostrils and the ingredients were then absorbed percutaneously (Daems, 2001). However there is evidence that the S*pongia somnifera* was ineffective (Priorschi, 2003). This monastery was also associated with the medical school at Salerno (see Salerno 1140 AD).

808 AD Japanese authors wrote *'Datong Leiqi Fang'* [A generalisation of the ancient native herb formulas] (Dharmananda, 2008) www.itmonline.org/arts/kampo.htm. Accessed 26th June 2008.

Abu Hasan 'Ali ibn Sahl Rabban at-Tabari who was born in 808. He wrote several medical books, the most famous of which is his *'Paradise of Wisdom'*, completed in 850. He warned that one mithqal (about 4 grams) of opium or henbane causes sleep and also death. (http://islqamset.com/heritage/pharmacy/3rd&9th. html Accessed 23rd August 2009).

813–873 AD Ibn Wahshiyah wrote '*Kitab al-sumum*' [Book on poisons]

Henbane '*This is a drug in which there is an injurious poison which is fatal through cold and dryness, drying of the blood and its clotting in the heart and veins...it is fatal in one to two days..his mind becomes disordered, his tongue swells so that it fills his mouth, he raves and then he is perplexed, he is lazy and lethargic, his sight is darkened and a violent vertigo affects him. He has difficulty in breathing, a continuous snoring in his throat, redness of the cheeks, shivering, violent coldness, and extreme sluggishness. The extremities become cold, the entire body acquires a yellowishness and the teeth chatter. When he sleeps and snores, his soul is about to leave.*'

Hellebore '*There are three kinds of hellebore. One is white. The black is the worst of them, and the most lethal and most penetrating. The third kind is blue... Whoever eats or drinks it experiences a serious quinsy in his throat, swelling of the tongue, trembling, palpitation of the heart, intense shivering, and he is cold so that he thinks he is in snow, his mind is disordered, often serious prostration befalls him, he vomits frequently. It is thus not useful for him but, on the contrary, it injures him. Often many (humoral) mixtures arise so that his soul departs.*'

Black hellebore '*black hellebore kills dogs and cats especially whilst white hellebore kills birds.*'

White hellebore '*When a man smells it, he coughs continuously...it produces a strong thirst, drying of the palate and throat, burning in the stomach, itching of the rest of the body, persistent tickling, excessive vomiting to such a degree that it seems to him that his stomach is drawn upward and the contents of his belly plucked upward, and perhaps one or both of his hands dry up.*' (Levey, 1966).

857 AD Annales Xantenses for the year 857: '*Great plague of swollen blisters consumed the people by a loathsome rot, so that their limbs were loosened and fell off before death.*' This is possibly the first account of ergotism.

865–925 AD Abu Bakr Muhammad Ibn Zakariya al-Razi (Latin: Rhazes) was born at Rayy in Persia. He wrote '*Kitab al-Hawi fi al-tibb*' [The comprehensive book of medicine] that has become known in Latin under the title '*Continens Medicinae*'. It consisted of 23 volumes. He tried proposed remedies first on animals in order to evaluate their effects and side effects. He advised '*If the physician is able to treat with nutrients, not medication, then he has succeeded. If, however, he must use medication, then it should be simple remedies and not compound ones.*' (Tibi, 2006). He was the first to produce sulphuric acid? He was instrumental in making Arabian authorities appoint a 'mutasib', whose duties included the supervision of the makers of drugs and syrups to ensure the purity of their wares. '*It is essential that the mutasib make them fearful, try them, and warn them against imprisonment. He must caution them with punishment. Their syrups and drugs may be inspected at any time without warning after their shops are closed for the night.*' He used mercurial compounds as topical antiseptics. Al-Razi was the first to include in the pharmacopoeia the white-lead ointment, later on known in the Middle Ages in Europe as Album Rhases, and the first to use mercury as a purgative and also tested it in monkeys (Abramowitz, 1934).

868 AD The use of woodblock printing came in during the Tang Dynasty in 868 AD.

9th Century AD '*The Medical use of opium in 9th century Baghdad*' by Selma Tibi, 2006. '*Dizziness, hiccups, dimmed vision, choking, body chills, severe convulsions, deep sleep and a smell of opium when the body is scratched.*' These adverse effects were extracted from six books:

'*Al-Aqrabadhin*' [Medical formulary] of Abu Yusuf Ya'qub ibn Ishaq al-Kindi (c800–870 AD).

'*Al-Aqrabadhin*' [Medical formulary] of Sabur ibn Sahl (d.869).

'*Kitab al-ashr maqalat fi al-'ayn*' [The book of the ten treatises on the eye] by Hunain ibn Ishaq (870–892 AD).

'*Firdaws al-hikma*' [Paradise of wisdom] by Ali ibn Sahl Rabban al-Tabari.

'*Kitab al-Dhakhira*' [The book of treasure] by Thabit ibn Qurra.

'*Kitab al-Hawi fi al-tibb*' [Liber continens] by Abu Bakr Muhammad ibn Zakariyya' al-Razi (b.865 AD) (Tibi, 2006).

900–950 AD *Leechbook[29] of Bald in three parts. 'For a woman's chatter taste at night fasting a root of radish that the chatter cannot harm*

---

[29] leechbook = book of a member of the healing profession

them.' No mention of adverse effects. It included details from the work of Gariopontus' predecessors from the Salerno medical school, showing that Anglo-Saxon medical practice was in no way inferior to its continental neighbours (Talbot, 1965).

918 AD The first book of medicinal herbs written by a Japanese author appeared in 918. It is *'Honzou-wamyou'* which means drugs of natural origin.

930–994 AD Haly Abbas (Ali Ibn 'al-Abbas al-Majusi), author of *'Kitab-al-Malia'* (Liber Regius) *'Kitab Kamil al-sina'a al-tibbiyya'* [The complete book of the medical art] also called *'Al-Kitab al-Malaki'* [The royal book] It is one of the most comprehensive and well-organized compendia in early medical literature. In Europe the treatise was known as 'Liber Regius' or Pantegni and the author as Haly Abbas. He divided his encyclopaedia into two large books, one on theoretical principles and the other on practical aspects. Each book had 10 chapters, with divisions and subdivisions under these, typical of the elaborate organizational format of medieval Arabic writings. One of the chapters was on therapy with simple drugs; He says that the patient should be treated if possible with diet, not with drugs. If he can be treated with simple drugs he should not be administered compound ones, nor indeed strange or unknown ones.

955–1015 AD There were at least three physicians named 'Mesue':

Mesue Major; Yuhanna ibn Masawaih (777–857 AD). He wrote 42 works especially on the eye. His *'Kitab al-Nawadir al-Tibbiya'* contained 132 aphorisms including:

Not a physician in the whole world
Escapes death when his time comes.
Strange, isn't it, that escape it can't
In spite of drugs that were so good for others.
Obviously death all who with drugs deals
will get. Those who prescribe, those who use,
Those who sell, and those who them import.

(Sterpellone and Elsheikl, 1995)

Mesuè the Younger. He was an Italian physician who had taken the name of the Pseudo-Mesue, after Mesue Major. Johannes Mesue, Masawaih al-Hardin of Damascus

(924–1015 AD). He wrote a book on purgatives and emetics *'De medicins laxativis'* [Concerning laxative medicines] and on the complete pharmacopoeia in 12 parts called the *'Antidotarium sive Grabadin medicamentorum'* [Of antidotes or of Islamic medicines] and *'De medicinis universalibus et particularibus'* [About universal and specific medicines] a book of medicine containing numerous recipes for jams and sweets written in Latin between the 11th and 12th centuries. The Mesue treatise on purgatives divides the latter into laxative (tamarinds, figs, prunes, cassia), mild (wormwood, senna, aloes, rhubarb) and drastic (jalap, scammony, colocynth). In the second section instructions are given on how to improve drugs that are too weak or too strong, avoid harmful side effects and direct the drugs to the organ intended. It passed through more than 30 editions up to 1581, and has influenced all later pharmacopoeias.

Mesue the youngest from the first half of the 13th Century (Prioreschi, 1996).

973 AD The first printed Chinese herbal was *'K'ai-pao hsiang-ting pen-ts'ao'*. It was printed from blocks (Hummel, 1941).

'Taiping Shenghuifang' [Prescriptions from the pharmacy of harmonious assistance] was commissioned by the government and written by Wang Huaiyin at the end of the tenth century. It lists a total of 16,834 prescriptions and gives details of the prescription, drugs used, syndromes and pathology.

10th Century The *'Kitab-al-Saydanah Fi Al-Tibb'* [Book on pharmacy and materia medica] by Al Biruni (973–1048). He describes 700 simples in 1197 entries.

Second half of 10th century

'Kitāb al-Aqrābādhīn' [Book on compound remedies] 'by Abū Bakr Hāmid Ibn Samajūn, who was working in Spain, is primarily known for an important compendium on materia medica entitled *'al-Jami' li-aqwal al-qudama' wa-al-muhdathin min al-atibba' wa-al-mutafalsifin fi l-adwiyah al-mufradah'* [The compendium on simple drugs with statements of ancient and modern physicians and philosophers]. In it the medicinal substances are presented in alphabetical order, and the treatise is notable for the large number of authorities quoted

by the author (Islamic Medical Manuscripts at the National Library of Medicine). The treatise begins with recipes useful for forgetfulness (which was the topic of the preceding item in the volume). Subsequent recipes are said to be useful for a wider range of ailments, though complaints of head and brain dominate.' (www.nlmnih.gov/hmd/arabic/). Accessed 15th November 2009.

980–1037 Avicenna (Ali Ibn Sina) author of '*Kitab ash-shifa*' [Book of healing] and '*Canon of Medicine*'. He recommended the testing of a new drug on animals and humans prior to general use (Carr, 1995). Ibn Sina's protocols required the following tests be done on any "new" product:

1. The drug must be free from any extraneous accidental quality, e.g. heat or cold.
2. It must be used on a simple, not a composite, disease, i.e. only a single disease entity.
3. The drug must be tested with two contrary types of diseases, because sometimes a drug cures one disease by its essential qualities and another by its accidental ones.
4. The potency of the drug must correspond to the strength of the disease. For example, there are some drugs whose "heat" is less than the "coldness" of certain diseases, and therefore would have no effect on them.
5. The time of action must be observed, so that essence and action are not confused.
6. The effect of the drug must be seen to occur constantly or in many cases, for if this did not happen, then it only constitutes an accidental effect.
7. The experimentation must be done with the human body, for testing a drug on a lion or a horse might not prove anything about its effect on man (Tschanz, 1997).

In his '*Canon of Medicine*' paragraph 355 Avicenna says:

'*There are four orders of medicaments–whether eaten, or taken in the fluid state, or whether given by inunction:*

The first degree. The action of the quality of a medicament on the body is imperceptible to the senses. Thus warming or cooling effects not perceived by the senses unless it is given repeatedly, or in large doses.

The second degree. A greater degree of action, without perceptibly interfering with the functions of the body or changing their natural course (excepting incidentally, or because given in large doses).

The third degree. There is evident interference with function, but not markedly enough to produce breakdown or death of tissue.

The fourth degree. Destruction or death of tissue is produced. This is the degree produced by poisons. A poison is lethal in all respects (that is, in all parts of its "substance").'

The four drugs are mentioned: hyoscyamus, hellebore, mercury and opium (Gruner, 1930).

c1000 The Arabs introduced the pulped paper process, which they had learned from their Chinese prisoners captured in Samarqand, at the onset of the tenth century.

Abu Al-Qasim Al-Zahrawi (936–1013) wrote a 30 volume treatise on medicine and surgery *'Al-Tasrif li-man 'ajaza 'an al-ta'lif'* [The guide for him who cannot compose]. The 28th volume was translated in 1472 as *'Liber Servitoris'* (Sneader, 2005).

1019 Ibn Hindu (Abu al-Faraj Ali ibn al-Husayn) died 1019, wrote *'Miftah al-Tibb wa-minhaj al-tullab'* [The key to the science of medicine and the students' guide] He quotes *'While walking through the fields, a group of boys picked laurel seeds, and one of them tasted some. He was later bitten by a snake and, when he did not suffer any symptoms, it was realised that the laurel seeds had saved him. This was proof of their usefulness as an antidote and, from that day, they were included in the antidotes for poison.'* (Nasser and Tibi, 2007).

1040 The use of woodblock printing, although in existence since the Tang Dynasty in 868 AD, was further improved by Bi Sheng in 1040 AD with the invention of movable type.

1061 *'Ben Cao Tu Jing'* [Atlas of materia medica]. Song Dynasty (960–1279). It was written by Song Su (1020–1101).

It was said that in order to evaluate the effect of genuine Shangdang ginseng, two persons were asked to run together. One was given the ginseng while the other ran without. After running for approximately three to five li [equivalent to 1500 to 2500 meters], the one without the ginseng developed severe shortness of breath, while the one who took the ginseng breathed evenly and smoothly. An early clinical trial. (http://www.jameslindlibrary.org/index.html)

High Middle Ages

1082–1117 Important prescription texts in the Song Dynasty (960–1279 AD).

1082 *'Zhenglei Bencao'* [Classified materia medica] by Tang Shen-Wei, listed 1,558 drugs.

1107–1110 Chen Shiwen wrote *Taiping Huimin Heji jufang* [Prescriptions from the pharmacy of harmonious assistance] This work lists 788 prescriptions and gives information on how to prepare and use drugs. It represents the first government-published prescription book in the world. The Imperial Bureau of Medicine established the department of drug manufacturing.

1116 *'Ben Cao Yan Yi'* [Extension of materia medica] by Kou Zong-Shi.

1111–1117 Cao Zongxiao and other medical officers of the Song dynasty wrote *'Shengji Zonglu'* [General catalogue of divine assistance] This book lists 20,000 prescriptions and describes the causes, symptoms and cures for different illnesses (http://www.shen-nong.com/eng/history/chronolgy.html accessed 10/2/2010).

1100s Variolation was developed, which involved the inoculation of children and adults with dried scab material from smallpox patients. Variolation was practiced in Turkey, Africa, China, and Europe.

c1123 Foundation of St Bartholomew's Hospital in London.

1140 The *'Antidotarium Salernitanum'* [Remedies from Salerno] is one of the more famous works of the first Medical School at Salerno in Southern Italy–Schola Medica Salernitana, which was founded in c820 AD. It is a rich collection of recipes for the preparation of medicines, their application and action. It was not only the basis for all later pharmacopoeias, but also the first witness on the separation of medicine and pharmacy. The *'Antidotarium Nicolai'* [Nicolaus's book of antidotes] was written in two versions (for physicians and for pharmacists) by an unknown Salernitan[30] physician, Nicolaus Salernitanus, about 1140. Also at Salerno there was a monk from Carthage, Constantinus Africanus (1020–1087) who translated Arabic and ancient Greek works into Latin, including *'Viaticum'*. Roger of Salerno wrote *'Practica Chirurgiae'* [Practice of surgery] in 1180 and described the use of quicksilver (argent vif) in ointment for chronic skin diseases (Jovic, 2004; Abramowitz, 1934).

Regimen Sanitatis Salernitanum

> *The willow's juice kills worms when poured into their ears;*
> *Its bark cooked in vinegar cures warts; (salicylic acid is still used for warts).*
> *The juice of the fruits and the flower are harmful to human reproduction.'*

It also mentions hellebore and henbane.

Roger II, King of the Two Sicilies[31], promulgated the first known law in Europe for the regulation of medical practice *'whosoever will henceforth practise medicine let him present himself to our officials and judges to be examined by them'*. He used mercury as an external remedy and Abramowitz says *'Toxic symptoms such as foetid breath, stomatitis, angina, intestinal and nervous manifestations had already been noted by the Arabs.'* (Abramowitz, 1934).

1151–1158 Hildegard von Bingen (1098–1179), the abbess known as the 'Healer of the Rhine', authored the *'Liber subtilitatum diversarum naturarum creaturarum'* (A book of the diverse fine distinctions between natural creatures), between 1151 and 1158. Her work contained about 140 herbs and described their medicinal uses. Soon after Hildegard's death it was divided into two parts, known as the *'Physica'* (Natural history), also known as *'Liber simplicis medicinae'* (Book of simple medicine), and the *'Causae et Curae'* (Causes and cures), also known as *'Liber compositae medicinae'* (Book of compound medicine). This reflects the traditional division of the materia medica into

---

'Simplicia' and 'Composita'. Liber simplicis medicinae, called *'Physica'* The Physica consists of nine sections or books, the first and longest comprising accounts of more than two hundred plants. There were books devoted to the elements (earth, water and air), trees, precious stones, fish, birds, mammals, reptiles, and metals. The medical uses of these objects described in a predominant way—however, with descriptions often being reduced to statements of their four cardinal properties - that is, whether they are hot, dry, wet, or cold *'In what way are the fruits of nature advantageous or disadvantageous to my health, help at healing its brokenness and in what way are they to be used for that purpose?'* She provided recipes for over 2000 remedies (Milot et al, 1998).

1151–1162 *'Kitāb a-Munjih fi al-tibb wa-al-tadāwī min sunuf al-Amrad Wa-al-Shakaua'* [Success in medicine and in therapy among the categories of diseases and complaints] by Ibrāhīm ibn Abī Sa'īd ibn Ibrāhīm al-'Alā'ī. This was a medical treatise with 28 chapters. Within each chapter the medicaments are listed that begin with the given letter, and, for each item, 16 categories of information are supplied: 1. name, 2. quality, 3. type, 4. preferred state, 5. temperament, 6. strength, 7. usefulness for parts of the head, 8. usefulness for respiratory ailments, 9. usefulness for the digestive organs, 10. usefulness for the body as a whole, 11. manner of production, 12. how much is to be used, 13. harmful properties, 14. antidote, 15. substitute, and 16. number assigned the medicament in the treatise (a total of 550). The last category is omitted in those copies that are not written in the form of tables. A random page referred to five drugs, but with no harmful properties mentioned. The text area of a page was about the size of A5 paper and with only 71 pages and 550 drugs and each drug having 16 categories would allow only a few words per category.

There were two major Greek sources for medicinal substances available through Arabic translations: Discorides' treatise on materia medica, which described approximately 500 substances, and Galen's treatise on simple remedies. (www.nlm.gov/hmd/arabic/). Accessed 26th June 2008.

1181 Lord Guilhem VIII signed an edict declaring that anyone, regardless of religion or background, could teach medicine in Montpellier, thereby creating the oldest operating medical school in the Western world.

1190 The first written document that recommended mercury as a treatment was in the *'Circa-instans'* (A shortened version of the full title *'Circa instans negotium in simplicibus medicinis'*) [About the present business with the medicinal simples]. It was also known as the *'Liber simplici medici na'* [Book with simple medicines] or *'Secreta salernitana* [Secrets known about in Salerno] of Matthaeus Platearius of Salerno. In it the early herbals plants were referred to as 'simples' meaning single plants or 'compound' meaning mixtures of more than one plant. No mention of ADRs.

Adulteration of Drugs

The fear of adulteration of drugs is a constant theme in the laws governing medicines and continues today with traditional Chinese medicines (TCM), which may contain unmentioned western drugs such as cortisone. There have been numerous similar laws throughout the world continuing until the present time. There are six possibilities:

1. The drug was of poor quality, i.e. too little of the active drug, which was accidental and affected efficacy, e.g. the quinine content of different chinchona barks varies from 0–4% for C. calisaya, C. officinalis 2–7.5%, C. ledgeriana 3–13%, C. succiruba 4–14 %.

   The measured amounts of St John's Wort (*Hypericum perforatum*) varies considerably from those claimed on the labels, from 0% to 109% for capsules and from 31% to 80% for tablets (Draves & Walker, 2003).

2. The drug was formulated with excipients, which might alter the efficacy or safety of the active principal, e.g. diethylene glycol still used in 2006 in Panama mixed with glycerine for a cough mixture (News, 2007).

3. The drug was diluted with an inert substance, e.g. water or chalk, which was deliberate and affected efficacy. Linguistic references: 'as different as chalk and cheese' – the commercial adulteration of dairy products with chalk, used to disguise rancidness, to whiten watered-down milk and to increase the weight of cheeses; 'sincere', sans cere (without wax) – Roman bakers' advertising that their bread was not bulked out with wax.

4. Diluted with an active substance, which was added deliberately and which affected safety. Some modern Chinese traditional medicines contain modern drugs such as cortisone and phenylbutazone.

5. Contaminated accidentally and affected safety. In 1902, 19 Punjabi villagers given an experimental plague vaccine died of a tetanus contaminant. (Ross, 1991) and in 1906 an American scientist in the Philippines inoculated 24 prisoners with an experimental cholera vaccine that inadvertently had been contaminated with plague. 13 of the men died (Chemin et al, 1989).

6. Contaminated deliberately and affected safety, e.g. in 1982 in the US seven people purchased a bottle of Extra Strength Tylenol (paracetamol), which had been laced with cyanide. They all died.

Medical philosophies

Presumably ancient physicians or healers tried to balance the benefits of treatment against its possible adverse effects for each individual patient. In doing so they would have used the knowledge from their and others' past experience as to the benefit of the treatment. However, this would have been tempered by the current medical philosophy, e.g. one of these philosophies was the Doctrine of Signatures. The main categories of the doctrine uncovered were: similarity between the substance used and the human organ; resemblance in shape or behaviour to a specific animal; correlation between the colour of a substance and the colour of the symptoms; similarities between the substance and the patient's symptoms and the use of a substance that might produce symptoms of a particular disease in a healthy person to remedy those same symptoms in one who is sick. Put succinctly *'Every natural substance which possesses any medicinal virtue, indicated by an obvious and well marked external character, the disease for which it is a remedy, or the object for which it should be employed'* (Paris, 1820). An early philosophy was that disease was caused by demons and the treatment or preventive measure was to use incantations and amulets to expel the demon from the body. This was slowly replaced by the theory that it was that the ill balance of the body humours that caused diseases and restoring that balance was the aim of all medicines. The idea that an excess of a humour was the cause of a disease led to the practice of increasing the excretion and secretion of body fluids via the bodies orifices, hence purging, sweating, emesis, salivation, blood-letting, etc. Empedocles thought that there were four elements: water, fire, earth and air. This merged with Hippocrates's idea of four humours: blood (sanguine), yellow bile (choleric), black bile (melancholic) and phlegm (phlegmatic). Galen added four temperaments: warm, cold, dry and moist. Had these philosophies confined themselves to working out the mechanisms by which the medicines achieved their goal, i.e. retrospectively, they would have caused little harm; but, unfortunately, these philosophies were used prospectively to decide on future treatments and millions of patients have been purged, made to vomit, bled, etc. to their detriment. The urge to purge has remained to this day and my contempories can recall the weekly Saturday purge given whether constipated or not. The philosophy lingers on in colonic irrigation. The salivation caused by mercury was welcomed as showing that the evil was being washed away and the dose of mercury was increased until the required amount of salivation had occurred. Two of the marker drugs: black hellebore and white hellebore were used as emetics and purges respectively and perhaps they fell into disuse partly because of the change in philosophy. These early pseudo-philosophies meant that treatments were designed to cause adverse drug reactions and not only caused misery but would have hastened the death of many patients. Towards the end of the 19th century new pseudo-philosophers, e.g. homeopathy and some so-called complimentary medicines, have replaced the old with the disappearance of those adverse reactions and the appearance of other problems detrimental to patients, such as delay in receiving an accurate diagnosis and the correct treatment and the expenditure of large amounts of money, which might be better spent. The public, however, seems to have a need for them and they still thrive in a scientific world beguiling patients with placebo treatments. Galenic principles still linger in 1992. The Hausa tribe in Northern Nigeria treat stomach ache by promoting vomiting, purgation and diuresis–all signs of egress, so they use salicylates as well as plants to cause abdominal distress and later use antibiotics to produce diarrhoea, i.e. egress (Etkin, 1992).

Summary

The phrase 'combined with other medicinals to reduce or eliminate toxicity' in 220 AD suggests that the Chinese knew about interactions, but then there is a gap until 1667 when there is the quotation *'The mixing of things which are harmless sometimes produces a poison'*. I have found no other references until 1880 when the interaction of sympathetic neurotransmitters combined with chloroform anaesthetic was discovered to be potentially fatal. This is more likely to be due to the inadequacy of my research rather than an absence of reports. During this period Pliny, Discorides and Galen refer to the marker drugs, but then with the exception of Ibn Wahshïya in the

8th century I found no further mention of them—a silent period of 300 years. There was tremendous progress in the first 1000 years after Christ, first by the Romans and then the Arabs as they started to explore the use of drugs and lay down the principles for their study.

Chapter 3. 1200 AD–1500 AD

Covering the end of the High Middle ages, the Late Middle Ages and the start of the Renaissance.

1215 The 5th Lateran Council, named after the Papal palace in Rome, instructed physicians to summon the physician of souls before administering bodily medicines.

FI 1220–1240 Bartolomaeus Anglicus[32] wrote in *'De Proprietatibus Rerum'* [Concerning the properties of items], a 19 volume encyclopaedia, commenting on henbane: *'This herb is called insana wood, for the use thereof is perilous; for if it be eaten or drunk, it breeds woodeness, or slow likeness of sleep; therefore the herb is commonly called Morilindi, for it takes away wit and reason.'* (Gordon, 1977).

1224 The Hohenstaufen[33], Emperor Frederick II, ordered the regular inspection of the drugs and mixtures prepared by apothecaries, and ruled that the life of the seller of a poison, magic elixir, or love potion would be forfeit if the consumer died (see below).

1241 Edict of Salerno (sometimes called the Constitution of Salerno) Emperor Frederick II, Hohenstaufen, Holy Roman Emperor (1194–1250) made the first legally fixed separation of the occupations of physician and apothecary: *'no one who claims the title of physician, shall exercise the art of healing or dare to treat the ailing, except such as have beforehand in our University of Salerno passed a public examination under a regular teacher of medicine and been given a certificate'*... *'Apothecaries must conduct their business with a certificate from a physician according to the regulations and on their own credit and responsibility, and they shall not be permitted to sell their products without having taken an oath that all their drugs*

---

[32] Bartolomaeus Anglicus = Geoffrey Launde Bartolomaeus, an English monk, who later became a professor of Divinity in Paris
[33] Hohenstaufen = dynasty of Germanic King (1138–1254) also King of Sicily. It is near Göppingen.

have been prepared in the prescribed form, without any fraud'. In addition, the edict provided official supervision of pharmacy practice and ordered pharmacists to prepare drugs reliably– 'forma curiae', according to skilled art, and in a uniform, suitable quality ' *We decree also that the growers of plants meant for medical purposes shall be bound by a solemn oath that they shall prepare their medicines conscientiously according to the rules of their art'.* One regulation which should still be applied today is '*He* (the regularly licensed physician) *must not enter into any business relations with the apothecary nor must he take any of them under his protection nor incur any money obligations in their regard'* (Walsh, 1908; Almuete, 2000).

1197–1248 Abdullah ibn Ahmed ibn al-Baytar, from Malaga in Spain, wrote a pharmacopoeia '*Kitab[34] al-Jami` li-mufradat al-adwiyah wa-al-aghdhiyah'* [The comprehensive book on materia medica and foodstuffs], which was an alphabetical guide to over 1400 'simples[35]' taken from his own observations as well as from 150 written sources that he names. He composed a book on medicinal substances entitled '*Kitāb al-Mughni fī al-adwiyah al-mufrada'h'* [The ultimate in materia medica].

1249 An early Chinese herbal printed in blocks '*Zheng-lei Ben-c'ao'* [materia medica arranged according to pattern] by T'ang Shen-wei.

1253 *Yan Yonghe* wrote '*Jishen fang'* [Prescriptions for saving life]. This was an individually published text. The decoction known as '*gui pi tang'* is still used today.

1256 Saint Albertus Magnus (1193–1280), also called Albert the Great, a German scholastic theologian and scholar. His treatise, '*De vegetabilibus libri VII, historiae naturalis pars XVIII'* [Seven books about vegetables, Natural history Part 8] was written before 1256. He has paraphrased the ten books of Aristotle's natural histories.

c1205–1298 The Bishop of Cervia[36], Theodoric, was the first to attribute salivation to mercury (Abramowitz, 1934).

---

[34] kitab = book
[35] simples = single herbs as opposed to 'compound' meaning a mixture
[36] Cervia = city in Emilia-Romana, Italy

13th century An oath for apothecaries in Basle, Switzerland, was published; it included the line that drugs should be *'of such good quality and of such usefulness that he knows, upon his oath, that it will be good and useful for the confection what the physician is making'* (Mez-Mangold, 1971).

1250–1306 Lanfranco of Milan, who later moved to Paris, wrote *'A most excellent and learned work of chirurgerie, called 'Chirurgia parua Lanfranci Lanfranke of Mylayne' his brief: reduced from divers translations to our vulgar or usual phrase, and now first published in the English print by John Halle chirurgien. Who has thereunto necessarily annexed. A table, as well of the names of diseases and simples with their virtues, as also of all other terms of the art opened. ... And in the end a compendious work of anatomy ... An historical expostulation[37] also against the beastly abusers, both of chyrurgerie and physick in our time: with a goodly doctrine, and instruction, necessary to be marked and followed of all true chirurgie[n]s. All these faithfully gathered, and diligently set forth, by the said John Halle.'* Date: 1565.

Henbane: *'There are three kinds: the black, the yellow, and the white. The black is our common kind: whose seed causes madness, and is not allowed. The yellow grows in my garden, the seed whereof was given me, of master Roger Lee Doctor of phisick: which is better than the black, but yet to be eschewed[38] as hurtful. That whose flower and seed is white, I never saw as yet. It is only allowed wholesome, being cold in the third degree, and is a narcotic, or stupefactive[39] medicine: assuaging pain, and represses the inflammations of the eyes: helps the gout, and assuages[40] the swellings of the breast and stones.'*

Opium: *'...brought by art into a mass, must needs be like in temperament to the poppy, whereof it is made: and is sayeth Galen the mightiest among narcotic medicines, and causes dead sleep, but ought rarely, in great extremities (and then warily) to be used. For it strangles, and vehement pains are often eased therby (being used alone) for some small time: after the which it returns more violently then before. But in every doubt of this and his use: let master Turner be to you a sufficient satisfier.'*

---

[37] expostulation = a protest
[38] eschewed = avoided
[39] stupefactive = make stupid
[40] assuages = relieves

Digitalis, mercury, willow and Hellebore foetides mentioned in *'The Physicians of Myddvai; Meddygon Myddfai'*, or the medical practice of the celebrated Rhiwallon and his sons, of Myddvai, in Caermarthenshire (Wales), physicians to Rhys Gryg, Lord of Dynevor and Ystrad Towy, about the middle of the thirteenth century. No mention of side effects.

1270 A treatise on antidotes for poisons was written in 1270 in Syria by 'Ali ibn 'Abd al-'Azim al-Ansari. The treatise provides information regarding medical learning in the Crusader States as well as the plants that the author describes as having been found in Syria at the time. Moreover, al-Ansari incorporated into the study extensive quotations from other treatises on plants and antidotes *'Dhikr al-tiryāq al-fārūq'* (MS A 64) [Memoir on antidotes for poisons]).

1271 The Medical Faculty of Paris forbade the prescribing of medicines except by qualified physicians. Apothecaries were to prepare only those drugs prescribed by the physicians (Prioreschi, 2001).

1275 Ether ($C_4H_{10}O$) discovered (no firm evidence) in 1275 by Spanish chemist Raymundus Lullius, but it was used for topical application only.

Late 13th century

Gilbert Anglicus reported that pouring quicksilver into the ear produces the most distressing symptoms: severe pain, delirium, convulsions, epilepsy, apoplexy and, if the quicksilver penetrates to the brain, ultimate death (Handersen, 1918).

1214–1294 Roger Bacon wrote *'Tract on the tincture and oil of antimony.'* It causes a sweat *'that is very inconstant, viscous and thick, that smells and tastes quite sour and offensive'*. He used it for gout, leprosy, apoplexy or stroke, dropsy, epilepsy, hectic[41] fever and pestilence. He also wrote *'De Erroribus Medicorum'* in which he explained the 36 errors committed by physicians. He starts by saying *'The ordinary doctor knows nothing about simple drugs, but entrusts himself to ignorant apothecaries, concerning whom it is agreed by these doctors themselves that they have*

---

[41] hectic = consumption

no other purpose but to deceive'. The fourth defect he mentions is *'as to the dosage of a harmful drug, which is unknown as regards the human body in this age, as with scammony, opium and the like. For there is no method prescribed or known as to the quantity men of this age should take, and how much ought to be given according to ages and epochs. And therefore death or bodily wasting very often follows, and various infirmities, and scammony brings man to dysentery or death, and opium produces idiocy'.* He finishes by exhorting doctors to prove their assertions by experiment *'Now follows "scientia experimentalis", whose prime dignity, as I have insisted before, is that it possesses in itself complete verifications as to conclusions of other sciences.* (Withington 1924).

1250–1326 Guglielmo da Brescia, who was a physician and professor in Padua and Bologna, singled out opiates in his long list of cures as having dangerous side effects. Vigilance was the watchword when it was used for, *'Sed cave a succo papaveris et mandragore propter fortem stupefactiones [sic] utriusque. Si non cogat vigiliarum instantia vuti utrisque'.* [but beware the sap of the poppy and of mandragora on account of the strong stupfying effect of either. If not it may cause pressing moments of sleeplessness]. He was also concerned about the use of purgatives. Noting that purgatives were both dangerous and prematurely aging, he argued that there were less potentially deadly means of expelling surfeit[42] humours, including regimen, massage, gentler medicines, and phlebotomy[43].

1316 The ordinances of the Guild of Pepperers of Soper Lane, London, wrote the first code of quality control (Penn, 1979).

1322 College of Medicine of Paris determined that the apothecaries of Paris had to have a copy of *'L'Antidotaire Nicoli'* by Nicholas le Myrepsos of Alexandria, written in Greek about 1300. This formulary was one of the first printed books (Venice, 1471), which prepared the way for the independent development of pharmacy.

---

[42] surfeit = excess
[43] phlebotomy = taking blood from a vein.

c1330 The Venetian Republic founded the first national health service in Europe, and obliged licensed practitioners to attend an annual course in anatomy (ref. Norwich, Venice, p.298). In 1368 they were required to attend monthly meetings to exchange notes on new cases and treatments (http://www.fphm.org.uk) accessed 15th November 2009.

1339 The '*Dynameron*' by Nicholas Myrepsos and other medical texts copied by Kosmas Kame consisting of more than 2500 Greek, Roman, Arab, Jewish and Christian remedies.

1347 The Bubonic plague reached England via Italy from China and was called 'The Black Death'. It killed 25 million people. The English population was approximately 6 million in 1300 dropping to 2.5 million in the 1450s only climbing again to 6 million in the 1700s. Life expectancy dropped from 31.3 years to 17.3 years between 1348 and 1375 rising to 32.8 years in 1436 to 1450 (Russell, 1948).

1353 August A French Royal Ordonnance forbade anybody from preparing all medicaments unless he knows how to read a prescription and dispense and confire[44] (Bouvet, 1937).

1363 '*Ungentum Saracenicum*' (containing Quicksilver) was recommended for scabies by Guy de Chauliac (1300-1367) in '*Grande Chirurgie*'. He said that it caused salivation, loosened teeth and gave him pains in the belly (Abraham, 1948). He also said that '*Spongia somnifera could cause asphyxia, congestion and death*'.

Francesco Petrarca in a letter to Bocaccio, Rerum Senilium V.3
   'I solemnly affirm and believe, if a hundred or a thousand men of the same age, same temperament and habits, together with the same surroundings, were attacked at the same time by the same disease, that if one half followed the prescriptions of the doctors of the variety of those practicing at the present day, and that the other half took no medicine but relied on Nature's instincts, I have no doubt as to which half would escape'.
(www.jameslindlibrary.org).

---

[44] confire = preserve

1380 Chaucer started writing 'The Canterbury Tales'.

Sompnour was with us in the place,	*A summoner[45] was with us in this place,*
That had a fire red Cherubins face,	*That had a fiery-red cherubic face,*
For saufleme he was, with iyen narow,	*For pimpled he was with narrow eyes,*
All hot he was, and lecherous as a Sparow,	*He was hot and lecherous as a sparrow.*
With scaled brows blacke, and pilled berde:	*With black and scabby brows and scanty beard:*
Of his visage Children were fore afferde.	*Children were afraid of his face.*
There nas quicksilver, litarge, ne brimstone,	*There was no mercury (Hg), lead oxide (PbO), nor sulphur (S),*
Borage, Ceruse, ne oile of Tartar none,	*Borax, lead carbonate ($PbCO_3$), nor Potassium Carbonate,*
Ne Ointment that would cleanse or bite,	*No ointment that would cleanse or remove,*
That him might helpe of his whelks white,	*That might help him with his white pimples,*
Ne of his knobbes sitting on his Chekes:,	*Nor his lumps on his cheeks:*
Well loued he Garlike, Onions, and Lekes,	*He loved garlic, onions and leeks,*
And for to drink strong wine, as red as blood,	*And for drink strong red wine,*
Then would he speak, & cry as he were wood.	*He would ask and cry for as if he was mad.*

The 'ceruse', $Pb(OH)_2 2PbCO_3$, whitelead, was the white make-up that can be seen on Queen Elizabeth's portraits.

---

[45] summoner = official responsible for calling people before a judge by issue of a summons.

1423 The 'Commonality of Physicians and Surgeons of London' appointed two apothecaries to inspect the shops and bring any that offended in the quality of their wares be brought before the Mayor and Aldermen of the City of London.

College of Physicians and Surgeons founded in London, but ceased after a few years (Warren, www.chronology.ndo.co.uk).

1440 Printed books from movable type began in Europe and heralded the start of the books on herbal medicines.

1443 A Leechbook, manuscript 136 at the Medical Society of London, mentions the use of quicksilver for scabs. It also refers to a mixture, which acts as an anaesthetic for 'cutting': *Gall of a swine 3 spoonfuls: Juice of Hemlock root 3 spoonfuls: Vinegar 3 spoonfuls all mingled and the add a spoonful or two of the mixture to a gallon of wine or ale. The dose of the latter was one spoonful'* (Warren R Dawson 1934).

1462 First Royal Charter of the Barbers Guild; the Guild was concerned with the treatment of the sick and hurt by outward applications; its functions were restricted to the City of London and one mile around (Warren www.chronology.ndo.co.uk).

1477 First German Pharmacopoeia (Artzneibuch) by Ortoloff von Bayrlaṉt.

William Caxton set up a printing press in the precincts of Westminster Abbey (Warren. www.fphm.org/resources/atoz/r_chronology_of_state_medicine.pdf).

1480 *'Regimen Sanitatis Salernitanum'* [The healthy way of living prescribed by Salernian knowledge] commonly known as *'Flos medicinae'* [The flower of medicine] or *'Lilium medicinae'* [The lily of medicine]. The first work is an anonymous poem on hygiene, drink, diet, and the beneficial properties of plants, with extensive commentaries. The woodcuts show people at the dinner table, wine casks, people drinking and vomiting, various edible plants and animals, and the production of foods and drinks. The poem dates back to at least the thirteenth-century and is associated with the famous school of medicine at Salerno in southern Italy. There is little grounds for its ascription to Jean de Milan, or to Arnauld de Villeneue (c1240–1311) who is supposed to have added many of the notes. It appeared in print many times, beginning c1480 and usually under the title, '*Regimen Sanitatis Salernitanum*', but in 1551 Christian Egenolph at Frankfurt published a new edition under the present title, with woodcut illustrations and revised by Johannes Curio (d.1561).

1481 '*Herbarium Apulei Plato*' [The Herbal of Pseudo-Apuleius] by Nici ad Marcum Agrippam : from the Ninth-Century Manuscript in the Abbey of Monte Cassino (Codex Casinensis 97): Together with the first printed edition of Joh. Phil. de Lignamine (Editio princeps Romae, 1481; Stearn, 1979).

1484 '*Herbarius Latinus*', first published in Mainz in 1484, is an anonymous herbal compilation from classical Arabic, and medieval sources.

'*Établissement de la profession d'apothicaire. Une déclaration de Charles VIII rend obligatoire l'appartenance à une corporation pour exercer la profession d'apothicaire. Mais ces mesures furent très relativement respectées.*' Establishment of the profession of apothecary. A declaration of Charles VIII makes it obligatory to adhere to a corporation in order to exercise the profession of apothecary, but these measures were only respected up to a certain point.

Start of Renaissance

1485 The first printed illustrated herbal in the German Language was '*Gart der Gesuntheit*' [The Garden of Health] published in Mainz by Peter Schoeffer.

1488 The next herbal was written in 1488: '*Herbarium vivae eicones*' [Living images of plants] by Otto Brunfels and was published at the time of his death in 1534 in three parts between 1530 and 1536.

1491 '*The Fasciculus Medicinae*' [The handbook of medicine] of Johannes de Ketham. Translated by Luke Demaitre, Section XVI: '*Hellebore (Helleborus niger) is dangerous to those who possess rigid fibres because it produces convulsions.*' Section V: '*Convulsions produced by hellebore are fatal.*' Section VII-XXV: '*Convulsions after a purgative are fatal.*' (Demaitre,1988).

'*Hortus Sanitatis*' or '*Ortus sanitatis*' [The origin of health], printed by Peter Schöeffer in Mainz, and went into several reprints and was also translated. It was of paramount importance to the development of the herbal in German speaking countries. It had 8 sections, the first on herbs and plants and the last *'Tabula medicinalis cum directorio generali per omnes tractus'* [A medicinal catalogue with a general listing of every work]. The Hortus sanitatis is a greatly expanded Latin version of the *'Gart der Gesundheit'* [Garden of health], which is sometimes attributed to Johann von Cube. However, it should be regarded as a separate work as it covered nearly a hundred more medicinal plants than the *'Gart der Gesundheit'* and also included extensive sections on animals, birds, fish and minerals, as well as a treatise on urine. The authorship of this lavishly illustrated herbal is unknown but it is generally believed to have been compiled by its printer, Jacob Meydenbach. It was first printed in 1491 in Mainz and is therefore the last major medical work to cover medicines from the Old World only.

1493 Mercury was introduced for the treatment of syphilis. *'Now none, I think, will deny, that the French disease is new, seeing it was never heard of in Europe, before the year 1493. but then brought by Christopher Columbus, and his associates, from India to Italy, and there communicated to the Italian women, who bringing victual[46] to the French soldiers in the Neapolitan siege, with their bodies communicated their disease to the men; which the men retaining after conquest, gave also to other Italian women: from whom their returning husbands, persolving the debt of matrimony, catch'd it of their own wives, who had got it of the Frenchmen, the French of Italian women, and they of Columbus his soldiers.'* (Renodæus, 1657). On the expedition with Columbus there were two brothers (Pinzon) from Palos de la Frontera, Spain: Martin Alonso, the elder, commanded the *'Pinta'* and died at his home from syphilis in Palos a few weeks after his return from the West Indies (Haiti). On the return journey across the Atlantic, early in 1493, the *'Pinta'* separated from the other remaining vessel in an Atlantic storm and put in at Bayona on the northwestern Spanish coast, before sailing on to Palos. The first well-recorded outbreak of what we know as

---

[46] victual = food

syphilis occurred in Naples in 1495. There is some documentary evidence to link the return of Columbus' crew, in 1494 from Haiti, to the outbreak. This is called the Columbian theory. Although some hold that syphilitic symptoms were described by Hippocrates in its venereal/tertiary form (Aphorisms book 3, chapter XX): *'that in the summer ulceration of the mouth, skin eruptions, and mortification of the privy parts occurs'*). Some passages in the Bible could refer to syphilis, especially Exodus 20:5 where the sins of the father are visited unto the third and fourth generation. The idea that syphilis or another treponema–yaws, spread from Saharan Africa and then either, became more virulent or that there was an alteration in the organism of yaws is called the Unitarian theory (Waugh, 1982). The subject is debated fully in *'The Origin and Antiquity of Syphilis: Paleopathological Diagnosis and Interpretation'* (Baker & Armelagos, 1988).

'In the Month of December, (as Nicholaus Leonitius reports, *writing of this disease* [syphilis]) *when K. Charles the viij. of France besieged Naples with a puissant* [powerful] *army, where he remained certain months, some of the Spaniards came to him, of the which Christophorus Columbus was chief, and spread this pernicious seed, and termed it the Indian sickness, which, has had his course since, not only amongst the Spaniards, who call it the Italian sickness, but also among the Italians, who call it the malady of Naples, not without cause: for it began first to flourish in Naples. Amongst the Frenchmen it is called the Spanish sickness, in England the Great Pox, in Scotland the Spanish Fleas, and that for two causes, the one, because it first occurred amongst the Spaniards'.*

1495 Syphilis broke out for the first time in an epidemic fashion during the 1496 siege of Naples by Carlo VIII, King of France. Gasparẹ Gaopon Torella, a Spanish physician to Pope Alexander VI, wrote in November 1497 referring to the disease as 'pudendagra'[47] described five cases treated with mercurial ointment (Waugh, 1982). Until Italy was a leading nation, syphilis was called 'French disease', but when Italy declined, the French appellation: 'Neapolitan illness' prevailed (http://

---

[47] pudendagra = syphilis

pacs.unica.it/biblio/lesson2.htm) accessed 15th November 2009. Other synonyms: 'Morbus gallicus'. There is some evidence that syphilis was present in Asia Minor prior to 1412. There were nine tracts published in Latin on syphilis between 1495 and 1498 (Sudhoff, 1925).

1497 Alessandro Benedetti (1460–1525 or?1450–1512), a professor of anatomy and surgery at Padua, described shaking, paralysis and loss of teeth with mercury (Quétel, 1992).

Gaspar Torella (c1452–1520) wrote *Tractus cum consilis contra Pudendagra, seu morbum Gallicum'* [A work with descriptions of syphilis, or the French disease] and he said that syphilis was known in Avignon in 1493 and also that he relied on mercurial ointment for its treatment, but later on he rejected it.

1498 The first official European Pharmacopoeia '*Nuovo Receptario composto dal famossisimo chollegio degli eximii doctori dell arte et medicina della inclita cipta di Firenze': Impresso Nella inclyta Cipta di Firenze per la Compagnia del Dragho; 1498.'* [New recipe book composed by the most famous college of the distinguished doctors of the art and medicine of the illustrious chapter of Florence, by the Florentine Guild of Physicians and Pharmacists.] It acknowledges many previous authors, e.g. Mesue, Nicholas, Avicenna and Galen. It covers all sorts of things used as medication: metals, viscere and flesh of animals, salts, and precious stones. The universal panacea – Mithridato contains 109 ingredients including laudanum[48]. There is no mention of ADRs.

Francisco Lopez de Villalobos, author of '*Sumaria de la medicina en romace trovado con un tractado sobre las pestiferas bubas';* ['*Sur les contageuses et maudites bubas histoire et médecine Salamanque'*]; [With an account of harmful swellings, and an account of contagious and deadly swellings and medication from Salamanca].

Natale Montesauro, a doctor of Verona, who was himself infected with syphilis, wrote: '*De dispasitionibus quas vulgares mal Franzoso appellant'.* [Concerning the different conditions which ordinary people call the French disease] 1498.

---

[48] laudanum = tincture of opium

Dispensatories

These also contained non-herbal remedies such as minerals, metals, animal products, precious stones, etc. They contained prescriptions for medicines and occasionally mention of adverse effects, Dispensatories were commercial ventures, which generally offered commentary and material additional to that found in pharmacopoeias, and with a wide readership, many had a significant influence on the standardization of medicines.

Pharmacopoeias

The term 'pharmacopoeia' first appears as a distinct title in a work published at Basel in 1561 by Dr A. Foes, but does not appear to have come into general use until the beginning of the 17th century. As these were official lists of drugs allowed they did not mention adverse effects but kept to ingredients and method of preparing various products. Individual cities produced their own pharmacopoeias:

1498 Florence *'Nuovo Receptario Composto'*
1535 Barcelona *'Concordia Pharmacolorum Barcinoesium'*
1546 Nuremberg *'Dispensatorium Valerii Cordis'*
1559 Mantua
1564 Ausberg
1565 Cologne
1574 Bologna
1580 Bergamo
1583 Rome
1618 London *'Pharmacopoeaia Londinensis'*
1634 Blois *'Pharmacopoea Blaesensis Blaesis'* – pour eviter les fraudes, abusey malversations qui se peuvent commetre en la composition des poudres' [In order to avoid the frauds, abusive malpractices which can be commited in the composition of powders.]
1638 Paris *'La Pharmacopoea Parisiensis–Codex Medicamentarius.'* It was ordered in 1598 and was delayed for 41 years.
1641 Brussels *'Pharmacopoeia Bruxellensis'*
1652 Gent *'Pharmacia Antverpiensis'*
1660 Antwerp
1686 Stockholm *'Pharmacopoeja Holmiensis Galeno-Chymica'*
1697 Brugge
1699 Edinburgh
1807 Dublin

1732 Paris. *'CODEX Medicamentarius seu Pharmacopoea Parisiensis'*

1778 Ratisbonne, Le Hague, Madrid and Liège. These were updated at irregular intervals.

Similarly national pharmacopoeias were published.

1581 Spain

1775 Sweden *'Pharmacopoea Svecica'*

1778 Russia

1818 France

1820 USA (There had been an army Pharmacopoeia in 1778)

1864 Britain,

1872 Germany

1886 Japan

The World Catalogue lists 729 pharmaceutical works prior to 1880. It was not possible to study all these for traces of pharmacovigilance, so a selection of herbals, dispensatories and pharmacopoeias has been made. The early works prior to 1 AD contained between 240 to 700 different drugs. The Chinese works contained over 1,000 drugs; one reaching 20,000 drugs. After 1 AD the numbers varied between 100 and 2,850 drugs. It is clear that with these large numbers space for adverse effects would have been very limited. Pharmacopoeias written by individuals will be mentioned later in the chapter.

483-1682 The Age of Herbals and Dispensatories

A herbal has been defined as a book containing the names and descriptions of herbs, or of plants in general, with their properties and virtues. The word is believed to have been derived from a mediaeval Latin adjective 'herballs'; the substantive 'liber' being understood. It is thus exactly comparable in origin with the word 'manual' in the sense of a hand-book. Herbals are compendious descriptions of therapeutic plants and their uses in medicine as well as general descriptions of plants, often accompanied by numerous illustrations depicting the various plants, Facts are often accompanied by superstitions. The term 'herbal' (herbarium) usually refers to early printed books of the fifteenth and sixteenth centuries on the therapeutic properties of plants used in medicine. However, it can be applied to earlier works dealing with the same topic, from their prototype, *'De materia medica'* by the Greek Dioscorides (first century AD), to late-medieval compilations such as the early fourteenth-century *'Liber de herbis'*.

In their medieval canonical form, herbals usually consisted of a list of plants whose parts (roots, twigs, leaves, flowers, fruits, and seeds) were used as primary ingredients (that is, drugs) for the preparation of medicines, be they simple or composed. A chapter was devoted to each plant and all such chapters were ordered alphabetically by plant name. Each chapter usually contained the following:

(a) The most commonly used Latin name of the plant and its synonyms

(b) A description of the plant

(c) The part or parts of the plant or plants to be used for therapeutic purposes (i.e., the drug or drugs), and their state (fresh or dry)

(d) The preparation of the drug and, when appropriate, the proper ways to store it, that is, the type of container necessary for good conservation, without interaction between the drug and the substance of the container itself, and the maximum possible length of conservation without alteration of the drug and its properties

(e) The properties of the drug, usually expressed according to Galen's system, that is, according to the four primary qualities (hot and cold; dry and humid) and their grade (on a scale of four degrees)

(f) The disease or diseases for the treatment of which the drug was used

(g) A drawing of the plant, more or less developed or schematic. After the translation period and the assimilation of Arabic texts into Western medical sciences, the schema above was modified to include a list of synonyms that included the Greek and Arabic names of plants transliterated into the Latin alphabet and often adapted to Latin phonetics but which was deformed by mistakes of all kinds. The list of diseases was very often preceded by long quotations from previous authors' works. Such citations were attributed and ordered according to the probable chronological sequence of the authors, be they Greek (known through their Arabic versions themselves translated into Latin) or Arabic (in Latin translation). A further innovation was the inclusion of medieval commentaries on these authors; these might contain the text of the primary author, divided into thematic sections.

After Guttenberg's invention of printing in 1452 the first herbal 'Das Buch der Natur' was published in 1471, followed by the'Herbarium Apuleii Platonici' in 1481, but it wasn't until the 1550s that the production of herbals, etc. really took off.

Apothecaries (UK)

Etymology: Middle English *apothecarie,* from Medieval Latin *apothecarius,* from Late Latin, shopkeeper, from Latin *apotheca* storehouse, from Greek *apothēkē,* from *apotithenai* to put away, from *apo-* + *tithenai* to put — more (Merriam-Webster Dictionary).

1180 The Pepperers' Guild (Gilda Piperarorium) was founded, which included drug sellers, e.g. apothecaries. They were a company of traders or merchants in Soper's Lane, London, who imported medicinal and other kinds of spices, together with drugs, from the shores of the Red Sea and various Eastern ports.

1316 This guild merged with the Spicers' Guild in Chepe, London, which was concerned with retail sales and the compounding of medicines, and together they made common regulations.

1318–1328 Some Grocers (Grossarii, meaning those that sold 'en gros') joined the Pepperers' Guild.

1345 The Guild became known as the Fraternity of St Antony.

1357–1373 Between these dates the Guild adopted the title of The Grocers' Company.

1429 The Grocers' Company were given a charter by Henry VI.

1607 The Apothecaries were members of a separate section of the company.

1617 The Worshipful Society of Apothecaries of London was incorporated by royal charter on 6 December 1617 by James I (Whittet, 1968).

1793 The Apothecaries formed the General Pharmaceutical Association to combat the growing power of the chemists.

1796 *'Of all branches of the medical profession that of the apothecary, without doubt, is of most consequence to the health of the nation at large. In this city, where a physician attends one patient, an apothecary attends twenty; and, in the country, this proportion is more than double'* (Good, 1796).

1802 An Act of Parliament imposed a tax on nearly all medicines, which the apothecaries and the chemists attempted to have repealed, but without success.

1804 Movements to reform the profession were started.

1812 Parliament imposed an exorbitant tax on glass. The apothecaries were exasperated by this further imposition.

1812–1815 Various attempts were made to protect the public from the dangers of unorthodox practitioners and to improve the character and respectability of the surgeon-apothecary. The General Pharmaceutical Association framed a bill to form a fourth body to examine apothecaries,

surgeon apothecaries, accoucheurs, mid-wives dispensing chemists and assistants, but it was opposed by the Colleges of Physicians and Surgeons and was not supported by the Society of Apothecaries. Finally the Society of Apothecaries prepared a bill that became the Apothecaries Act 1815.
1815 The Apothecaries Act. (McConaghey, 1967).

Summary

Although there are many references to herbs in the Chinese and Arab works they do not give much information on ADRs. The 'laws and regulations' main theme was that the writing of prescriptions should be undertaken by physicians and the preparation of mixtures by pharmacists. After printing became established in Europe in 1440 and in England in 1477 many books on drugs were produced. The distinction between herbals, dispensatories and pharmacopoeias becomes rather blurred. Sometimes words in other languages are translated as 'Pharmacopoeia', i.e. kitab. The end of the century saw the arrival of syphilis and its various treatments would occupy both physicians and surgeons, and trouble patients until the twentieth century.

Chapter 4. 16th Century

The Renaissance. The introduction of syphilis into Europe sets off a vain search for a cure.

Several writers, Pedro Pinctor[49], Marinarus Brocardus[50] and Juan Almenar[51] warned of the dangers of stomatitis from the use of mercury (Abramowitz, 1934).

1503   Joseph Grünpeck (1470–1531), who suffered greatly from the adverse effects of mercury, wrote *'De la mentulagre[52] ou de mal Français'* [Treatment of the pestilent syphilis or the French disease containing its origins and its treatment] and *'Tractus de Pestilentiali Scorra[53] sive Mala de Franzos: originem Remediaque Eiusdem Continens'* [An essay on dangerous flux or the French disease: containing the origins and remedies for the same] Nuremberg: Kaspar Hochfeder, 1496 (Translated by Dr A Corlieu, Published by G Masson, 1884) .

c1504   A book appeared in Paris, entitled, the *'Grand Herbier'*, which carried the first mention of belladonna, although the term *'Solatrum minus'* [Lesser deadly nightshade] used by Saladinus[54] about 1450, is presumed to refer to it. *Le Grand Herbier en Francoys: Contenant les Qualitez, Vertus & Proprietez des Herbes, Arbres, Gommes & Semences,* [The Great Herbal in French containing the qualities, vertues and properties of herbs, gums and seeds]: Extract of several medical tracts from Avicenna, Razie, Constantin, Plataire, It was newly printed in Paris by Jaques Nyverd, 1521. Anonymous compilation including most of the *'Circa Instans'* of Matthaeus Platearius as well as extracts from other authors. First edition (c1486–88)

---

[49] Pedro Pinctor = (1423–1503) physician to Pope Alexander VII. From Valencia. Wrote *'De Morbo fœdo et occulto bis temporibus affligente'* in 1500.
[50] Marinus Brocardus = wrote *'Dissertatio de Morbo Gallico'*. Lived in Venice 1516–1567.
[51] Juan Almenar = physician to Pope Alexander VII. From Valencia. Wrote treatise on the Morbo Gallico in 1502
[52] mentulagre = maladie du membre viril = diseases of the penis
[53] scorra = syphilis
[54] Saladinus = Saladinus Asculanus author of *'Compendium aromatariorum'*. Bonon, 1488. Flourished 1441–1463 in Ascoli, Italy. Also known as Ferro Saladino.

published under title: '*Arbolayre*'. Paris. 1521.

1505 '*Ben Cao Pin Hui Jing Yao*' [Essentials of Materia Medica] by Lu Wen-Tai, et al. Written, but not published until 1700.

1505/6 Incorporation of the Barber Surgeons of Edinburgh [Warren www.chronology.ndo.co.uk).

1506 Angelo Bolognino, professor of surgery at the University of Bologna first used fumigations in the treatment of syphilis.

Giovanni (Joannes) da Vigo (1450?–1525), a Spanish surgeon who was physician to Pope Julius II, wrote in '*The most excellent workes of chirurgerie*'. London, Thomas East for Henry Middleton 1571 Folio, ff. (vi) 270 (xv), describing the first use of mercury for the French Pox (syphilis) (see 1525 AD). He advocated mercury red precipitate and used mercury plaster and Neopolitan Cream.

In his '*This lytle practice of Iohannes de Vigo, in medicine, is translated out of Latin into Englyshe, for the health of the body of ma'n*, 1564.

'*For the French Pox*

Take of black turpentine i.d, oh.[55] Bolear moniacke i.d, Alum three groats weight, and as much of Argentum Vif (Quicksilver), and mingle them all with fasting spittle, and it will flee. Give Seraphine, three groats weight, give Armoniac as much Popillion, a spoonful and a half, Verdigris as much as of your gumes, and anoint the body and keep him close, and give him to drink the juice of Galles often, for it will drive them out of the body, and if there be any unkind sore that will not heal, cast there upon powder of Mercury sublimed, but it is painful, and Popillion will slake the pain, and some men after their healing two or three years break out of scabs and great sores on their body, and in the soles of their feet, and will not heal for no medicine. Then take the root of Clecompana, and pare it fair, and beat it as fine as you can, then take fair swines grease fresh, and beat them strongly together, and anoint the place in two or three days it is whole. Also I have seen men broken out in the face, full of small quadelles like scabs, and that have I beat dib..illed with the powder of Alum, and Verdigris and Popillion'.

---

[55] id., oh = the same, every hour

1508 Guaiacum (guaiac, legno sancto) was first imported from the West Indies and later used for the treatment of syphilis.

1511 *'Concordia Apothecariorum Barchin'*, [Collection of the Apothecaries of Barcelona] was printed in Barcelona. It was the first edition of a pharmacopoeia, written by the guild of apothecaries of Barcelona and the first one published in Spain. The name of *'Concordia'* referred to the unanimous agreement reached by the apothecaries of Barcelona that the book might be used as the official work of reference for their formulas, the so-called 'compound' medicaments. The 1511 edition was followed by several works of a similar nature: two also printed in Barcelona (in 1535 and 1587), two in Saragossa (in 1546 and 1553) and two others in Valencia (in 1601-3 and 1698), though under the title of *'Officina Medicamentorum'* [Recipes for making medicines]. A Benedictine monk, Henricus Breyell, finished in 1511 for a Benedictine nunnery, a textbook, containing a herbal. His herbal was found to be an adaptation of the *'Gart der Gesuntheit'*, the first printed illustrated herbal in the German language of 1485.

Physicians and Surgeons Act (3 Hen. VIII, c.1 1) ...in the Parliament holden at Westminster in the third year of the King's most gracious reign, amongst other things, for the avoiding of sorceries, witchcrafts, and other inconveniences, it was enacted, that no person within the city of London, nor within seven miles of the same, should take upon him to exercise and occupy as physician or surgeon, except he be first (examined approved and admitted) by the Bishop of London and the Dean of St Paul's Cathedral, with the assistance of four physicians or surgeons. For the rest of England the examination was to be conducted by the bishop of each diocese in a similar manner. Oxford and Cambridge universities retained their rights to issue licences to practice (Warren. www.chronology.ndo.co.uk).

1518 Thomas Linacre founded the College of Physicians.

1525 Banckes Herbal is a compilation of herbal treatises from anonymous sources that was published by Richard Banckes in 1525. It was the first printed English herbal. It contains a copy of the famous discourse on the virtues of rosemary sent by the

Countess of Hainault to her daughter Queen Philippa, wife of Edward I (1239–1307). No mention of ADRs.

'There was never no such disease known,' as Giovanni da Vigo put it in 1525, *'wherefore it was needful for the curation of this disease, to search out new remedies. And to say the truth, the medicines lately invented are better in this disease then the medicines of old writers.'*

1526 The great herbal which gives perfect knowledge and understanding of all manner of herbs [and] their gracious virtues which God ordained for our prosperous welfare and health, for they heal [and] cure all manner of diseases and sickenesses that fall or misfortune to all manner of creatures of God created, practised by many expert and wise masters, as Avicenna and others. Also it gives full perfect understanding of the book lately printed by me (Peter Trevris) named the noble experience of the virtuous handwork of surgery. Imprinted at London in Southwark: By me Peter Treueris, dwelling in the sign of the wodows, In the year of our Lorde God. M.D.xxvi. the xxvii. day of Iuly]. This is a copy of the French 'Grand Herbier'. No mention of ADRs.

1527 The first description of a chronic mercurialism in Idrija (Mercury mining town in Slovenia started in 1490) was from Theophrastus Paracelsus in his book *'Von der Bergsucht und anderen Krankheiten'* (On the Miners' Sickness and Other Miners' Diseases). He had published *'De morbi gallici curandi ratione, dialogus'* [A dialogue about an account of the French disease] (Bologna, 1530), a traditional examination of the origins and treatment of syphilis (in which he was either the first or one of the first to recommend mercury as a cure).

'A fume to cleanse the body of foul and filthy scabs proceeding of the pox. Recipe. Cinabrij {ounce}.j. mercuric. sublimati {dram}. j. myrrhae, masticis, thuris, styracis calamine. ana[56].{scruple}. v. gummi iuniperi, terebint. laudani ana.q.s[57]. Fiant trochisci' (Banister, 1589).

Paracelsus burnt the works of Galen and Avicenna on the 27th June 1527, St John's Day, because he opposed the theories put

---

[56] ana = of each, one
[57] q.s. = quantum sufficiendum = sufficient quantity

forward by the ancients and preferred the use of chemicals (see 1541).

1530 Girolamo Francastoro (1478–1553), who was born in Verona, wrote of the topical mercurial treatments for syphilis, '*Patients, a truce to the disgust which may be caused by this remedy! For [if] it is disgusting, the disease is still more so'. Besides, your cure is at this price… Very soon you will feel the ferment of the disease dissolve themselves in your mouth in a disgusting flow of saliva.'* He also used guaiacum for syphilis (Stratman-Thomas, 1930)

He also wrote '*Syphilis sive morbus Gallicus'* [Syphilis or the French Disease].

'A shepherd once (distrust not ancient fame)
Possest these downs, and Syphilus his name…'

This was the origin of the use of the word 'Syphilis' for the venereal disease.

He first wore buboes[58] dreadful to the sight,
First felt strange pains and sleepless past the night;
From him the malady receiv'd its name,
The neighboring shepherds catcht the spreading flame.
The greater part, and with success more sure,
By mercury perform the happy cure;
A wondrous virtue in the mineral lies….
This done, wrapt close and swath'd, repair to bed,
And there let such thick cov'rings be o'erspred
Till streams of sweat from ev'ry pore you force:
For twice five days you must repeat this course;
Severe indeed but you your fate must bear,
And signs of coming health will streight appear.
The mass of humours now dissolv'd within,
To purge themselves by spittle will begin,
Till you with wonder at your feet shall see
A tide of filth, and bless this remedy'.

1533 '*De Medicina Guaiaci[59], et Morbo Gallico; Liber uno'* [About the Guaicum medicine, and the French disease; Book 1] by Ulrich von Hutten (1488–1523) mentions ulcerated throat, palate, cheeks, and tongue due to mercury as well as loose

---

[58] buboes = tender and large lymph nodes in axilla or groin
[59] guaici = guaiacum wood or resin from the West Indies. It was used from the 16th century as a cure for syphilis

teeth and swollen gums all of which gave a flow of saliva and an unbearable stench so that they were unable to eat. Some developed vertigo and tremors whilst others went insane or died (Abramowitiz, 1934). As this is a translation I have changed some of it into modern spelling. Symptoms of mercury poisoning are in bold italics.

'How men at the beginning resisted this infirmity, the French pox. Capit. iiij.

*When the physicians were thus amazed, the surgeons came forward in the same error, and put to their hands: and first they began to burn the sores with hot irons. But for as much as it was an infinite labour to touch them all, they went about to anoint them by ointments, but divers men used divers ointments, and all in vain, except he added quicksilver thereto, they beat for this use the powders of myrrh, of mastic, of ceruse[60], of bayberries, of alum, bolli Armenian[61], cinnabar, of vermillion, of coral, of burned salt, of rusty brass, of leddrosses[62], of rust of iron, of resin, of Turpentine, and of all manner of best oils, oil of bay, oil of pure roses & terebinth, oil of juniper, of great effect, oil of spike, swine's grease, fat of ox feet and butter, made specially in May, tallow of goats and harts, virgins honey, powder of red worms dried into dust, or consumed with oil and beaten, camphor, euphorbia & castor: & with two or three of these foresaid things mingled together they anointed the sick man's joints, his arms, his thighs, his backbone, his neckbone, with other places of his body. Some anointed them once a day, some twice, some thrice, some four times. The patient was shut in a stufe[63], kept with continual and fervent heat, some twenty and some thirty whole days: And some were laid in a bed within the stewe[64] and anointed, and covered with many clothes, and were compelled to sweat. Part of them at the second anointing **began to faint marvellously**. But yet the ointment was of such strength & effect, that what so ever disease was in the higher part of the body it drew into the stomach, & from thence up into the brain, & thence the disease **annoyed both by the nose and the mouth**,*

---

[60] ceruse = white lead
[61] bolli Armenian = Armenian clay containing aluminium silicates and iron oxides used, in the treatment of inflammation, allergy and tumours, by Galen and Avicenna
[62] leddrosses = This is probably litharge, lead monoxide (PbO) in its crystalline form, which is red
[63] stufe = bath-house
[64] stewe = steam bath

*and did put the patient to such pain, that except they took good heed, **their teeth fell out, all their throats, their tongues, their roofs of the mouths, were full of sores, their jaws did swell, their teeth were loosened, and continually there annoyed the most stinking scum and matter,** that could be, and what so ever it ran upon, by and by it was polluted and infected whereby their lips so touched gathered sores, and within forth their cheeks were grievously pained. Al the place, where they were, did stink. Which manner of curing was so painful, that many had lever[65] die than so to be eased. How be it scantly the hundreth person was eased, but shortly after fell down again: so yet his ease lasted very few days whereby men may estimate, what I suffered in this disease, that proved this manner of curing eleven times, with great jeopardy & peril, wrestling with this evil nine years. And yet in the mean time taking what so ever thing was thought to withstand & resist it. For we used baths & herbs lapped about then, & drinks & caresses, And for this we had arsenic, ink, calcantun[66], verdigris, or aqua fortis, which wrought in us so bitter pain, it they might be judged very desirous of life, it had not lever die than so to prolong their life, but though curings were most bitter & painful, which were made with ointments, And was also so much the more dangerous because the ministers of it, knew not the operation thereof. For the surgeons only did not use it, but every bold fellow went about playing the physician, giving to all manner of men one ointment, either as he had seen it ministered to other, or as he had suffered it himself. And so they healed all men with one medicine, as the proverb said, 'One shoe for both feet'. If ought happened amiss to the sick, for lack of good council, they knew not what to do or say. And these men tormenters were suffered to practise on all persons what they would while the physicians were done as in an universal error & ignorance. And so without order or rule, with torment of heat and sweat plenty, all were cured after one fashion, without regard of time, habit, or complexion. Neither these ignorant anointers had not so much knowledge, as with laxatives to take away the matter, which caused the evil, or to diet them, or appoint any diversity of meat: but at length the matter must come to this*

---

[65] lever = rather
[66] calcantum = iron sulphate

*point, that they should **lose their teeth**, for they were loosed, **their mouth was all in a sore,** & through coldness of the stomach & **filthy stench**, they **lost appetite**. And although **their thirst was intolerable**, yet found they no kind of drink to help the stomach, **many were so light in their brain, that they could not stand, & some were brought into a madness & not only their hands trembled & shook thereat**, but also their feet & all the body: **some mumbled in their speaking as long as they lived**, & could have no remedy. And **many I have seen die** in the middle of their curing. And one I know did so his cure, that in one day he killed three husbandmen, through immoderate heat which they suffered patiently, shut within an hot stewe, trusting that they should the sooner obtain their health till through vehement heat their hearts failed them, and perceived not themselves to die, and so were wretchedly strangled. Other I saw die, when their **throats were swollen in the interior, that first the filthy matter**, where they should have annoyed in **spitting** could find no way out, and at length **their breath was like wise stopped**, and an other sort, **when they could not piss**, Very few they were that got their health and they passed through these jeopardises, these bitter pains, and evils'.*

Elyot, Thomas Sir, 1490?–1546. *'Of the knowledge [sic] which makes a wise man.'*
Opium: *'…and the juice of Poppy, called Opium, to them which by some unnatural cause be let from sleep, do profit much, if they be measurably taken: contrary wise if they be taken by him that is much fleumatike* (phlegmatic)*, and of nature disposed to sleep very soundly, and also the medicine exceeds his portion, he brings the patient in to so deep a slepe that he never awakes.'*

1534 Otto Brunfels (1484–1534) wrote '*Herbarium vivae eicones*' [Living images of plants] with beautiful pictures of plant by Hans von Weiditz.

1536 Gerolamo Cardano (1503–1576) wrote '*De malo recentiorum medicorum usu libellus*' [A short treatise on the damaging use of more recent medicines], Venice, The common medical practices that Cardano vehemently denounced were seventy-two in number. He attacked the premise that in every case of illness immediate recourse should be had to powders and potions. *'To do nothing with physic is far better than to do too much, and a physician desiring to act rightly should consider a great number of things before setting down prescriptions for the pharmacist to manufacture'*. He denounced other practices, *'the result of the tribal insecurities of men who banded themselves together and showed to the world a surface of pomp and learning that satisfactorily concealed from the beholders the depth of ignorance beneath'*.

1539 *'Here beginneth a good boke of medecines called the Treasure of pore men.'* London: imprynted by Robert Redman dwelling at the sygne of the George nerte to Saint Dunstan's Church. This is one of the earliest English medical books. It contains numerous homely prescriptions, mainly consisting of herbs, for instance: *'for stopping of the Spleen. Take the Elder root and seethe (boil) it in white wine unto the third part & drink therof for it cures marvellously.'* It mentions henbane but I could not find hellebore or opium. No mention of ADRs.

1540 *Digitalis purpura* was originally discovered in the 16th century by Leonard Fuchs (1501–1566), who named the plant 'digitalis'. Unfortunately, due to severe toxicity and the deaths of some patients, digitoxin was rejected and forgotten until 1775, when it was rediscovered by William Withering.

Early English Statute: (Apothecary Wares Drugs and Stuffs Act 32 King Henry VIII, c40 For Physicians and their privileges) empowering physicians to appoint four inspectors of 'Apothecary Wares, Drugs and stuffs' (Goodall, 1684; Penn 1979).

Henry VIII amalgamated the Barbers Company of London and the Guild (or fellowship) of Surgeons to form the Company of Barber-Surgeons.

1541 Konrad Gessner (26 March 1516–13 December 1565) Swiss *'Enchiridion historiae plantarum'* [Handbook of the history of plants] (1541) and the *'Catalogus plantarum de remediis secretis liber secundus'* [Book 2, the catalogue of secret plant remedies]

Paracelsus–Philippus Aureolus Theofrastus Bombasto di Hohenheim (1493–1541) alias Paracelsus. *'The Third Defence Concerning the Description of the New Receipts.'* is one of seven defences presented as replies to the accusations of Paracelsus's enemies, published posthumously in 1564: *'If you wish justly to explain each poison, what is there that is not poison? All things are poison, and nothing is without poison: the Dosis alone makes a thing not poison.'* ['*Alle Ding sind Gift und nichts ohn Gift; alein die Dosis macht das ein Ding kein Gift ist'*.]

'Die Grosse Wundartzney' (Greater Surgery) by Paracelsus had been translated into French by Pierre Hassard of Armentières as early as 1566 while Jacques Gohory had prepared a Compendium of Paracelsian theory the following year (Debus, Chemical Philosophy, 1, pp.145-173).

'The several kinds of diseases are divided into various boughs, branches, and leaves, but yet the cure is but one: For example, Consider a Mercurial disease, and you shall find that the Mercurial Liquor does likewise pass into many branches and leaves; so 'tis in the small pox, or pustules, all the kinds thereof are under Mercury, for the disease it self is mercurial: Some French-pox are under common Mercury: some pustules are under a metallic Mercury, some are under an ebony wood Mercury, some are under a Mercury…'Tell me, how comes it to pass that mercury heals the French pox and the filthy scab? Why do you command the miserable sick persons to annoint themselves with quickesilver as shepherdesses grease their sheep? How happens it (I say) that mercury is the special best remedy against these diseases….'

'A hundred and fourteen experiments and cures of the famous physician Philippus Aureolus Theophrastus Paracelsus;' translated out of the German tongue into the Latin. Whereunto is added certain excellent and profitable works by B.G. a Portu Aquitano (Portuguese in Aquitaine). Also certain secrets of Isacke Hollandus concerning the vegetable and animal work. Also the spagericke[67] antidotarie for gun-shot of Iosephus Quirsitanus.' Collected by Iohn Hester, 1596.

---

[67] spagericke = distiller

*¶19 *'One had two Pushes (pustules?) as it were warts upon the yard[68], which he got by dealing with an unclean woman, so that for six months he was forsaken of all Physicians, as uncurable, the which I cured by giving him* Essentia Mercuriale, *and then mixed the oil of vitriol, with* Aqua sophiae, *and laid it on warm with a suppository for ten four days.'*

¶53 *'A certain man being long sick of the pox had two tumours and an ulcer in his nose, at the which every day there came forth great quantity of stinking and filthy matter, in whose nose I cast this decoction with a syringe. R. Hony {ounce} iiij. the juice of Calendine, Common salt prepared {dram} ij. Aloes washed {ounce} ss. mix them together. Inwardly he was purged with* Oleum Mercurij.'

¶57 *'One called Gallenus had lost his speech by means of a hole that he had in the palate of his mouth coming of the pox, the which I cured with* Mercurius Dulcis diaphoreticus *cast in by a syringe, and so the flesh grew again and was made whole.'*

¶95 *'One had a hard swelling in the flesh of his leg caused of* (Morbus Hispanicus) *whom I cured with* Oleum Antimoni, **3** *ii. Mercurie mortified according to our order* **3** *i. mixed into an ointment.'*

These are typical examples of his style. He had, it seems, a 100% success and no adverse effects to report. He earned his name 'Bombastsus'. He also introduced the use of some mineral remedies, e.g. antimony and he named 'Tincture of Opium', 'Laudanum'.

Later in 1590 there was published *'An exalted treatise teaching howe to cure the French pockes: with all other diseases arising and growing thereof, and in a manner all other sicknesses drawne out of the bookes of that learned and Prince of Physicians, Theophrastsus Paracelsus'* compiled by the learned Phillipus Hemanni, 1590.

The patient being confined to a fumigation chamber with cinnabar heaped on the coals he describes the results: *The patient then begins to sweat the mercury with his whole substance, creeps into him in such sort, that it causes all the slime in his body to ascend into his mouth, infecting and corrupting all parts of the patient in such sort, that it is pitiful*

---

[68] yard = penis

80

to behold, so that the one after long martyrdom at length creeps into his grave, the other becomes cripple and deformed, the third toothless and such like miserable accidents which are befallen them, that it would grieve a man to see, how they have handled a number of their patients.

For mercury being used corporallie[69], has this nature, that it both draws all the corrupt matter of the pockes into the mouth, and because they have dealt so disorderly therewith, taking more of it than they ought, they have therewith, all drawn the corruption into the mouth in such abundance that it could not have sufficient egress, but for want thereof is returned, and has sought a place in the entrails, as in the liver, the lungs, the milt[70], and the stomach, etc. So that some are fallen into the diseases of the lungs, as pleurisies, shortness of breath, coughs, consumptions, and such other, almost altogether incurable diseases. Other are fallen into diseases of the stomach, as vomitings, queasiness, great and intolerable pains, and apostoms[71] of the stomach, not being able to digest any good nourishment. Others are fallen into diseases of the liver, as the yellow jaundice, or ictteritia[72], the dropsies, the bloody flux, hot fiery agues and such like. And some into the diseases of the milt, as the fever quartaine[73], the canckers[74], the woolfe[75], the leprosy, to all which diseases they were not any way subject or inclined, until such time, as they were brought thereto by the unskilfulness of foolish surgeons, and all these aforesaid diseases, are altogether in manner incurable, and in the end deadly. Wherefore I would wish every man to take heed, not to deal with mercury in any such sort as is before expressed. But if you will use it in any such order as hereafter shall be shown you, it shall not only not be hurtful, but you shall also therewith perform that which the you promised to your patient, that is also to say the curing of his disease.'

---

[69] corporallie = orally
[70] milt = spleen
[71] apostoms = abscesses
[72] ictteritia = icterus
[73] fever quartaine = quartan fever = fever occurring every four days usually caused by Plasmodium malariae.
[74] canckers = ulceration of the mouth
[75] woolfe = probably Lupus vulgaris (tuberculosis of the skin)

1542 **Henry VIII Charter** so called Herbalists' Charter

Annis Tricesimo Quarto and Tricesimo Quinto. Henry VIII Regis. Cap. VIII. (Thirtythird and thirtyfourth year of the reign of Henry VIII) An act that persons, being no common surgeons, may administer outward medicines. Were in the Parliament holden at Westminster in the third Year of the King's most gracious reign, amongst other things, for the avoiding of sorceries, witchcrafts, and other inconveniences, it was enacted, that no Person within the City of London, nor within seven miles of the same, should take upon him to exercise and occupy as physician or surgeon, except he be first examined, approved, and admitted by the Bishop of London and other, under and upon certain pains and penalties in the same act mentioned: Since the making of which said act, the Company and Fellowship of Surgeons of London, minding only their own lucres, and nothing the profit or ease of the diseased or patient, have sued, troubled, and vexed divers honest persons, as well men as women, whom God hath endued with the knowledge of the nature, kind and operation of certain herbs, roots, and waters, and the using and ministering of them to such as been pained with customable diseases, as women's breasts being sore, a pin and the web in the eye, uncomes[76] of hands, burnings, scaldings, sore mouths, the stone, strangury[77], saucelim[78], and morphew[79], and such other like diseases; and yet the said persons have not taken anything for their pains or cunning, but have ministered the same to poor people only for neighbourhood and God's sake, and of pity and charity: And it is now well known that the surgeons admitted will do no cure to any person but where they shall be rewarded with a greater sum or reward that the cure extendeth unto; for in case they would minister their cunning unto sore people unrewarded, there should not so many rot and perish to death for lack or help of surgery as daily do; but the greatest part of surgeons admitted been much more to be blamed than those persons that they troubled, for although the most part of the persons of the said craft of surgeons have small cunning yet they will take great sums of money,

---

[76] uncomes = whitlows
[77] strangury = painful passing of little urine.
[78] saucelin = tumour possibly a facial swelling with inflammation
[79] morphew = scaly eruption, probably derived from Morphea, its latin translation, which is a localised form of scleroderma

and do little therefore, and by reason thereof they do oftentimes impair and hurt their patients, rather than do them good. In consideration whereof, and for the ease, comfort, succour, help, relief, and health of the King's poor subjects, Inhabitants of this realm, now pained or diseased: Be it ordained, established, and enacted by authority of this present parliament, That at all time from henceforth it shall be lawful to every person being the King's subject having knowledge and experience of the nature of herbs, roots, and waters, or of the operation of the same, by speculation or practice, within any part of the realm of England, or within any other the King's dominions, to practice, use, and minister in and to any outward sore, uncome wound, apostemations[80], outward swelling or disease, any herb or herbs, ointments, baths, poultices, and plasters, according to their cunning, experience, and knowledge in any of the diseases, sores, and maladies beforesaid, and all other like to the same, or drinks for the stone, strangury, or agues, without suit, vexation, trouble, penalty, or loss of their goods; the foresaid statute in the foresaid third year of the King's most gracious Reign, or any other act, ordinance, or statutes to the contrary heretofore made in anywise, not withstanding.' (Stone and Matthews, 1996).

1542 Leonhart Fuchs *'New Kreüterbuch'* [new book of herbs] *'De historia stirpium'*[81] [Concerning the history of plants], Basel. Describes 400 German plants.

Mandrake (*Mandragora officinarum*), which also contains tropane alkaloids. ...*'The apples as you sniff and taste them, bring about the sleep. Such power has also their juice. But you shall not use too much, because otherwise they kill.... Because the internal use of mandrake is very dangerous, it is better to bring about the sleep, if need be, using the apples and fruits of it by just tasting them and not taking them into the body.'*

Nightshade (*Atropa Belladonna*) which contains tropane alkaloids...*'The other one we named Maddening Herb* [deadly nightshade]. *Others call it Swine Herb and think it is the woody nightshade; but not without great error as this herb is a deadly plant and cannot be ingested without harm, as is possible with*

---

[80] apostemations = process of suppuration (Weber's Dictionary, 1913) (see footnote 69)
[81] stirpium = plants

the woody nightshade. However, it might be the third sex of mandrake…. Without doubt the Maddening Herb has the power of the fourth nightshade, which makes mad and foolish because it is a deadly herb for human, as given by experience. I also know certainly of two children, who have eaten the berries, which taste quite sweet and they died soon thereafter, although they had been lively and healthy before'….

Henbane (*Hyoscyamus niger*), which also contains tropane alkaloids.

'*The green henbane leaves, the seeds and juice, which not only make man mad and foolish; but also the beasts, must not be used internally; but only externally to stop the pain and to bring sleep, and if used at all then only with good modesty*' (Dioscorides, 1544). '*Many call henbane also Swine Beans and Sleeping Herb…. Henbane ground freshly alone / or mixed with malted barley and applied / takes away all sorts of pains. The juice pressed from the herb / a handkerchief wetted therein / and put onto the hot / running and painful eyes / quenches the heat / stops the flow and their pain. The juice or the seed oil put into the ears / quenches the stinging therein / and the pain. But use these with great care…. A foot bath made from henbane / brings sleep…. The roots of Henbane boiled in vinegar and held in the mouth for some time / takes away the great and bad aches of teeth. In summary / the green Henbane leaves / the seeds / and juice / which not only make man mad and foolish / but also the beasts / must not be used internally / but only externally to stop the pain / and to bring sleep / and if used at all then only with good modesty.*'

1544 '*Les Commenteires de Monsieur Pierre Andre Matthiole, médecin Seinois, sur les six livres de la matière médicinale de Pedacius Dioscorides*' [The comments of Ms Pierre Andre Matthiole, a Swiss physician, on the six books on medical matters by Pedacius Dioscorides] by Pietro Andrea Mattioli: (1501–1577). Written in 1544 and translated into French in 1680.

Henbane: he quotes Scribonius Largus and Galen: '*Both black seeds and red are dangerous and poisonous, but the white is very good in medicine.*'

Mercury: *'There are those who often use (red mercury) by mouth from 4 to 8 grains (518 mgm) in order to excite the flow from the syphilitic mouth; but it is hazardous to the patient and burns the viscera if one gives it without correcting it.'*

Opium: *'It ulcerates the mouth and tongue. It makes one sleep a long time. Opium used as an eye lotion make some almost lose their sight, others become deaf because of putting poppy juice in their ears.'*

1546 Valerius Cordus (1515–1544), a Nuremberg physician writes the *'Dispensatorium'*, the first German pharmacopoeia (*Das Dispensatorium des Valerius Cordus: Faksimile des im Jahre 1546 erschienenen ersten Druckes durch Joh. Petreium in Nurnberg)* [The Dispensatorium of Valerius Cordus: a facsimile of the 1546 First Edition by Joh. Petreium of Nuremberg] by Valerius Cordus; Ludwig Winkler. Publisher: Mittenwald (Bayern): Buchdruckerei und Verlag Arthur Nemayer, 1934). Composed of prescriptions. He described the synthesis of ether and named it 'sweet vitriol'. At about the same time, Swiss physician and alchemist Paracelsus discovered the hypnotic effects of ether.

'Medicine makes people ill, mathematics makes them sad, and theology makes them sinful.' Martin Luther (1483–1546).

'Kreüter Buch' [Herbal book] by Hieronymus Bock (1498–1554) published by Wendel Rihel in 1546. Classified 700 plants by characteristics and medicinal use.

Henbane: *'Henbane flowers and seeds are of a cold nature, should seldom be ingested for this plant when ingested is harmful, not alone to man, but also to all cattle. This can be seen from the fish in the water when the fish are tricked by tramps with henbane and Rokilien[82] grains, that they are made crazed by it, leap up, and finally turn whit side up that in such stupor they may be caught with the hands. The hens on the eaves fall down when they are exposed to the smoke of henbane. Such artful tricks are dome by the gypsies and their folk.'*

'Henbane flowers and seeds serve for sleep, calm pain, but

---

[82] rokilien = Despite extensive searches I have been unable to find the meaning of this word. It might be related to 'Rauke' rocket which has been used in India as an aphrodisiac or to 'Roggen 'rye' if the latter, then henbane mixed with rye grain would be a fish bait

too much used make one wild and crazed"In summary, green henbane leaves, its seeds and essences, should only be taken externally to calm pain and to promote sleep.'

'A lytel herball of the properties of herbes', newly amended and corrected, with certain additions at the end of the book, declaring what herbs have influence of certain stars and constellations, wherby may be chosen the best and most lucky times and days of their ministration, according to the Moon being in the signs of heaven, the which is daily appointed in the almanacke, made and gathered in the year of our Lord God. M DL the XII day of February, by Anthony Askham, Physician.' This work, which is generally called Askham's Herbal, is directly derived from Banckes' Herbal, with the addition of some astrological lore. No mention of Henbane or Hellebore and no mention of ADRs.

1552 Aztec Herbal, published in 1552 is the earliest treatise on Aztec pharmacology *'Medicenalibus Indorum Herbis.'* [About the mediaeval plants of India]. Written by Martin de la Cruz, an Aztec doctor, it was later translated by Juan Badiano, an Indian doctor from Xochimilco, Mexico. It was discovered in the Vatican library in 1919 and has become known as the Badiano Codex. The book was a compendium of 250 medicinal herbs used by the Aztecs.

1553 John XXI Pope (d1277) wrote ' *The treatise of Health containing many profitable medicines gathered out of Hippocrates, Galen and Avicenna, by one Petrus Hyspanus [and] translated into English by Humfre Lloyde who has added thereunto the causes and signs of every disease, with the aphorisms of Hippocrates, and Jacobus de Partybus redacted to a certain order according to the members of mans body, and a compendious table containing the purging and conforting medicines, with the expostion of certain names [and] weights in this book contained with an epistle of Diocles unto King Antigonus.'* 'In Fleete street at the sign of the Rosegarland by Wyllyam Coplande, [Imprinted at London] : 'Petrus Hyspanus was a Portuguese physician who practised in Sienna and who in his last years was made John Pope XXI'.

Opium: *'If opium, henbane seed, & mandrage be mingled with wax & oil, in the which they have soaked, and the members therewith be anointed and a plaster therof being made, & bound unto the coddes[83], it taketh away the desire of copulation.'*

Henbane: *'Let the fume of the matter be drawn downward with a suppository or clister[84], and with moderate rubbing of the hands and feet, then put a sponge dipped in the decoction of Henbane or a whelp or a cock wrapped over the belly upon the head, or the lungs of a swine, also bind the arms and legs of the patient, and let him smell opium, camphor, henbane, basil, saffron or wax mingled with rose water, afterwarde anoint the ears, eyes and nodle with myrrh, storax, castoreum, or wash, the head, with henbane or smalage[85] that have been soaked in sweet wine.'*

Mercury: *'Against the French Pox, take of brimstone. {dram} ii. of nesyng[86] powder, quicksilver, & cumin, of each {dram} i. of staphisagre[87] {dram}. And a half and incorporate there with .{dram} vi. of stale hog's grease, by this means every evil disease or sickness is for a surety healed, except it be of glandules or kernels[88] which must be cured after an other means.'*

Willow: *'The juice of sallow or willow root mixed with oil of roses is wonderful good for the hot gout.'* (Galen).

1554 A celebrated herbal *'Cruyderoek'* by Rembert Dodoens (1517–1585) was printed in the Lowlands in 1554 (see 1586 and 1619).

1657 The Expert Doctors Dispensatory says in its introduction concerning drugs: *'They must be safe, that if they do no remedy they may no wise predjudice the party, although in desperate diseases desperate medicines may be used with an exquisite judgement'.*

1564 The *'Horti Germani'* [German Gardens] of Konrad Gesner, a Swiss naturalist, was printed in 1561. *'Epistolarum medicinalium'* [About accounts of medicines], a collection of Gesner's scientific correspondence published with the first monograph on aconites and hellebores in 1557. He had also published a *'Historia Plantarum* [History of plants], 1541, *'Of Mercurie precipitate, which serves and is a remedy against all*

---

[83] coddes = testicles
[84] clister = enema
[85] smalage = *Apium graveolens*, which acts as a diuretic.
[86] nesyng = sneezing
[87] staphisagre = *Delphinium staphisagre*, a species of larkspur, also known as lousewort. The seeds contain diterpene, an alkaloid which is a powerful emetic and cathartic.
[88] kernels = testicles

sicknesses and diseases, caused of the rottenness of humours.' Chapter LXXXX.

1564 Gabriele Fallopius (1523–62) used mercury for syphilis, but preferred guaiacum, China root and sarsaparilla (Waugh, 1982).

1566 The Paris Faculty of Physicians forbade antimony use by physicians charging that antimony in any form was a dangerous poison that should not be taken internally. This would seem to be the first official withdrawal of a drug from the market. The ban was lifted 100 years later after it had been given the credit for saving the King's life. This was a result of a long and bitter controversy between the Galenic school in Paris and the Paracelsian school of Montpellier.

1568 William Turner *'The first and second parts of the Herbal of William Turner, Doctor in Phisick, lately overseen, corrected and enlarged with the third parte'.* (Cologne, 1568).

'A New Herball: Wherein are contained the names of herbs in Greek, Latin, English, Dutch, French, and in the apothecaries and Herbaries Latin, with the properties, degrees and natural places of the same. A new herbal, wherin are contained the names of herbs...' (London: imprinted by Steven Myerdman and solde by John Gybken, 1551) is the first part of Turner's great work; the second was published in 1562 and the third in 1568, by Arnold Birckman of Antwerp. It was mainly copied from Leonhart Fuchs's 1542 *'De Historia Stirpium'* [Concerning the history of the families of plants] Cologne. (Chapman & Tweddle, 1995). Turner like many other herbalists gave credit to his predecessors: Pliny, Theophrastus, Dioscorides and Galen.

<u>White hellebore</u>: *'tells us, that in his time it was an ordinary receipt among good wives, to give hellebore in powder to ii.d. weight, and he is not much against it. But they do commonly exceed, for who so bold as blind Bayard[89], and prescribe it by pennyworths, and such irrational ways, as I have heard myself market folks ask for it in an apothecary's shop: but with what success God knows; they smart often for their rash boldness and folly, break a vein, make their eyes ready to start out of their heads, or kill themselves.'*

---

[89] Bayard = An old blind horse

Poppy: '*He that has eaten opium has a great sluggishness and a disposition to sleep and all the body is encumbered with a sore itch.*'

Mangora: '*Because this has diverse ways, taken is very jeopardous for a man, it may kill him if he eat it, or drink it, out of measure, and have no remedy for it... Mandraga be taken out of measure, by and by sleep ensues and a great lowering of strength with a forgetfulness, but If a man takes to much of it will kill him.*'

1571 Petrus Severinus, physician to the Danish king, wrote that the effects of antimony were '*Vomare, cacare, sudare*' (to vomit, to defaecate, to sweat) [Severinus, 1571].

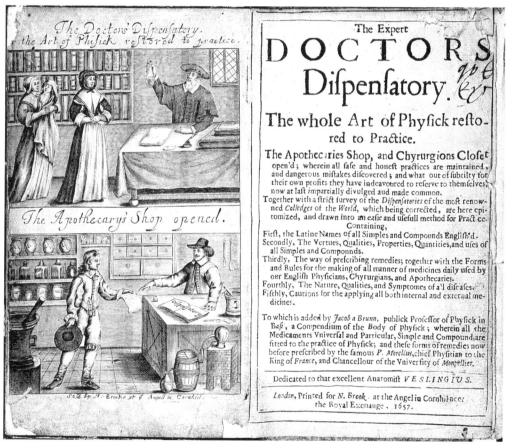

Figure 2. The Expert Doctor's Dispensatory

1564–1616 Shakespeare, as one would expect, mentions herbal treatment and its adverse effects:

Friar Lawrence: *'Within the infant rind of this weak flower,*
Poison hath residence, and medicine power
For this, being smelt, with that part cheers each part;
Being tasted, slays all senses with the heart.'
Romeo and Juliet, Act 2, Scene 2.

Banquo: *'Were such things here as we do speak about?*
Or have we eaten on the insane root
That takes the reason prisoner?'
Macbeth Act I, Scene 3.
(Henbane was also known as 'insina' mad).

'Trust not the physician
His antidotes are poison, and he slays
More than you rob.'
The Life of Timon of Athens (Timon at IV, iii).

Cornelius *'I do not like her. She doth think she has*
(physician) *Strange lingering poisons: I do know her spirit,*
And will not trust one of her malice with
A drug of such damn'd nature. Those she has
Will stupefy and dull the sense awhile;
Which first, perchance, she'll prove on cats and dogs,
Then afterward up higher: but there is
No danger in what show of death it makes,
More than the locking-up the spirits a time,
To be more fresh, reviving. She is fool'd
With a most false effect; and I the truer,
So to be false with her.'
Cymbeline Act 1, Scene 5 .

Macbeth: '*Throw physic to the dogs, I'll none of it!*'

                                            Macbeth & Doctor at V, iii Tr.

Hamlet: '*Upon my secure hour thy uncle stole,*
            With juice of cursed hebenon in a vial,
            And in the porches of mine ears did pour
            The leprous distilment whose effect holds
            such an enmity with blood of man.'

                                            Hamlet, Act 1, Scene 5.

The logic of poisoning via the ear is explained by Basilio Kotsias (Kotsias, 2002).

It has also been suggested that Shakespeare suffered from syphilis and the resulting mercury toxicity: '*Shakespeare's late-life decrease in artistic production, tremor, social withdrawal, and alopecia were due to mercury poisoning from syphilis treatment. He may also have had anasarca due to mercury-related membranous nephropathy*' (Ross, 2005).

1579 '*Bullein's bulwark of defence against all sickness, soreness, and wounds that do daily assault mankind: which bulwark is kept with Hilarius the gardener, [and] Health the physician, with the chirurgian, to help the wounded soldiers.*' '*Gathered and practised from the most worthy learned, both old and new: to the great comfort of mankind: by William Bullein, Doctor of Phisick. 1562. Date: 1579*'.

'*With this Quicksilver and Sal Armoniac, is made Mercury sublimate, which must be kept in a closed vessel, adjusted in a oven, or burnt until it come to the colour of white Sugar, which Mercury sublimate is used of Chirurgians for to cleanse foul ulcers and sores, and is a poison inwardly to be taken, except with all speed after the same a vomit be taken of oil or Azarabaccha[90]. If Quicksilver be taken inwardly, it is also perilous, and nothing better to help it, than to drink Wormwood wine with the seed of Clary[91] boiled therein. Marvellous things be done by means of Quicksilver as the Chemists do know, and yet for all that we see little Gold multiplied thereby. Thus*

---

[90] arabaccha = *Asarum european* = Hazel wort or wild nut
[91] clary = *Salvia sclarea*

to conclude, Quicksilver may be conveniently ministered in ointments, to heal the Pox.' A reference to the use of mercury for venereal disease.

Jean Fernel d'Amiens (1497–1558), Chief Physician to Henri II, in *'Le meilleur traitement du mal vénérien'* [The best treatment for Syphilis] *1579* maintained that all the late symptoms of syphilis were due to mercurial poisoning (Abraham, 1948). He also attacked the use of mercury, not because it was ineffective, but because of its empirical nature. He favoured guiacum for the treatment of syphilis (Sherrington, 1946). He said *'beaucoup de malades aiment mieux mourir du Mal que de chercher la guérison dans un traitement si dangereux et si cruel* (Many patients prefer to die of syphilis than to look for a cure with such a dangerous and cruel treatment'].

However, he also noted a curious case of mercury poisoning in a painter of Anjou. This individual was *'seized first with palsy of the fingers and hands, later with spasms in these parts, and the arm too was similarly affected; this disorder next attacked his feet; finally he began to be tormented by pain in the stomach and both hypochondria, so violent that it could not be relieved by clysters, fomentations, baths or any other remedy. When the pain came on, the only thing that gave him any relief was for 3 or 4 men to press with their whole weight on his abdomen; this compression of the abdomen lessened the torture. At last, after about three years of this cruel suffering, he died consumptive'.* Fernel stated that the most imminent physicians of his day disagreed violently as to the true cause of this terrible disorder. And when Ramazzini read Fernel's case study, he stated, *'I admired the frank confession of Fernel; "we were all beside the mark and completely off the track." However, Fernel went on to say that since this painter was "in the habit of squeezing the color from his brush with his fingers and worse still was imprudent and rash enough to suck it, it is probable that the cinnabar was carried from the fingers to the brain by direct communication and so to the whole nervous system; while that which he took in by the mouth infected the stomach and intestines with the mysterious and malignant qualities, and was the occult cause of those violent pains"* (Fernel, 1579).

1580 It took approximately 2,000 years before the work of Shen Nung and his followers were documented in a book called '*Shen Nung Pen Ts'ao Ching*'. Chinese medicine seems to have reached its peak during the Ming dynasty (1368-1644) when Li Shih-chen wrote his '*Pen ts'ao kang mu*' (The Great Herbal). This pharmacopoeia, which summarizes what was known of herbal medicine up to the late 16th century, describes in detail more than 1800 plants, animal substances, minerals, and metals, along with their medicinal properties and applications.

1580 '*Approved medicines and cordial recipes with the natures, qualities, and operations of sundry samples. Very commodious and expedient for all that are studious of such knowledge.*' by Newton, Thomas, 1542-1607. There is no mention of hellebore or willow.

Opium: '*taken in excesse it does refrigerate so much, that it stupifieth, and makes the body without sense or feeling: but taken in a convenient quantity, it doth cease pains, and provokes sleep.*'

Henbane (*Herba Apollinaris, Iusquiamus vulgò*)

'*The kind of henbane that has the white flower & the white seed is used in physick, to cease vehement pains and distillations of the head, and the eyes: given in a convenient quantity it provokes sleep, the other kinds are not to be used, for they be stupefacient and perilous.*'

1581 The first Spanish Pharmacopoeia.

1586 '*A New Herball or Historie of Plants*' by Rembert Dodoens, physician to the Emperor. Imprinted in London by Ninian Newton. Originally written in German it was translated into French and this was translated into English by Henrie Lyte. Each herb is described under the headings: the kinds, the description, the nature, the virtues and the dangers. This one of the earliest herbals to deal systematically with the adverse effects.

Opium: The dangers '*The use of poppy is very evil and dangerous, and especially opium, the which taken excessively, or too often applied upon the flesh outwardly, or otherwise without good consideration and advice, it will cause a man to sleep too much, as though he had the lethargy, which is the forgetful sickness, and brings foolish and doting fancies, it corrupts the sense and understanding brings palsy, and in time it kills the body.'*

Hellebore *'White hellebore, which some call sneezing-powder, a strong purger upward, which many reject, as being too violent: Mesue and Averroes will not admit of it, "by reason of danger of suffocation," "great pain and trouble it puts the poor patient to," saith Dodonæus.'*

The *'de plantis ... epitome'* [Summary of plants] of J. Camerarius in herbal by Rycharde Banckes.

'Historia generalis plantarum' [A general history of plants] and *'Historia plantarum Lugdunensis'* [A history from Lyon of plants] by Jacques d'Aléchamps (1513–1588) of France.

1588–91 *'Neuw vollkommentlich Kreuterbuch'* [New Compleat Herbal] by Iacobus Theodorus Tabernaemontanus (1522–1590). First edition probably 1613.

Another noteworthy herbal was the last great German work of its kind printed in the 16th century, the *'Neuw Kreuterbuch'* (1588-91; further editions: 1613, 1625) by Theodorus, which also included plants endemic to non-German regions.

Clowes, William, c1540–1604. *'A prooued practise for all young chirurgians, concerning burnings with gunpowder, and woundes made with gunshot, sword, halbard, pyke, launce, or such other Wherein, is delivered with all faithfulnesse, not onely the true receipts of such medicines as shall make them bolde, but also sundry familiar examples, such, as may leade them as it were by the hand, to the doyng of the lyke.* Heereto is adioyned a treatise of the French or Spanish pockes, written by Iohn Almenar, a Spanish physition. Also, a commodious collection of aphorismes both English and Latin, taken out of an old written coppy. Published for the benefyte of his countrey, by Wylliam Clowes, mayster in chirurgery. Seene, and allowed, according to the order appoynted. 1588'.

'Certayne difficulties are dissolved which may be propounded touching this disease.' Chap 6.

'So this disease is readier to be first taken in the yard then in the neck, head, shoulders, and not in other places. Therefore the

influence at that time was an enemy to the head and yard. And if it be demanded why it has the termination by the mouth? it may be aunswered, that this procéeds of the property of Quicksilver, which doth draw humours to those parts: or better thus, that Quicksilver by his heat doth warm, and make thin the humours thus prepared, to expell them by the uppermost parts: therefore Paulus affirms it to be hot and moist in the fourth degrée, to whom, I do rather stick then to Avicenna, who maks it cold in the second degrée. And if it be demanded, why the mouth doth stink? It may be answered, that this comes of the Quicksilver, whose fume hath property to make the mouth stink as Avicenna saith, can. 2. cap. 2. Hereupon also comes pain in the head, and hurt in the mouth, as it may be gathered of the nature of it, unto this may be added the burnt, putrified ill humour, which may make the same accidents, and therefore it is no marvel if there be so great pains. Now the especial remedy is, that when the humour begins to be expelled by the mouth, it be diverted by medicines ministred upward and downward, to bring it to the lower parts. If it be demanded, wherefore some persons being apt to melancholic diseases, both in regard of complexion and ill order, are not infected? I say that perhaps their bodies are more firm, and consequently do more hardly receive an impression then others, or by some other property, which in divers bodies is found to be divers, as saith Avicenna. 1. 1. And if it be demaunded why Quicksilver helps, or is more available than other medicines, except the distilling of Triacle[92] before mentioned? it must be answered, to come of his property, or rather manifest quality, because it is hot and moist in the highest degrée, and the disease cold and dry.'

For Galen *saith, 9. de tuenda sanitate. It is hard to finde such an helpe as hath no hurt in it.'*

1589 Spenser's *'Fairy Queen'*.

'Faire Venus sonne . . . Lay now thy deadly Heben bow apart and with thy mother mild come to mine aid.'

Mammon's garden: 'Of direful deadly black, both leaf and bloom fit to adorn the dead, and deck the dreary tomb, There mournful cypress grew in greatest store, and trees of bitter gall, and Heben sad.'

---

[92] triacle = Venetian treacle = Therica + Mythridatum (see 120 BC)

Arthur 'Till that they spied where towards them did pace an armed knight, of bold and beauteous grace, Whose squire 'bore after him an heben lance, and covered shield.' (Warriors used to dip the ends of their arrows and lances in henbane to kill the prey).

1590 Paré, Ambroise, (1510?–1590). *'The workes of that famous chirurgion Ambrose Parey'* translated out of Latine and compared with the French by Th: Johnson, 1634.

Henbane: *'drunken, or otherwise taken inwardly by the mouth, causes an alienation of the mind like drunkenness; this also is accompanied with an agitation of the body, and exultation of the spirits like sowning[93]. But amongst others, this is a notable symptom, that the patients so dote, that they think themselves to be whipped: whence their voice becomes so various, that somtimes they bray like an ass or mule, neigh like a horse, as Avicenna writes.'*

'We will first declare what the general signs of poison are, and then will we descend to particulars, whereby we may pronounce that one is poisoned with this or that poison. We certainly know that a man is poisoned, when as he complains of a great heaviness of his whole body, so that he is weary of himself; when as some horrid and loathsome taste sweats out from the orifice of the stomach to the mouth and tongue, wholly different from that taste that meat, howsoever corrupted, can send up: when as the colour of the face changes suddenly, somewhiles to black, sometimes to yellow, or any other colour, much differing from the common custom of man; when nauseousness with frequent vomiting, troubles the patient, and that he is molested with so great unquietnesse, that all things may seem to be turned upside down. We know that the poison works by the proper, and from the whole substance, when as without any manifest sense of great heat or coldness, the patient sownes often with cold sweats, for usually such poisons have no certain and distinct part wherewith they are at enmity, as cantharides have with the bladder. But as they work by their whole substance, and an occult propriety of form; so do they presently and directly assail the heart, our essence and life, and the fortress and beginning of

---

[93] sowning = fainting

the vital faculty. Now will we show the signs whereby poisons, that work by manifest and elementary qualities, may be known. Those who exceed in heat, burn or make an impression of heat in the tongue, the mouth, throat, stomach, guts, and all the inner parts, with great thirst, unquietness, and perpetual sweats. But if to their excess of heat they be accompanied with a corroding and putrefying quality, as arsenic, sublimate, rose-ager[94] or rats-bane[95], verdisgris[96], orpiment[97], and the like, they then cause in the stomach and guts intolerable pricking pains, rumblings in the belly, and continual and intolerable thirst. These are succeeded by vomitings, with sweats some-whiles hot, somewhiles cold, with sounings, whence sudden death ensues. Poisons that kill by too great coldness, induce a dull or heavy sleep, or drowsiness, from which you cannot easily rouse or waken them; sometimes they so trouble the brain, that the patients perform many indecent gestures and antic tricks with their mouths and eyes, arms and legs, like as such as are frantic; they are troubled with cold sweats, their faces become blackish or yellowish, always ghastly, all their bodies are benumbed, and they die in a short time unless they be helped; poisons of this kind are hemlock, poppy, nightshade, henbane, mandrage, mercury. Some have devised a fourth manner of curing the Lues venerea, which is by suffitus or fumigations. I do not much approve hereof, by reason of sundry malign symptoms which thence arise, for they infect and corrupt by their venimous contagion, the brain and lungs, by whom they are primarily and fully received, whence the patients during the residue of their lives have stinking breaths. Yea many while they have been thus handled, have been taken hold of by a convulsion, and a trembling of their heads, hands, & legs, with a deafness, apoplexy, and lastly miserable death, by reason of the malign vapours of sulphur and quicksilver, whereof cinnabaris
(sulphide of mercury) *consists, drawn in by their mouth, nose, and all the rest of the body.'*

1595 Henry Lyte's Herbal. *'New herbal, or history of plants wherein is contained the whole discourse and perfect description of all sorts*

---

[94] rose-ager = roseager = realgar = As_2S_2 = disulphide of arsenic
[95] rats-bane = arsenious oxide = As_2O_3 = white arsenic
[96] verdisgris = verdigris = green rust = cupric acetate (correct definition) or a sulphate ($CuSO_4.3Cu(OH)_2$, or a carbonate ($CuCO_3.Cu(OH)_2$ or an acetate in maritime regions = atacamite $CuCl_2.3Cu(OH)_2$
[97] orpiment = a sulpharsenide (As_2S_3)

of herbs and plants: their divers and sundry kinds: their names, natures, operations, & vertues: and that not only of those which are here growing in this our country of England but of all others also of foreign realms commonly used in physick. First set forth in the Dutch or Almaigne (German) tongue, by that learned D. Rembert Dodens, physcian to the Emperor: and now first translated out of French into English, by Henry Lyte Esquire (1529–1607).'

Henbane *'It is so hurtful and venimous that such as only sleep under the shadow thereof become sick and sometimes die.'* In 1578 he published his *'Niewe Herball'*, a translation from the work of the Flemish herbalist, Dodoens, and dedicated to Queen Elizabeth I. The book, which became known as *'Lyte's Herbal'*, was a best seller and was still being reprinted in 1678.

1596 Peter Lowe (c1550–1612) wrote *'An easy, certain, and perfect method to cure and prevent the Spanish sickness Wherby the learned and skilful chirugian may heal a great many other diseases.' Arellian: 1596.*

'you shall use a decoction of salsparil[98]*, or gaiac, according to his temperature, and some liniment particular on the part affected, as also on the parts adjacent: the which liniment shall be composed of axungie[99], rosat Mesues, or butter, adding such quantity of mercury as you shall find expedient. By this liniment and the decoction, you shall have a great help in the cure.'*

'Of the nature of Quick-siluer*, and the true preparation thereof.'*

The 10. Chapter. Of the nature of Quick-siluer, and the true preparation thereof.

'I find great diversity of opinions amongst the ancients, touching Quicksilver, for the most part esteem it to be cold and humid. Avicenna in his second canon, notes it to be cold and moist in the second degree. Gulielmus Placentinus[100], Arnaldus de villa novae[101], and Placarius[102], thinks it to be cold in the fourth degree, which may easily be perceived, for it is truth that it repels the humour from the circumference to the centre, &

---

[98] salsparil = sarsparilla, *Smilax ariistolochiaefolia*, Introduced into European medicine in 1536 from Mexico as a treatmenr for syphilis.
[99] axungi = lard
[100] Gulielmus Placentinus = Guglielmo da Saliceto (c1216-1280) born Saliceto near Piacenza, Italy. Wrote *'Summa Curationis et conservationis'*
[101] Arnaldus de Villa Nouae = Alchemist,astrologer and physician from Valencia (c1235-1311)
[102] Placarius = I can find no trace of this person.

causes by the great coldness hereof, palsy and trembling, and the members to be inflexible, as says Pliny, Dioscorides, and Palmarius. Avicenna says, that it causes a stinking breath, with dimness of the sight, falling of the teeth, which we see to be true in such as have this sickness, and have often been rubbed therewith. Some esteem it to be hot and dry, but few approved authors are of that opinion. There are two kinds of it, natural and artificial, the natural is found in the veins and dens of the earth, as says Pliny and Dioscorides, and is called by them, Hydargirus. It is found also amongst metals, as reports Dioscarides in his first book. The artificial is made of Minium, and scrapings of marble, as writes Vitruvius[103] in his seventh book of his architecture. Some of it is found & drawn out of lead, and is easily known from the other, being of colour brown, and black, and of substance thick, leaving some rest behind, like the excrements of lead, which is not meet for this purpose. That which is clean white and subtle is good. Nevertheless, having chosen the most proper for our use, it must be yet prepared and purified after this sort following. First you shall take so much of it as you will use, and boil it 6. or 7. hours in water, putting in such things with it as have the virtue to corroborate & comfort the parts, as also to purify it, like as sage, rosemary, camomell, melilot, tyme, with other natural herbs. That being done, strain it through a cloth, then after extinguish it, according to the manner which you shall hear hereafter; and incorporate it with a little swine's grease. Being well compounded, you must melt it on the fire, then taking it of, you shall perceive the Quicksilver separated from the grease: the excrement and leaden substance shall remain in the same grease: Having so done, you shall strain it through a piece of leather, to the end that it may be very pure, then after, extinguish it again, to the effect that you may the better incorporate it with other swines grease, or with such medicaments as you shall hear. If you will haue your ointment white, and neither black nor gray, you must make it after this order ensuing. Take your Quicksilver and beat it in a mortar with vinegar and salt, then pour out that vinegar and salt, and put in new, and so beat it with 3. or 4. sundry shiftings, and so

---

[103] Vitruvius – Marcus Vitruvius Pollio, writer, architect and astrologer (c80/70 BC – after 15 BC)

your ointment shall be white. But to extinguish the same, you must put into the mortar with it a little syrup of roses, or oil of petroly, or juice of lemons, or fasting spittle, or a little ointment wherein Quicksilver has been put, for that is the best, and will soonest extinguish it. Then beat them together, till such time as there be not any appearance of the Quicksilver, least that being not well extinguished, it should return to the old form. So being well quenched, as is requisite, you shall make your ointment (having likewise prepared the swine's grease) in this manner. Melt it on the fire, and boil it with the herbs before mentioned, or with others of like virtue, being all chopped small: then all being boiled together, you shall strain it through a cloth, and mingle with it a little Iris of Florence, which will take away the savour of the grease, then after, compose the ointment thus. "Recipe axungiae suilae lib. 1. olei Cammomillae, et Anetini an vnc. i. Radicum anulae parum contrito, unc. quat. therebentinae venetae, unc. ss. Argenti viui preparati, unc. quat. Incorporentur omnia simul spatio viginti quatuor horarum, fiat linementum ut decet".' [Take thou of pig's lard one pound, oil of Cammomile one ounce, and dill one ounce, anulae root, a little bruised, four ounces, Venetian terebinth half an ounce, prepared Quicksilver four ounces. Incorporate all together over 24 hours, make a liniment as befits].

'I use always instead of the swines grease, the ointment called Rosatum Meseuis, and put to one pound of this ointment, five ounces of Quicksilver, oil of bayes and aniseed, of either half an ounce, so with that I give every day one friction, or once in two days, according to the temperature and strength of the patient, the which must be considered by the skilful chirurgian.'

1596 Li Shi-Zhen wrote: '*Běncao Gāngmù*'; or '*Pen-ts'ao Kang-mu* 'or '*Ben Cao Gang Mu* '[The Compendium of Materia Medica] which is a 1596 pharmaceutical text written by the Ming Dynasty physician Li Shi-Zhen (1518–1592) in 1579. The Bencao Gangmu is regarded as the most complete medical book written in the history of traditional Chinese medicine. It describes 1892 drugs and includes 11, 096 prescriptions and lists all the plants, animals, minerals, and other objects that were believed to contain medicinal properties. It states: '*On account of the fact* *that sanqi is an herb belonging to the xue (blood) phase of the yangming and jueyin meridians, it can treat all diseases of the blood.'* There are two basic types of adverse responses reported. One is an oesophagitis that appears to occur as a result of consuming tablets of sanqi without drinking much water. The tablet may directly contact the tissues and cause some irritation or might lead to some acid reflux; there were two such cases reported. The other, more frequent, problem is with allergic reactions. These include dermatitis (allergic exanthema), shock, purpura, blisters, or other reactions of idiosyncratic nature. It warned that mercury could cause convulsions and gingivitis (Leung, 1990).

1597 John Gerard's (1545–1612) *'The Herball or General Historie of Plantes'*, 1404 pages.

'Organy cures them that have been poisoned by drinking Opium, or the juice of Black Poppy or Hemlock, especially if it be given with Wine and Raisons of the Sunne.' It has been said that most of his book was a translation of Dodoens Herball (above). First published in 1597, it was republished in 1633 revised and enlarged by Thomas Johnson in an edition that retained much of the original Elizabethan text. The 1633 edition contains some 2850 descriptions of plants and about 2700 illustrations. It was divided into three volumes including an appendix.

Deadly nightshade: Gerard called the plant the lethal olanum or sleepy nightshade (*Atropa belladonna*). He recounts three cases of poisoning with the berries and instructs the readers of his herball *'Banish therefore these pernicious plants out of your gardens, and all places near to your houses, where children or women with child do resort, which do oftentimes long and lust after things most vile and filthy; and much more after a berry of a bright shining black colour, and of such great beauty, as it were able to allure any such to eat thereof.* He also said, *This kind of nightshade causes sleep, troubles the mind, brings madness if a few of the berries be inwardly taken, but if more be given they also kill and bring present death.'*

Opium: *'It mitigates all kinds of pains: but it leaves behind it oftentimes a mischief worse than the disease itself, and that hard to be cured, as a dead palsy and such like.'*

Henbane *(Hyoscyamus niger):* *'The leaves, seed, and juice taken inwardly cause unquiet sleep, like unto the sleep of drunkenness, which continues long and is deadly to the party... To wash the feet in a decoction of henbane causes sleep, or given in a clyster it does the same; and as also the often smelling of the flowers.'*

1599 King James VI of Scotland issued a charter making provisions for the supervision of the sales of drug and poisons. The first inspector appointed was William Spang, who was responsible for approving *'droggis'* (drugs) offered for sale in the city of Glasgow. Letter of Gift by King James VI under his Privy Seal, whereby he granted full power to the chirurgians and professors of medicine within the city of Glasgow to examine all persons practising chirurgery, and to license such as should be found duly qualified; prohibiting such as do not hold the license of a university in which medicine is taught, or a license from the chirurgians of Glasgow, from practising in the city; prohibiting the sale of drugs in the city, except such as is sighted by the chirurgians, and prohibiting the sale of rat poison except by the apothecaries, who should be caution for the persons to whom the same was sold. Holyrood, 29 November 1599. (Acts of the Parliaments of Scotland, vol. viii, p. 184) (City of Glasgow, 1897).

Dose

It was difficult to use the correct dose with herbs since there were several factors which were unknown: there were several varieties of many herbs, their active principles were not known, the active principles depended on when they were harvested, where they were grown and which part of the plant was used. Then the conditions of storage might affect the active principle. Where mixtures were used there could be problems of interactions between the ingredients. Since many mixtures contained powdered leaves, stalks and roots there was the possibility that one ingredient would come to the surface and another to the bottom. One of the purposes of the herbals, dispensatories and pharmacopoeias was to standardise their usage. The only safe way was to titrate the dose (Huxtable, 1990). When the margin between the therapeutic dose and the toxic dose is narrow it is said to have a low toxic-therapeutic ratio or a low therapeutic index, e.g. digoxin. These are the drugs one would expect to have problems when the amount of the active principle is unknown. These drugs will have ADR, which should be picked up more easily due to their frequency. As mentioned earlier mercury dosage was increased until salivation occurred. Withering also increased the dose of digitalis until the patient vomited in the belief that this would ensure a diuretic effect. Quinine dosage was increased until there was singing in the ears. The principle of increasing the dosage until an adverse reaction occurred must have been common with drugs/herbs with a low therapeutic index. In the beginning the amount of herbs to be taken must have been measured numerically for berries and leaves, but roots and stems would have been more difficult.

Thompson says that the symbols were first employed by the Chaldeans (mathematicians or astrologers from Babylonia) and Babylonians, but that Alexander was the first to use the scruple and dragma. Before the 13th century they used 'a piece the size of a corn' and 'a pinch' (Thompson, 2003). In the Leechbook of 1443 a dose of a 'spoonful' is mentioned and De Vigo in 1506 refers to a 'groat's weight'. By 1527 a 'dram' and a 'scruple' were used in a prescription (Banister, 1589). Pope in 1553 said, 'The least of all weights (commonly used by physicians) is a barley corne, and xx (20) cornes make a scruple, three scruples make one drachme and eight drachms make one ounce'.

A corne = gra = G = a grayne = a grain

A scruple = Ɔ = scrupulus

A drachme = ʒ = dragma = dram

An unce = ℥ = unciam = ounce

A pounde = l = libra

A quarter = q

A half = s = ss = ß

A handfull = m

One = j (Pope, 1553).

However, in 1579 Thomas Cartwright was using handfuls of elder leaves, one spoonful of turpentine and also uses the phrase ' by as even portions as you can guess' Those prescriptions for medicines for external use often did not specify quantities, e.g. 'then take bramble leaves, elder leaves, mustard seeds, and stamp them all together' (Cartwright, 1579).

The amount of a drug in an ointment or in other preparations for external use could be less accurate in dose without causing serious harm, but for those drugs taken orally the possible variation in dose, when added to the inconstancy of the amount of active principle due to the difference mentioned above, might be fatal.

Dichotomy

In all people there is some dichotomy between believing and knowing; between the acceptance without strong evidence and rejection of anything that is not backed up by irrefutable evidence. This dichotomy varies with the different aspects of their lives. It is not unusual for a person to have a strong religious belief, but demand irrefutable evidence in their work. However, this dichotomy is not usually absolute and it is common that a person with a strong religious or other belief will allow it to permeate their scientific work and may, thereby, produce biased results. A scientist with a strong personality may dominate an institution to the extent that it reflects their view, eg. Montpellier. Pharmaceutical companies will try to promote a strong belief in its employees of its own integrity. They will also try to influence the regulatory authorities in the same way. Galen believed in the doctrine of humours, but at the same time undertook experiments to establish the facts. Again, this dichotomy exists today in that some qualified physicians also practise homeopathy.

'C'est le Galénism contre la médicine chimique, mais c'est aussi Paris contre Montpellier, sa rivale, nos docteurs-régents contre les médicins/ l'étranger (provincial) leurs concurrents et les apothecaries, c'est Gui Patin (Dean of the Paris faculty and a Galenist) contre les Renaudot'[104] Renaudot (c1586–1653) was a disciple of Paracelsus) (Lévy-Valenai, 1933). (See page 115).

It is Galenism against chemical medicine, but also Paris against Montpellier, its rival, our doctors against provincial doctors, their competitors and the apothecaries; it is Guy Patin (Galenist) against Renaudot (Paracelsian).

Summary

If there had been no syphilis in Europe before 1493 then the use of mercury as a treatment seems to have been almost instantaneous. It is therefore not surprising that the adverse effects of mercury dominated the early 1500s. The honour of introducing the disease was eagerly fought over with everybody blaming each other: Spaniards, Indians, French, Neapolitans, the Japanese, who in their turn blamed the Portuguese, the Tahitians who blamed the British and the Turks who blamed the Christians. Gradually the name, syphilis given by Fracastorius in 1530 took over and became the standard throughout the world. The availability of moveable type in the

---

[104] Renaudot = Theophraste Renaudot lost his permission to practice medicine in Paris, due to the opposition of Guy Patin and other academic physicians.

mid-1400s meant that there was an outpouring of books on all subjects. Authors of medical texts gave credit to their predecessors, e.g. Pliny, Galen and Avicenna. The statement by Paracelsus in 1541 that all things are poisonous but that it depends on the dose was an important step towards scientific assessment of side effects of drugs. The English physicians fighting to maintain their lucrative business lost the battle when the law allowing anybody to practise herbal medicine was passed, because the physicians treated their patients badly. The Scottish physicians fared better when a law was passed at the end of the century declared that only duly qualified persons could practise medicine.

Chapter 5. 17th Century

The end of the Renaissance and the start of the Age of Reason or Enlightenment, but alchemy was still a strong influence.

1603 The first Royal Spanish Pharmacopoeia, the work *'Officina Medicamentorum'* [Recipes for making medicines], a book of more than 400 pages that gathered the knowledge of the time on making medicines of vegetable, animal and mineral origin. It began to be written in 1601 by pharmacists from the Valencian Association of Apothecaries (Col. Legi dels Apothecaris de la Ciutat y Regne de Valencia), which is the oldest in the world and was finished in 1603. A year later it was distributed throughout the Spanish Territories which belonged to the crown of Aragon. This edition was authorised by King Felipe III and is considered to be the first Royal Spanish Pharmacopoeia (see 1581).

1604 *'Triumphal Chariot of Antimony.'* By Basil Valentine. Transcribed by Ben Fairweather. This was first published as *'Triumph-Wagen Antimonii... An Tag geben durch Johann Thölden. Mit einer Vorrede, Doctoris Joachimi Tanckii.'* Leipsig, 1604. His style of writing is extremely extravagant and he starts by giving his opponents' views before going to great lengths praising antimony's virtues, which I have represented by one of his more modest comments.

'And, to begin here I say, Antimony is mere Venom, not of the kind of the least Venoms, but such, as by which you may destroy Men and Beasts, so venomous a power is diffused through the whole Substance of this Mineral. Hence arises the common Exclamation of all men. For the People, unskilful Doctors, and all Those, to whom the ground of true Medicine is unknown, do with one mouth proclaim it Venom, Venom! Poison, say they (as I myself above confessed) lies in Antimony. For this Cause let us dissuade all men from its use; for it endangers the

Health and Life. Therefore Doctors resident in Princes Courts, admonish Monarchs, Princes, and other Potentates not to use Antimony. Other Scholasticks cry out, Beware, you in no wise admit Antimony into Medicinal Use; for it's mere Poison: these the Inhabitants of Cities and Villages follow. And this far spread Clamour so moves the greatest part of Mortals, as Antimony in these our Days is very ill spoken of, and no man dares put confidence in the Medicine thereof, which in it is found so various and unexpressible. For truly and holily I affirm (as truly as GOD is the Creator of all things visible, which are contained in Heaven or Earth, which either have come, or in time to come shall come unto our knowledge) that under Heaven, or by the Rays of the Sun, with the Guidance of Experience, can be found or demonstrated no greater Medicine, than is in this Mineral; yea, there is no Subject, in which so fluently and abundantly can be found such most certain Remedies for Health, as shall be declared (by sure and undeniable Experiments) to be in Antimony.

It causeth gentle Stools, and purgeth without Gripings of the Belly; and indeed if you have proceeded well in preparing, it renders the Blood agile, and is a Medicine apt for those who desire Gentle Purgations.'

(http://www.levity.com/alchemy/antimony.html)

Throughout the period from 1560–1670 there was a very polarised struggle between those in favour of antimony and those wishing to ban it, which is perhaps why Valentine was so vehermently in favour.

1607 King James I gave privileges to the Apothecaries as a section of the Grocers' Company.

1610 Markham, Gervase, (1568?–1637) *'Markhams master-piece, or, What does a horse-man lack containing all possible knowledge whatsoever which does belong to any smith, farrier or horse-leech, touching the curing of all manner of diseases or sorrances[104] in horses: drawn with great pain and most approved experience from the public practise of all the foreign horse-marshals of Christendom and from the private practice of all the best farriers of this kingdom: being divided into two books, the first containing*

---

[104] sorrances = disease or sores in horses

*all cures physical, the second whatsoever belongeth to chirurgerie,
with an addition of 130 most principal chapters and 340 most
excellent medicines, receipts and secrets worthy every man's
knowledge, never written of nor mentioned in any author before
whatsoever: together with the true nature, use, and quality of every
simple spoken of through the whole work : read me, practise me,
and admire me,* written by Geruase Markham gentleman.

<u>Henbane:</u> *'squiani which we call henbane, is cold in the fourth
degree: it astonieth, and benumbeth'.*

1611 *'L'eau de Melisse des Carmes*[105]*'* a digestive with 14 plants and
9 spices was made originally by the monks of the Carmelite
monastry in Bordeaux. It is still available in 2008. We know
that two toxic plants (muguet and primevère) were removed
from it and that there have been many different versions. It was
probably a secret remedy to start with (Renou, 2005).

1612–3 *'I find the medicine worse than the malady.'* Francis Beaumont
and John Fletcher, Love's Cure (Act III, Sc 2).

1617 King James I gave the apothecaries a charter as 'Master, Warden,
and Society of the Art and Mistery of the Apothecaries of the
City of London'. They agreed not to supply cathartics[106], vomits
or sudorifics[107] without the knowledge of a physician; or opiates,
hypnotics or abortifacients without a prescription; and also not to
supply poisons without a signed prescription (Penn, 1979).

A Spanish Royal Decree of 1617 concerning the examination of
physicians and surgeons.

*'1, Firstly, That the professor read the works of Galen,
Hippocrates and Avicenna aloud to the students, the professor
having the book in his hand and the students one in theirs so
that they can understand him.'*

1618 First edition of the London Pharmacopoeia appeared on the 7th
May. Although other editions of the London Pharmacopoeia
were issued in 1621, 1632, 1639 and 1677, it was not until
the edition of 1721, published under the auspices of Sir Hans
Sloane, that any important alterations were made. It contained

---

[105] l'eau de Melisse des Carmes = alcoholic balm obtained from the distillation of fresh mélisse (*Mélisse Officinalis*) leaves
with alcohol made by the White Friars (Carmelites)
[106] cathartics = laxative
[107] sudorifics = causing sweating

712 compound remedies and listed 680 crude drugs used in these remedies. A Royal proclamation led to it being recognised as Europe's first national pharmacopoeia. It applied to '*all and singular apothecaries of this our Realm of England or the dominions beyond thereof.*' No mention of ADRs. It still mentions 'Mithridatum', but now it only has 44 ingredients.

1619 '*A new herbal, or history of plants wherein is contained the whole discourse and perfect description of all sorts of herbs and plants: their divers and sundry kinds, their names, natures, operations, and vertues: and that not only of those which are here growing in this our country of England [sic], but of all others also of foreign realms commonly used in physick.* First set forth in the Dutch or Almaigne (German) tongue, by that learned D. Rembert Dodoens, physician to the Emperor: and now first translated out of French into English, by Henry Lyte Esquire. Imprinted at London: By Edward Griffin, 1619'. 564 pages.

For all the drugs there is a section for their 'vertues' and also for many there is also a section 'Dangers' such as:

Black Hellebore: '*Although black hellebore is not so vehment as the white, yet it cannot be given without danger, and especially to people that have their health: for as Hippocrates saith, Carnes habentibus sanas, Helleborus periculsus, facie enim Convulsions, that is to say, to such as be whole, hellebore is very perilous, for it causes shrinking of sinues: therefore hellebore may not be ministered, except in desperate causes, and that to young & strong people, and not at all times, but in the spring time only, yet ought it not to be given before it be prepared and corrected.*'

Poppy: he used identical words to those used by Dodoens in 1586.

Black Henbane: '*The leaves, seed, and …. Of henbane, but especially of the black henbane, the which is very common in this country, teken either alone or with wine, causes raging, and long deep sleep, almost like unto drunkenness, which remains a long space and afterwards killeth the party.*'

(http://0-eebo.chadwyck.com.libsys.wellcome.ac.uk/works/search?action=searchorbrowse&search=viewselectedrecords&somtype=viewselrecs).

1624 Already in 1624 Wihelm Fabry alias Fabricius Hildanus (1560–1634) had clearly expressed in letters his disappointment at the confrontations with all the 'pseudo-chemists' that administered potent substances imprudently without bothering about the toxic effects that could have arisen in the patients. Hildanus, apart from pointing out some cases of death occurring immediately after taking a drug, acutely observed that the toxicity of some substances could manifest themselves a long time after their administration, at times with fatal outcomes. The battle against the abuse and the bad use of medicaments, continued with stubbornness by Hildanus, was not enough to make the medical profession aware of the problem: his remained for a long time a lone voice.' (Borghi & Canti, 1986; Fabry von Hilden, 1936) (The life and works of Quilhelmus Fabricius Hildanus [1560–1634] by Ellis Jones) In 1646 Fabricius Hildanus (1560–1634) wrote '*Opera observationum et Curationum medico-chirurgicarum quae extant medico omnia*' [All existing medical accounts of observations and medico-surgical cures].

1625 First recorded use of the thermometer for studying disease (Sanctorius, 1625).

1628 William Harvey published '*Exercitatio anatomica de motu cordis et sanginis in animalibus*' [An anatomical treatise concerning the movement of the heart and the blood in living things] describing the circulation of blood.

1630 A possible treatment for malaria was found in the forests of the Andes Mountains. In that decade, an Augustinian monk published a notice regarding the treatment, burying it in a work on the Augustinian Order. '*A tree grows which they call "the fever tree" in the country of Loxa* (Equador)*, whose bark, of the colour of cinnamon, made into powder amounting to the weight of two small silver coins and given as a beverage, cures the fevers and tertian* (Vivax malaria)*; it has produced miraculous results in Lima*', wrote the monk, Antonio de Calancha. He was describing the bark of the cinchona tree; the bark contains the alkaloid quinine along with several other alkaloids effective against malaria (Burba, 2007).

1637 Baltasar Gracian. Spanish Philosopher in *'The art of worldly wisdom cxxxviii. The art of letting things alone'*. *'The more so the wilder the waves of public or of private life. There are hurricanes in human affairs, tempests of passion, when it is wise to retire to a harbour and ride at anchor. Remedies often make diseases worse: in such cases one has to leave them to their natural course and the moral suasion of time. It takes a wise doctor to know when not to prescribe, and at times the greater skill consists in not applying remedies. The proper way to still the storms of the vulgar is to hold your hand and let them calm down of themselves. To give way now is to conquer by and by. A fountain gets muddy with but little stirring up, and does not get clear by our meddling with it but by our leaving it alone. The best remedy for disturbances is to let them run their course, for so they quiet down.'*

1640 *'Theatrum Botanicum, The Theater of Plantes or An Universal and Compleate Herball'*, composed by John Parkinson, Apothecary of London and the King's Herbalist. London. This vast book of 1756 pages each 12½ inches by 8 inches follows the precedence of Dodoen's herbal in having sections on the virtues of each plant, but does not have any section on the dangers of each plant. Under virtues of opium he says '... *but Galen, and divers others in the former as well as in our times, have forbidden such medicines, as too dangerous for the eyes, and even any other ways used inwardly, it is not to be taken, but with good correction and great caution...*' Parkinson, who died in 1650, was the last of the great herbalists in England.

Age of Reason or Enlightenment

1648 Simon Paulli, *'Flora Danica'* 1648 *'Among other herbs which are poisonous and harmful, henbane is not the least, so that the common man, not without fear should spit at that herb when he hears its name spoken, not to mention when he sees it growing in great quantity where his children are running at play.'*

1649 *'A physicall directory'* or A translation of the London Dispensatory made by the Royal College of Physicians in London by Nicholas Culpeper, Gent. This small book has details of preparation, but no mention of ADRs.

Hyoscyamus &c. '*Henbane, the white henbane is held to be cold but in the third degree, the black or common henbane and the yellow, in the fourth, they stupify the senses and therefore not to be taken inwardly, outwardly applied they help inflamations, hot gouts, applied to the temples they provoke sleep.*'

1651 '*Mataeotechnia medicinae praxeōs. The vanity of the craft of physick. or, a new dispensatory. Wherein is dissected the errors, ignorance, impostures and supinities[108] of the Schools, in their main pillars of purges, blood-letting, fontanels[109] or issues, and diet, etc., and the particular medicines of the shops. With an humble motion for the reformation of the Universities, and the whole landscape of physick, and discovering the terra incognita of chemistry by Noah Biggs. The Marquess Spinetti had been sick with epilepsy but cure by Dr Helmont. The College of Physicians on the following morning prescribed him a scruple of white hellebore with as much aniseed. Half an hour later he vomited. In vain implored the help of his physician, being absent, accursed his murderers and saying "My Helmont, You told me the physicians would kill me". He held his peace and after two hours his stomach first suffered a convulsion and then his whole body, he dieth in a swound.*'

1652 Culpeper, Nicholas, (1616–1654). '*The English physitian: or an astrologo-physical discourse of the vulgar herbs of this nation.*' London: Peter Cole, 1652. It acknowledges the work of 43 previous authors. Each herb is dealt with under: description, place, vertues and use.

Briony: '*The Roots of the briony purge the belly with great violence, troubling the stomach, and hurting the liver, and therefore not rashly to be taken, but being corrected is very profitable for the diseases of the head, as falling-sickness[110], giddiness, and swimmings, by drawing away much phlegm and rheumatic humours that oppress the head, as also the joints and sinews, and is therefore good.*'

Wild Poppy: '*Galen said the seed (wild poppy) is dangerous to be used inwardly.*'

---

[108] supinities = acts which are mentally or morally inactive
[109] fontanels = an outlet for body secretions
[110] falling-sickness = epilepsy

Common Nightshade:'*This common nightshade is wholly used to cool all hot inflammations either inwardly or outwardly, being no way dangerous to any that shall use it, as most of the rest of the nightshades are; yet it must be used moderately.*'

Henbane (Hyoscyamus): '*This herb must never be taken inwardly, outwardly, as oil, ointment or plaster of is most admirable*'. *The poisonful qualities of hemlock, henbane, nightshade, mandrake, or other such like herbs that stupify or dull the senses, as also the lethargy, especially to use it outwardly to rub the forehead and temples in the lethargy, and the places bitten or stung with beasts, with a little salt.*'

Poppy (White) or opium *Papaverus somniverum*: '*An over dose causes immodesty, mirth or stupidity, redness of the face, swelling of the eyes, relaxation of the joints, giddiness of the head, deep sleep, accompanied with turbulent dreams and convulsive starting, cold sweats and frequently death.*'

Foxglove is mentioned but only for external application. Other than these type of statements there is little about the adverse effects of the plants. He includes flowers, vegetables, trees and fruits.

The hellebore is not mentioned, but he does mention it in his '*School of Physick or the experimental practice of the whole art*' in 1659: black hellebore: '*that black hellebore rightly used is a hurtless media and may safely be given to a child; have a care of women with child and other weak bodies.*'

1546
1656 Nuremberg Pharmacopoeia was published; the first dispensatory or list of drugs. This was based on the work of Valerius Cordus, which he had written, basing it on the writings of the most eminent medical authorities.

Christopher Wren and Robert Boyle performed the first intravenous injection of opium into a dog using a pig's bladder and a sharpened quill. It noted that the dog appeared extremely 'stupified'. This paved the way for pharmacology (Scarborough, 1945). Boyle, although not a physician, wrote a great deal on medical matters and criticised Galen's practices.' *These helps are bleeding, vomiting, purging, sweating, and spitting; of which I briefly observe in general that they are sure to weaken or discompose when they are employed but do not certainly cure afterwards'* and physicians did not escape lightly ' *When a poor patient lies sick of a dangererous disease, the aim of his recourse to a physician is, to be cured by him, or at least to be relieved. But if he desired no more than that the physician should do him no hurt, his surest course were not to send to a physician at all; For then he need not fear to be killed by him.'* (Boyle, 1663; Hunter, 1997).

1657 Morel, Pierre, Johannes Jacobus Brunn, and Nicholas Culpeper. 1657. *'The expert doctors' dispensatory the whole art of physick restored to practice : the apothecaries shop and chyrurgions closet open'd ... : together with a strict survey of the dispensatories of the most renowned colleges of the world ... : to which is added by Jacob A. Brunn ... a compendium of the body of physick, wherein all the medicaments universal and particular, simple and compound, are fitted to the practice of physick. London: Printed for N. Brook.'*

Black hellebore: '*Where note, that black hellebore rightly used is a hurtles medicine and may be safely be give to children, have a care with women with child or other weak bodies.*' (identical words to those used by Culpeper in 1652).

Nature's Cabinet Unlock'd, wherein is discovered the natural causes of metals, stones, precious earths, juices, humors, and spirits' by *Sir Thomas Browne, Dr of Physick*. '*Some plants are enemies, pernicious and hurtful, and that either to the whole body, or part: to the whole they prove fatal, by everting the continuity of union, and depraving of life, or stupefy or benumb part of the body: as henbane to the head.... One and the same plant, is sometimes salutary to one man but noxious and death to another, by reason of the peculiar constitution of the individuum.'* Printed for Edw. Farnham in Popes-And: head alley near Cornhill, 1657.' A reference to personal idiosyncrasy.

'*A medicinal dispensatory, containing the whole body of physick discovering the natures, properties, and vertues of vegetables, minerals, & animals: the manner of compounding medicaments, and the way to administer them. Methodically digested in five books of philosophical and pharmaceutical institutions; three books of physical materials galenical and chemical. Together with a most perfect and absolute pharmacopoea or apothecaries shop. Accommodated with three useful tables.'* Composed by the illustrious Renodaeus, chief physician to the monarch of France; and now Englished and revised, by Richard Tomlinson of London, apothecary'. London: printed by Jo: Streater and Ja: Cottrel; and are to be sold by Henry Fletcher at the three gilt Cups neer the west-end of Pauls, 1657. (See page 104).

'Every medicament does more or less offend nature, as its faculty is stronger or weaker: by so much it causes more molestation.'

'Those which by a certain antipathy, and special potency impair the principles of life, spirit and heat, consume the flesh, and destroy the integrity of sanity, must not be exhibited without extraordinary care and prudence; as vipers flesh against the pestilence or leprosy, the reins[111] or rather the flesh of the loins of Stincus[112] to provoke to venery, Cantharides against the retention and obstruction of urine; for these cantharides rightly prepared and mixed with fit medicaments, and administered in a small quantity, do move urine without harm.'

Quicksilver: *'Often causes palsy, stupour and tremblings... move salivation...hurt the nerves, and sometimes cause strangulation.'*

Opium:..*'and much discommend it, if unduly used; for it does not only induce tremour and palsy, but leads to perpetual sleep.'*

Hellebore: *'it excites vomit in the assumer, and its powders adhibited at the nostrils, moves sternutation[113]'...'it is perilous to the sane, imbecil, and young.'*

Henbane: *'because such as are maddened with henbane, torment themselves with brawling and altercation, as if they were excited by Phoebus his fury. Matthiolus saw some boys who by eating henbane seed were so desipient[114] that many thought they were deluded by the Devil.'*

---

[111] reins = kidneys
[112] stincus alias Sincus = North African sand fish used in medicine
[113] sternutation = sneezing
[114] desipient = dissolute

1662 Van Helmont Jan Baptiste (1579–1644). '*Oriatrike*[115], *or physick refined: the common errors therein refuted and the whole are reformed and rectified.*' Lodowick-Loyd: London. This was a translation of his 1648 work '*Ortus Medicinae: id est Initia physicae inaudita. Progressus medicinae novus, in morborum ultionem, ad vitam longam*' [The dawn of medicine: That is, the beginning of a new Physic. A new advance in medicine, a victory over disease, to [promote] a long life].

'*Let us take from of the itinerants' hospitals, from the camps, or from elsewhere, 200, or 500 poor people, with fevers, pleurisy, etc. and divide them in two, let us cast lots, that half of them fall to me, and the other half to you. I shall cure them without blood-letting or perceptible purging. You will do so according to your knowledge (nor do I even hold you to yout boast of abstaining from phlebotomy or purging) and we shall see how many funerals each of us will have: the outcome of the contest shall be the reward of 300 florins, deposited by each of us: thus shall your business be concluded.*' *... let the trial be made for the public good, in order to know the truth, for the sake of your life and soul and for the health of all the people, sons, widows, and orphans.*' (Rose, 1982). The first proposed randomised controlled trial (Holland) involving adverse events, but it was not performed.

'The sixth book of practical physick of occult or hidden diseases; in nine parts

Part I. Of diseases from occult qualities in general

Part. II. Of occult, malignant, and venemous diseases arising from the internal fault of the humours

Part III. Of occult diseases from water, air, and infections, and of infectious diseases

Part IV. Of the venereal pox

Part V. Of outward poisons in general

Part VI. Of poisons from minerals and metals

Part. VII. Of poisons from plants

Part VIII. Of poisons that come from living creatures

Part IX. Of diseases by witchcraft, incantation, and charms

By Daniel Sennertus, N Culpeper, and Abdiah Cole, Doctors of Physick. 1662'.

---

[115] oriatrike = I cannot find a translation but as it is supposed to be an English translation of 'Ortus Medicinae' it should mean the birth or development of medicine.

Opium: '*is hot, which Scaliger Exercit[116] affirms, calling it by the name of Amphiam or Aphioure, and also Vesalius Mercurialis, and* Capivaccius[117]*, and* Erastus[118]*, and they confirm it by reasons:*
1. *Its inflaming and burning quality*
2. *Its strong scent*
3. *The bitter taste*
4. *Its burning the mouth and lips*
5. *Its causing thirst*
6. *Its heating the mind*
7. *It provokes venery*
8. *It causeth itching*
9. *It causeth sweat.*'

Hellebore: '*If it be taken in great quantity without preparation; it purges violently upwards and downwards, and causes great pains in the stomach and guts, hickets[119], suffocation, difficult breathing, trouble of mind, sudden weakness, heart-beating, and they die by convulsions or suffocation.*'

1664 '*A brief examination and censure of several medicines of late years extol'd for universal remedies and arcana's of the highest preparation*' by George Starkey. '*No less dangerous is that mercurial preparation not more famous about town and country, for its monstrous price, then infamous for its salivative quality, of which an ounce of fine gold is but the perchase of eight grains (518 mgm), and that quantity exceeds a single dose but one grain (65 mgm)*'...

'*It would confirm the old scandal, that hath been from the beginning thrown upon Chymical medicines, to wit, that they are full of danger, and quickly Kill or Cure.*'

1665 '*Medicina Instaurata or: a brief account of the true grounds and principles of the art of physick*' by Marchmount Nedham, London, John Starkey, 1665. '*The time and motion of a disease, one of so great moments in the giving of physick, that the very same remedy which saved a man's life to-day may in the same disease, at a different time, kill another to-morrow.*'

---

[116] Scaliger Exercit = Julius Caesar Scaliger (1484–1558) an Italian physician wrote 'Exotericarum exercitationen' in 1557
[117] Capivaccius = Capivaccius, Hieronimus (or Girolamo) (1523–1589) wrote 'Opusculumde differentiis doctinarum logicis, philosophis, atque medicis pernecessarium'.
[118] Erastus = Thomas Erastus,(1524–1583) A Swiss Theologian
[119] hickets = hiccups

<u>White Hellebore</u>:*'That if anyone be but pricked with a needle infected with this juice he would be die within a few hours.'*

<u>Mercuries dulcis</u>—*calomeus: 'giving of it to some bodies and constitutions, been accompanied with very ill accidents.'*

The first issue of '*Philosophical Transactions of the Royal Society*' appeared in March 1665 and it included some medical articles.

The Great Plague of London was treated with Mithridatium and Galene.

1667 George Castle wrote '*The chymical Galenist. A treatise, wherein the practise of the ancients is reconcil'd to the new discoveries in the theory of physick; shewing, that many of their rules, methods, and medicines, are useful for the curing of diseases in this age, and in the northern parts of the world. In which are some reflections upon a book, intituled, Medela medicinæ;*' by George Castle, Dr. of physick, lately fellow of All-souls Colledge in Oxon.'

This little book of 114 pages mentions interactions: '*The mixing of things which are harmless sometimes produces a poison. Thus out of vitriol, salt, mercury, niter is made sublimate; of vitriol, niter and alum, aqua for to which though made of innocent ingredients, are mixtures most destructive to the body of man.*'

<u>Mercury</u>: Mercurius dulcis- calomelous...*'giving of it to some bodies, constitutions, been acccompanied with very ill accident.'*

<u>White Hellebore</u>: '*That if anyone be but pricked with a needle infected with this juice, he would die within a few hours.*' (Copied from Nedham 1665).

1669 Mercury is '*the hottest, the coldest, a true healer, a wicked murderer, a precious medicine, and a deadly poison, a friend that can flatter and lie*'. (Woodall, 1639).

1670 A French physician, Dr. Thuillier, put forth the concept that it (ergotism) was not an infectious disease, but one that was due to the consumption of rye infected with ergot that was responsible for the outbreaks of 'St. Anthony's Fire' (see 1725).

1671 *'Person of quality. Westminster-drollery, or, a choice collection of the newest songs & poems both at court and theaters by a person of quality; with additions.'* 1671. An anonymous work.

She then did bid me drop in her eyes
A sovereign water sent her that day,
But I had a liquor I more did prize,
Made of *Henbane* and *Mercury* steep'd in Whey:
I dropt it in and nointed her face,
Which brought her into a most devillish case:
For she rore and she ranted, and well she might;
For after that time she ne'er had sight.
  Then did get her a dog and a bell,
To lead her about from place to place:
And now 'tis, husband, I hope you are well;
But before it was cuckold and rogue to my face;
Then blest be that *Henbane* and *Mercury* strong,
That made such a change in my wives tongue.
You see 'tis a medicine certain and sure,
For the cure of a scold, but I'll say no more.

1672 The law of the 4th December 1672 in Denmark-Norway assigned physicians control over both apothecaries and midwives and physicians who were obliged to provide free medical care to the poor. At that time there were only 5 physicians in the country (Hubbard, 2006).

1673 *'Presque tous les hommes meurent de leurs remèdes, et non pas de leurs maladies.'* [Nearly all men die of their medicines, not of their diseases]. *'La Malade Imaginaire'*. Molière (1622–1673). Molière also observed that *'medicine is only for those who are fit enough to survive the treatment as well as the illness.'*

1676 Charas, Moyse, 1619–1698, *'Pharmacopée Royale Galénique et Chymique'* [Royal Pharmacopoeia for apothecaries and Chemists] *(A Paris, M.DC.LXXVI..)'* No mention of ADRs for opium, despite the fact that he experimented with opium on himself. He came to London as Hugenot refugee in 1680, but later converted to Catholicism and returned to France
  Mercury: *'… and because mercury passes for a medicament which is a great enemy of the nerves'* … *'although sometimes it*

excites the salivation in delicate persons'… from whence it can make a great ravage in the stomach.'

Henbane (semenis hyosciami albi) *'I admit also that the roots of henbane eaten in quantity upsets for a time the judgement and troubles the reason.'*

1678 *'Experiments and Observations of the Effects of Several Sorts of Poisons upon Animals, etc.'* Made at Montpellier in the Years 1678 and 1679, by the Late William Courten Esq; Communicated by Dr. Hans Sloane, Secretary of the Royal Society' in *'Philosophical Transactions'* (1683–1775), Vol. 27, 1710–1712, 485-500. This mentions that intravenous injections of opium caused violent convulsions and death. William Courten wrote of his experiments *'In the month of July anno 1678 we gave a dog'… 'two drachms of white hellebore (Hellebore Album) very much disordered him, and caused reachings, suffocations, vomiting, and voiding of excrements… often scratched the ground with his feet.'* (Sloane, 1710–1712).

1679 Lonicerus A. *'Kreuterbuch '*(1679). Reprinted by Verlag Konrad Kölbl, München, Germany. (1962) in which he described the plants particularly under medical-pharmaceutical aspects. He also wrote the first known record of the use of ergot by midwives as an ecbolic (hastens childbirth).

Johann Jacob Wepfer (1620–1695) Physician in Ordinary to several dynasties in Southern Germany: *'My sin will be less, if I explore the effects of poison in animals in order to be of benefit to me.'* Another example of animal toxicology.

1680 Thomas Sydenham brought opium into England in the form of laudanum and commented: *'Among the remedies which it has pleased Almighty God to give to man to relieve his sufferings none is so universal and so efficacious as opium.'* (Postler & Waisel, 1997). He was also renowned for writing very detailed clinical notes on his patients and has , thereby, given us figures for amounts involved in bloodletting and saliva extracted with mercury. For apoplexy he says he took 12℥ of blood from the arm and then a further 8℥ from the jugular vein, making a pint in all. In treating the French Pox with mercury he says *'The salivation ought to be so moderated, that the patient may spit 4 pints in 24* *hours'.* He was imbued with the belief in humours, but tempered it with concern for his patients. For gout *'yet bleeding does as much harm as it does good in the just mentioned'* (pleuritics and rheumatism) and again as for purging in gout *'Therefore I am fully persuade, having learnt by continual and repeated experience that all purging whether by gentle or strong medicine, such as are usually designed for purging the joints, do much hurt..'.* He was not disinterested as he himself suffered from gout (Sydenham, 1696).

1684 *'Dr. Willis's practice of physick being the whole works of that renowned and famous physician wherein most of the diseases belonging to the body of man are treated of, with excellent methods and receipts for the cure of the same: fitted to the meanest capacity by an index for the explaining of all the hard and unusual words and terms of art derived from the Greek, Latine, or other languages for the benefit of the English reader: with forty copper plates.'* (Willis, Thomas, 1684).

'Of vomiting and medicines that give vomits.

As to the distinction of vomits, and the several ways or reasons of their working, since they are commonly divided into two sorts, to wit, such as are more gentle, and those that are more strong; whereof the former carry their force, and power or virtue in view (as it were) declaring their irritative or provoking quality by manifest signs; as when a decoction of hyssop or carduus, an infusion of the roots of squills, or radish, disolved vitriol, warm water or water mingled with honey (if you drink a great draught of it) and the like (which upon the first sight or taste move the stomach) are given for vomits: and when they are given, it oftentimes is necessary for them to be aided by the irritation of the palate and throat in order to their producing of a vomit. Secondly, The stronger vomits (which are more properly so called) are such medicines, that if they are taken in a due quantity they move most people to vomit; as for example, white hellebore, nux vomica, vitriol, with many preparations of them and mercury: which though they are useful, yea very necessary in Physick, yet in their nature and virtues, wherein their vomiting quality consists, they seem to differ very little from poison: wherefore if they are taken in a dose too great, they often are the death of the patient.'

Archer, John, fl. 1660–1684. '*Secrets disclosed of consumptions shewing [h]ow to distinguish between scurvy and venereal disease : also, how to prevent and cure the fistula by chemical drops without cutting, also piles, haemorrhoids, and other diseases.*' by John Archer. 1684.

'*a person is afflicted with a Venereal Distemper, that for want of a skilful Doctor, takes Physick from the ignorant, who poisons the Body with Mercury; thence I frequently find bad and dangerous symptoms following, as pain in the Head, Neck, Back, Teeth, Deafnes, Dimness of Sight, Distillations, at length [...] Consumption; and without proper Medicines Anti-venereal and Anti-mercurial, the noble parts are assaulted and overcome, and so the do make the number of them in the Weekl[...] Bills of Mortality dead of a Consumption therefore to prevent Death before the accomplishment.*'

First medical journal '*Medicina Curiosa*' ceased publication after two issues.

1685 John Evelyn wrote in his diary that on the 4th February 1685 King Charles II had an apoplectic fit and that after he had been suitably bled, cupped, bled again, made to vomit and then purged he was said to be '*somewhat feverish; This they seem'd glad of, as being more easily allayed, & methodically to be dealt with, than his former fits, so as they prescrib'd the famous Jesuit's powder* (Quinine); *but it made his Majesty worse; and some very able doctors present, did not think it a favour, but the effect of frequent bleeding, & other sharp operations used by them about his head: so as probably the powder might stop the circulation, & renew his former fits which now made him very weak*' Next day they bled him again . He gave up the ghost at half an hour-after eleven in the morning, being the 6th of Feb.' This illustrates the problem of deciding on causality after multiple treatments over a short time, which have been followed by an adverse event. '*Post hoc ergo propter hoc*' [It happened afterwards therefore it was the cause], but which treatment?

1689 '*The London practice of physick: or the whole practical part of physick contained in the works of Dr. Willis.* Faithfully made English and printed together for the public good. London:

Printed for T. Basset, T. Dring, etc., 1689.

Opium: *'This excellent drug when taken by mistake, or otherwise, in too large a quantity, is converted into a poison.'* He then goes on to give the doses that should be used for mercury, hellebore and opium, e.g. Tinct. Opii Gutteae i ad vi; Opii purific grain ¼ (16 mgm) ad grains fi ad grains ij.

'General rule, particularly where active medicines are employed, to begin with small doses and gradually increase them to the extent the constitution will bear.' An example of dose titration until there are side effects.

1694 Pechey, John, (1655–1716). *'The complete herbal of physical plants containing all such English and foreign herbs, shrubs and trees as are used in physick and surgery...the doses or quantities of such as are prescribed by the London-physicians and others are proportioned: also directions for making compound-waters, syrups simple and compound, electuaries...moreover the gums, balsams, oils, juices, and the like, which are sold by apothecaries and druggists are added to this herbal, and their virtues and uses are fully described by John Pechey.'*

<u>White Ellebore, or Hellebore</u>, in Latin *'Helleborus albus'.*

'The root of white hellebore, which is only in use in physick, purges very violently upward and downward; yet it may be used, says Tragus[120], being infus'd twenty four hours in wine or oxymel, and afterwards dried: half a dram of it, so prepar'd, may be given in wine to mad and melancholy people. But either of the hellebores, says Gesner[121], may be used inoffensively, being boiled to a syrup with honey and vinegar; and are very useful for many phlegmatic diseases, especially of the breast and head; as, an asthma, difficulty of breathing, and the falling sickness. They wonderfully purge the belly, the urine, and all the passages. In the use of white hellebore two things are chiefly to be minded: First, that the diseases are very obstinate: and secondly, that the patient has sufficient strength to bear the operation. Wherefore the root ought not to be given to old men, women, or children, or to such as are weakly, and costive in the body: and the hellebore ought to be well prepar'd. The old way of giving of it was, with horse-radish, which they used three ways; for, either they stuck

---

[120] Tragus = Hieronymus Bock (1498–1554)
[121] Gesner = Conrad Gesner (1516–1565) a humanist bibliographer

the roots into horse-radish, and continu'd them in it twenty four hours; and afterwards, the roots being taken out, they gave the horse-radish: Or they infus'd the horse-radish, stuck with the roots, in oxymel, in B.M[122]. and gave only the oxymel: or, they left the horse-radish so prepar'd all night, and in the morning infus'd it in oxymel, having first cast away the hellebore; and then they gave the oxymel. But Parkinson[123] says, the best way of preparing it is, to infuse it in the juice of quinces; or to roast it under ashes, in a quince. If, upon taking hellebore, there is danger of suffocation, the eating of quinces, or the taking the juice or syrup of it, is a present.'

1697 First dispensary opened in the premises of the Royal College of Physicians in Warwick Lane, London, where the poor were offered free consultation and advice, and prescribed drugs dispensed from a special stock. Branches were opened later in other parts of the City. Closed in 1725 (Warren, http://www.chronology.ndo.co.uk).

By the late 17th century Chinese medicine entered a relative decline and Western medicine, via Jesuit priests, started to replace it (Hong, 2004).

1699 Sir Samuel Garth (1661–1719) Physician to George I. Canto IV 1699.

'Oxford and all her passing Bells can tell,
By this Right Arm, what mighty numbers fell.
Whilst others meanly ask'd whole Months to slay,
I oft dispatch'd the Patient in a Day:
With Pen in hand I push'd to that degree,
I scarce had left a Wretch to give a Fee.
Some sell by Laudanum, and some by Steel,
And Death in ambush lay in ev'ry Pill.
For save or slay, this Priviledge we claim,
Tho' Credit suffers, the Reward's the same.
What tho' the Art of Healing we pretend,
He that designs it least, is most a Friend.
Into the right we err, and must confess,
To Oversights we often owe Success.

---

[122] B.M. = Balneum Mariae = hot water
[123] Parkinson = John Parkinson (1567–1650) Apothecary to James I and James VI (see entry for 1640 AD)

Thus Bessus got the Battel in the Play,
His glorious Cowardise restor'd the Day.
So the fam'd Grecian Piece ow'd its desert
To Chance, and not the labour'd Stroaks of Art.
Physicians, if they're wise, shou'd never think
Of any other Arms than Pen and Ink.
But th' Enemy, at their expence, shall find,
When Honour calls, I'll scorn to stay behind.'

Journals, Tracts and Monographs

English: *'Philosophical Transactions'* (The Royal Society of London) started on 6th March 1665 and amongst other scientific articles there were some on medicine. *'Weekly Memorials* 'and *'Medicina Curiosa'* were both established in 1684 but the first was mostly non-medical and the latter was transitory only lasting for two issues. (Chalmers and Tröhler, 2000). *'Medical Observations and Inquiries'* (The London Society of Physicians) 1757–1784. *'Medical Transactions'* (Royal College of Physicians) 1768–1820, *'London Medical Journal'* (The Society for Improvement of Medical Knowledge & Lyceum Medicum Londinese) 1781–1790, which continued as *'Medical Facts and Observations'* until 1800. *'Memoirs'* (Medical Society of London) 1787–1805. *'The Lancet'* started in 1823 and the *'British Medical Journal'* in 1857.

German: 'Miscellanea Acta Eruditorum ' [Miscellaneous Journal for the Learned] founded in 1682 and *'Miscellanea Curiosa Medico-physica Academiae Naturae Curiosorum sive Ephemeridum medico-physicarum Germanicarum curiosarum.'* [A miscellany of medico-physical curiosities] (the journal of) [The Academy of natural curiosities or The German medico-physical curiosities journal] in 1670.

Italian: *'Giournale dei Litterati di Roma'* [Journal for well-read Romans] established 1668.

French: *'Journal des Sçavans'* [Scientists' Journal] was established in 5th January 1665, a few months before *'Philosophical Transaction. Histoire de l'Academie Royale des Sciences'* [History of the Royal Acadamy of Sciences] began in 1666. *'Nouvelles Découvertes sur toutes les Parties de la Médicine'* [New discoveries in all fields of medicine] first appeared in 1679 and folded in 1681, but it has been claimed to be the first medical journal (Nicholls, 1934), because *'Philosophical Transactions'* was *'certainly not a medical journal in the ordinary sense of that term.'* The author also claimed that *Journal des Savants* [Scholars' Journal] was not published until 1681 (Nicholls, 1934). *'Progrès de la Médicine'* [Medical Progress] ran from 1695 until 1700.

'*Journal de la Societé des Pharmciens de Paris*' published 1797 folded 1799.

Danish: '*Acta Medica et Philosophica Hafniensia*' [The Copenhagen Medical and Philosophical Journal] established 1673.

Dutch: '*Collectanea Medico-Physica*' [A Medico-Physical Collection] established 1680.

Scottish: '*Medical essays and observations*', revised and published by the Philosophical Society of Edinburgh. 1733–1744. '*Medical and Philosophical Commentator*' (Society of Physicians of Edinburgh) London 1774–1795).

United States of America: '*Medical Repository*' (Quarterly in 1824) Started on 26th July 1797 by T & J Swords. '*Philadelphia Medical Museum*' Quarterly September 17th 1804 until 1811. '*Philadelphia Medical and Physical Journal*'. November 1824–May 1899.

The increasing numbers of journals containing articles on medicine gave more opportunity for comments on specific drugs and their adverse effects, e.g. Rev Stone's on willow bark. The tracts and monographs varied from 20 pages to 315 pages.

Summary

The references to herbal ADRs are now more specific and several are mentioned for each drug especially for hellebore and opium. Authors frequently refer back to their predecessors such as Galen and their references to 'third degree' harp back to the theory of humours. The emphasis has changed from the Chinese and Arab works to European literature. The production of medical journals means that there is an outlet for the increased research which was undertaken.

Chapter 6. 18th Century

The Age of Enlightenment. The power of alchemy starts to fade as experimentation increases.

1704 William Rose, a liveryman of the Society of Apothecaries, was sued by the Royal College of Physicians for treating a butcher without using a physician as an intermediary. The physicians won the case. The defence said that *'selling a few Lozenges, or a small Electuary to any asking for a remedy for a cold, or in other ordinary or common cases, or where the medicine has known and certain effects, may not be deemed unlawful or practising as a physician, where no fee is taken or demanded for the same. Furthermore the physicians, by straining an act made so long ago, may not be enabled to monopolise all manner of Physick solely to themselves and be an oppression to the poorer families not able to go to the charge of a fee'*. On appeal to the House of Lords, the decision was reversed declaring that the public interest would be served if an apothecary dispensing a remedy gave medical advice, but that he would not be able to charge a fee for the advice (Mann, 1984). These apothecaries later became the general practitioners of today. As apothecaries were cheaper than physicians, advice was given to a far greater number of patients than before, but it meant that all patients were given drugs whether they were necessary or not.

1707 Sir John Floyer wrote the *'The Physician's pulse-watch; or an essay to explain the old art of felling the pulse, and to improve it by the help of a pulse-watch'*. He was the first to give pulse rates; *'In health there is about 75 beats in a minute, and in fever 100.'* (Floyer, 1707). He had had his pulse-watch especially made for him, which had a second hand. Later in the century we see Samuel Bard in 1765, William Withering in 1785 and Samuel Crumpe in 1793 all giving pulse rates, but Hahnemann doesn't mention them in his works in the early 1800s.

1711 Nicolas Boileau (1636–1711) wrote:

You say without reward or fee
Your uncle cured me of a dangerous ill:
I say, he never did prescribe for me;
The proof is plain, I'm living still.

John Marten wrote '*A treatise of the Venereal Disease*' (7th edition).

He mentions the following adverse effects of mercury:

Salivation, swelling of salivary glands, caries, acute bone pains, oppression about the hypochondria, extreme anxieties, faintness, difficulty in breathing, present danger of choking, prickings and twitchings, soreness, lameness, palsies, spasms, convulsions, apoplexy, thirst, giddiness in the head, trembling, impediment of speech, loss of hearing, decay of sight, loss of smelling, swollen tongue, fever, want of sleep, cold sweats, vomiting, dysentery, hair fell off, headache and, of course, death. '*Mercury as us'd , the body fills, With wholesome goods, or noxious ills, And quickly cures, or quickly kills.*' (Marten, 1711).

1712 '*A Compleat History of Druggs*' by Monsieur Pomet, Chief Druggist to the present French King, done into English, published in London.

<u>Mercury</u>: '*Quicksilver is a remedy for misery, in which the patient swallows a pound or more: It is voided by the stool, without any alteration*'. ... '*It is used in the composition of several unguents and plasters. It is one of the best remedies in physick, to dissipate and eradicate the grossest, most foul, malignant, and inveterate humours …*'

'*one of the most surprising effects that mercury produces is to raise a salivation, and so carry off the very radix or root of the distemper in all venereal foulnesses. To explain this, it must be considered, that the venereal virus conflicts in a humour that is salt or acid, tartarous and gross; which fermenting by degrees, corrupts the blood and other humours, and causes all the ill accidents that follow it….*'

'*Such a salivation is approved of, whereby about two or three pints of a viscous or glutinous humour are discharged every day, and which is fully accomplished in the space of twenty or twenty-five days, or a month at furthest.*'

'The head, the gums, the palate and the tongue are ulcerated: the salivary vessels relaxed.'

Opium—*Opium is narcotic, hypnotic and anodyne; it composes the hurry of the spirits, causes rest and insensibility, is comfortable and refreshing in great watchings and strong pains; provokes sweat powerfully; helps most diseases of the breast and lungs; as coughs, colds, catarrhs and hoarseness; prevents or allays spitting of blood, vomiting, and all Lasks[124] of the bowels; is specific in cholerick, pleurisies, and hysterical cases. Dose, from half a grain to three or four.'*

'It is proper to allay fermenting humours, to excite or procure sleep, to calm or appease pain… to stop looseness and vomiting, to provoke sweat' presumably an allusion to its constipating property. *'Apply'd to the eyes and ears it has caused blindness and deafness; and a plaster of it on the head has occasion'd death'.* He goes on to say *'Custom will bring people to bear great doses of it, but at first every one must begin with very small ones'* Obviously an acknowledgement of tolerance developing.' (Pomet, 1712).

1714 I sent for Radcliffe[125]; was so ill
The other doctors gave me over:
He felt my pulse, prescribed his pill,
And I was likely to recover.
But when the wit began to wheeze,
And wine had warmed the politician,
Cured yesterday of my disease,
I died last night of my physician.
'The Remedy Worse Than the Disease,' by Matthew Prior (1664–1721).

The Mercury thermometer was invented.

1715 Plough Court pharmacy, the forerunner of Allen and Hanburys Ltd and GlaxoSmithKline, is established in London by Silvanus Bevan.

1718 John Quincy (d1722). *'Pharmacopoeia officinalis & extemporanea; or, a compleat English dispensatory, in four parts'* London: A. Bell, 1718. 618 pp.

---

[124] lasks = looseness
[125] Radcliffe = This may be John Radcliffe (1652-1714) of the Radcliffe infirmary. Both he and Prior were members of parliament at the same time and both lived at that time in London. Perhaps Radcliffe's death allowed him to escape libel charges.

Ellibori Nigri: *'Parts do adhere to the fibres of the stomach causing gripings.'* Quincy's Lexicon (1787) defined it as a remedy used more to please than to heal persons.

Ellibori Albi: *'The violent operation has expelled it now from internal use–its mutations are so great.'*

Cinnabar (Mercuric sulphide): *'That it is extremely safe so that it may be given in considerable doses without any danger of the ruffles[126], which sometimes happens from mercurials especially salivation or any other tendency thereunto.'*

Mercurum sublimates dulcis: *'The consequences of this poison manifest somewhat like this to be the texture of its parts; for it occasions violent griping, distention of the belly, a flimsy froth by vomit, bloody stools and an intolerable heat and thirst with cold sweats, tremblings and convulsions, which symptoms demonstrate uncommon twitchings and vellications[127] upon the fibres and membranous parts and it terminates in a gangrene.'* (Quincy, 1718).

'The Modern Quack or Physical Impostor detected' ... *with a supplement displaying present Set of Pretenders to clap[134]- curing, giving Judgement upon Urine etc.* Printed for J Roberts near Oxford Arms in Warren Lane, London ... This is a violent diatribe against all quacks, by which he means all that are not members of the Royal College of Physicians. He finishes by giving a list of the latter to make sure the reader knows who to consult. ... *'And lastly, To instannce in no more, In the disease called an humoral Asthma, or where there is Catarrh, or great Defluxion of Rheum attending, especially that which is thick and troublesome to be hawk'd up: here, I say, a Dose of one of these sleep-procuring, or resting cordials (Opium) ... some Persons have been so quiet as never to wake more.'* (London Physician, 1718).

1720 The beginning of the Golden Age of Quackery aided by the newspapers, which were surplanting pamphlets as a means of advertisement (Kelly, 2008).

1722 Thomas Nettleton suggested the best method for testing the effectiveness of variolation (inoculation) against small-pox

---

[126] ruffles = wrinkles or disturbances
[127] vellications = muscle twitching
[134] clap = gonorrhoea

would be compare the mortality of smallpox and that of those inoculated. Of the 3,405 cases, he collected from the surrounding towns, of natural smallpox 636 died, whereas there were no deaths in the 60 patients he had inoculated (Boylston, 2008; Nettleton, 1724). An early cohort study.

1723 *'The practice of salivating shewn to be of no use or efficacy in the cure of the venereal disease, but greatly prejudicial thereto, or, The antivenereal virtue of mercury proved to be independent of any salival evacuation* by M. Chicoyneau ... Illustrated with notes and observations; and confirm'd with instances of the success of this method in England by C. Willoughby. London: J. Roberts, 1723.' Whereas it is apparent that most physicians used salivation as a marker for the correct dose, because they presumed the saliva washed out the syphilitic agent.

1725 Freind, John, 1675–1728, *'The history of physick; from the time of Galen, to the beginning of the sixteenth century. Chiefly with regard to practice; in a discourse written to Dr Mead* (London: Printed for J. Walthoe, jun. 1725). : Printed for J. Walthoe, jun. 1725).' He was physician to the Hanoverian Court, yet imprisoned for his Jacobite sympathies; Freind exerted a significant impact on contemporary medical theory and practice. There was no mention of the adverse effects of drugs. This was the first history of medicine.

Mercury: *'As to mercurial unction he condemned it as pernicious and takes notice how many persons General Quack had killed by this practice.'*

Hellebore alba: *' And even as to purges, tho' white hellebore be much cried up by the Alexander, famous amongst the ancients, it has grown into utter disuse.'*

Hellebore nigra; *'which he thinks more effectual than others, but not so safe.'*

Friedrich Hoffman (1660–1742). At the end of the 17th century Friedrich Hoffman described an epidemic of ergotism discovered in Germany and he attributed the responsibility to the alkaloid contained in the ergot of rye. In order to confirm his theory Hoffman conducted experiments on animals, which revealed without doubt the toxic action of the ergot. On the basis of this and other reports the Academy of Science in Paris prohibited the therapeutic use of rye in several European countries. The episode was significant as it represented the first identification of an adverse effect of a drug; whose gravity, confirmed on the basis of ad hoc studies, was such to require a resolute intervention on the part of government departments'. (Borghi & Canti, 1986).

'*Opera Medica*' in volume 15. 'Friderici Hoffmanni, Opuscula physico-medica antehac seorsim edita; iam revisa, aucta, emendata et delectu habito recusa denuò revisa...' [A short physio-medical work previously issued already revised, enlarged, corrected and with careful selection recently again revised] Ulmae: Bartholomai, 1725 Republished in 1788; another book by Hoffman is '*Medicina Medica*', in one volume.

1729 Sir Hans Sloane was consulted by a man concerning his four children who had taken some henbane seeds mistaking them for filberds[128]. Their symptoms were '*great thirst, swimmings in the head, dimness of sight, ravings and profound sleep; which last in one of them continued for two days and two nights*'. He had them bled, blistered, purged and made to vomit (Sloane, 1745).

1730 A German scientist, W.G. Frobenius changed the name of 'sweet vitriol' to 'ether' (*Spiritus vini aetherus*) (Frobenius, 1730; Belluci, 1982).

1732 '*An analytical enquiry into the specifick property of mercury, relating to the cure of venereal disease.... with Dr Chicanneau's method of curing this distemper without salivation.*' by Vincent Brest and Francois Chicanneau. This contains several lists of rules: First — That if the salivation rises plentifully three to four days after the first unction the cure will miscarry. Second — If gripes and looseness attend the patient and continue for six to eight days the patient dies, or at least the cure miscarries. He advocated small doses of Quicksilver ointment applied by friction. This was called the 'Montpellier Method'. (Brest, 1732).

Two UK acts bearing the title 'An act for preventing frauds and abuses committed in the making and vending unsound, adulterated and bad drugs and medicines' were approved in 1735 and 1762.

---

[128] filberd = hazel nut

1733 *'Poor Richard's Almanack'* by Benjamin Franklin, (1706–1790).
*'He's the best physician that knows the worthlessness of most
medicines.'*

James Alleyne's *'A New English Dispensatory'* (1733) He
repeats Quincy's comments on Cinnebar (HgS) and Mercurous
sublimates dulcis.

    Hellebore: *'white and black hellebore, the first of which brings
on such violent spasms, that a prudent physician will not venture
to prescribe it.'*

    Henbane: *'All authors agree that the use of them is not so
safe'..." The bad are those which produce a most profound sleep,
commonly ending in death; but if it happens to be shaken off,
there generally follows a depravation of the faculties of the mind;
and of this sort are the leaves, flowers, fruits, roots and juice of
both sorts of henbane; seeds of thorn-apple, which being taken to
$3\frac{1}{2}$ creates madness, and to 3 i is mortal.'* (Alleyne, 1733).

*'The Ancient Physician's legacy to his country being what he
has collected in forty-nine years practice or an account of the
several diseases incident to mankind, in so plain a manner, that
any person may know the nature of his own distemper, and the
several remedies proper for it, wherein the extraordinary effects of
mercury are more, particularly consider'd.'* by Thomas Dover[129],
1733. *'Iliac Passion*[130]*: You must go no further for the cure of this
fatal disease than to take a pound or a pound and a half of crude
mercury.'* (Dover, 1733). That should settle the patient for good.

    Yo-Ho-Ho. Pulv. Ipecac.Co (Dover's Powder)

    'Oh, Dover was pirate, and he sailed the Spanish Main.

    A hacking cough convulsed him; he had agonising pain.

    So he mixed hisself a powder, which he liked it more and more.

Ipecac. and opium and K_2SO_4'[131] (Anon, 1923; Weatherall, 1996)

*'Augustine Belloste, the author of this book "The Hospital
Surgeon containing several essays on mercury",* calls it (mercury)
the miracle of nature, and the greatest gift of God in the whole
Materia Medica. I appeal to the Reader, if such a person as I

---

[129] Thomas Dover = A Warwickshire physician who became a second captain on a privateer 'Duke' which sailed to South America in the years 1708-11.
[130] iliac passion = intestinal colic
[131] Dover's Powder = Ipecacuanha Root 10 Grammes; Opium 10 Grammes; Potassium Sulphate 80 Grammes, Dose 3 – 10 decigrams

lately mentioned, deserves the title of doctor. As for my part, though I am only but a poor bachelor of physick, I shall for ever scorn so much, so dishonourable a behaviour.' (Belloste, 1733).

'To procure the desired benefit from a salivation, it must be carried to excess, and the patient must be reduced to the last extremity. If he is weak, you must curb the Flux, and in thus favouring him, your end is lost'. (Belloste, 1721).

'Everyone is sensible that all countries abound with a great number of people of no service to the community, who are kept at a considerable expense in hospital, on account of several real and pretender Infirmities, which their manner of living, either in laziness, or in fatigue and misery has brought upon them who pass for incurable, and are really so at last, for want of using the only remedy which is capable of curing them speedily and with small expense. Cruel mercury taken at the mouth, would clear the hospital of them all, and re-establish number of slothful vagabonds in a condition of work, who under pretext of certain maladies, which they industriously cherish and prolong–until this becomes contagious infect whole cities and countries and extract alms, which they apply to evil use.' (Belloste, 1721). He was obviously full of the milk of human kindness.

'A Treatise on Mercury with some remarks on the ancient physician's legacy by Henry Bradley. Physical and Philosophical remarks on Dr Dover's late pamphlet, entitled The Ancient Physician's legacy to his country.'

'It is one thing to know how to bleed, purge, vomit, etc. and a quite different thing to know when and under what circumstances either the one or the other is to be chosen; how far to be allowed, and when or by what means to be moderated and restrained. The former may be got by reading, or learned by rote[132]; but the latter can only be obtained by a just acquaintance with that part of natural philosophy which respects the animal economy.'

<u>Mercury:</u> *'Very dismal symptoms often attend it; as fevers, violent colics, diarrhoea, dysenteries, swellings and erosions of the glands, terrible headaches, vertigo, tremors, delusions, convulsions and often death closes the rear'... 'salivation, some were grown mad, loss of sense, great weakness, emaciated,*

---

[132] by rote = learn by heart

rheumatism, effusion of lymph, livid colour, palsy, suffocated by an asthma.' (Bradley, 1733).

Mercury: *'an antidote, or some remarks upon a treatise on mercury by Thomas Harris. "A treatise on the force and energy of crude mercury proving the usefulness innocency of its intense application by a great many experts and history of cases acute and chronic"....* It also copies word for word from the 1733 Alleyne's dispensatory (Harris,1734).

1735 Hermann Boerhaave (1668–1738), who was made professor of Botany and Medicine at Leyden in 1709, wrote his aphorisms in 1728 and it was translated from the Latin in 1735. He is renowned as an outstanding bedside clinician and as a chemist. His therapeutic range was large and for epilepsy he advocated: *'Revulsions and dissipating means are useful, such as clear and depurate[133] the passages: Hence bleeding, purging, vomiting, burning, issues, fistules, a blister, a wound of the head, the trepanning of the skull, antihysterics and opiates are useful: which must be learned from the discovery of the proximate cause of the disease'.* He was still very influenced by the 'humours' and he describes epilepsy in the following terms: *' This disease wonderfully different in its many aspects does often appear so surprising that it has in all ages been attributed to the Gods, Devils, Divine wrath, Witchcraft and like causes above and greater natural ones'.* His treatment for madness was extreme: *'The greatest remedy for it is to throw the patient unwarily into the sea, and to keep him under water as long as he can possibly bear without being stifled'.* His mention of adverse drug effects is casual and they are only mentioned occasionally, e.g. *'the steam of arsenic, antimony, fresh quick lime, mercury, and other poisons, are able to cause a palsy'.* He recommend Peruvian bark for intermittent fevers, *'which, according to the fancy of the patient, he may give in powder, infusion, decoction, extract, or boiled up into a syrup; joining proper specifics and antidotes, according to the different symptoms, or its way of operating; 'for some people it will purge violently and others it will bind'.* (Boerhaave, 1735).

---

[133] depurate = purify

<u>White and Black hellebore</u> *'The form of which is not ventured upon by discreet physicians, on account of the violent spasms which it brings on, for being given to half a scruple it acts most violently.'* (Boerhaave, 1740).

John Astruc wrote *'A treatise of the venereal disease, containing an account of the original, propagation, and contagion of this distemper in general'*. Under the chapter heading *'Of the force and efficacy of mercury and mercurial medicines, and whence they proceed'* he gives: *'pulsations of the heart...is made stronger, and fuller secretions ...are plentifully promoted... as urine, sweat, liquids discharged by the glands of the stomach, and saliva; were so affected with the spitting, diarrhoea, ulcers in the mouth, and inflammation of the head, which attended it, that growing lean, pale, squalid, toothless, stammering, and not able to open their jaws, after long and severe sufferings he hardly got over it'.* (Astruc, 1737).

1736 Nicholas Robinson wrote *'A New treatise of the Venereal Disease'*. He refers to the ADRs of mercury: huge swellings in the head and face, in the throat and tongue...threatens the patient with a suffocation; tremors, faintings; convulsions; cold clammy sweats; salivation; blindness; deafness; contraction of the jaws; stubborn pains and weaknesses; violent hurries and intolerable headaches (Robinson, 1736).

Joseph Clutton wrote *'A true and candid relation of the good and the bad effects of Joshua Ward's pill and drop'*. He described 68 cases and one of these is given below:

'Case XXXVIII. Gilbert Jones, at the Butcher's Arms, in King-street, Westminster, aged 50 years, had a cough, was a little pthisical, and stuffed in his lungs, he was also troubled with rheumatick Pains, which made him go with two sticks.–A person (who seemed to be one of Ward's intimate Friends, and with whom, he said, he had been abroad in France) being in the house as a guest, and, observing the condition of Gilbert Jones, told him what wonderful Cures Ward had done there, and also in England, and therefore mightily persuaded him to try some of his pills, assuring him, if he would consent to try them, that he should throw away his Crutches in a Month's time. Gilbert

Jones, upon such Persuasions of this person, was prevail'd on, and he having some of these famous Pills about him, left Gilbert Jones two of them, one of which he took soon after, which had but little Operation, and thereupon he took the other, but without any Benefit, and afterwards he took one of his drops, (for which and what Pills he had then of him, he paid him a guinea) but this Drop strain'd, vomited, and purg'd him to so great a degree, that it brought upon him such dismal and frightful Symptoms, that his wife, who constantly attended him, declar'd she would not continue in the room, if he took another of these Drops, for twenty Pounds. After he had taken this Drop, he was never able to go out of his Room, and his Head was so much affected with the Violence of its Operation, that it was never well afterwards. R. Varley, an Apothecary, in the same Street, was about the 5th of April, 1735, sent for to him, who upon asking him what his Complaints were, Jones told him, that he had taken Mr. Ward's Medicines, and that he was much worse for them; that his Limbs were a great deal worse than before he took them; and, notwithstanding R. Varley the Apothecary's Endeavours, he grew daily worse and worse; and thereupon he desired a Physician might be advised with upon the Case, which was agreed to, and Dr. Williams, of Dartmouth–street, was sent for, but his whole Constitution was so much shock'd and impair'd by the Pills followed with this Drop, that, notwithstanding all the Endeavours of the Physician and Apothecary, they could not remove its dire Effects, and thereupon he died about the 20th Day of the following Month.' (Clutton, 1736). Clutton maintained that Joshua Ward's medication contained arsenic. This case illustrates the adverse effects of 'secret remedies' and the attitude of the medical profession towards them and the quacks that sold them. (see 1803).

John Douglas wrote '*A dissertation on the venereal disease*'. He quotes other authors on the problems with mercury: '*Deep sordid ulcers affect several parts of the mouth; whence spitting is continued….. the patient is gradually wasted, and at length turns consumptive… so fretted and teased with pain… a violent and dangerous looseness; which often turns into a bloody flux… the salivary, maxillary and parotid glands swell all of a sudden, grow hot and painful, the tongue is tumified and hangs out at the mouth; the face and the whole head are much swelled, whence great difficulty of swallowing and breathing; their speech is lost… deep sleep, lethargy, fever, etc… sickness and vomiting spasms of the members, fainting and cold sweats.'* (Douglas, 1737).

1740 The *'Remediorum Specimina ex praxi A.W.'*, or *'Examples of Remedies from the practice of Abraham Wagner'*, is a approximately 200-page octavo manuscript in German with clinical notes and patient observations and recipes reproduced both in Latin and in the extensive pharmaceutical notation of the period. Apparently begun in 1740.

1745 William Heberden (1710–1801) denounced Mithridatium as *'good for nothing'*. (Heberden, 1745).

An anonymous review of the London Dispensary gave an amusing account of many of the drugs within it:
'Mel Helleboratium (Honey of Hellebore) Seldom ventured on; seldom to be met with any good.'
'Oleum Lateritium (Oil of Brocks) Nonsense'
'Causticum Commune Mitius (Common mild caustic) Beneath all criticism'
'Pulvis Antilyssus Powder (Against the bite of a mad dog) A mere plaything and not dangerous in itself, but in the delay from other medicines.' (This comment could be applied to most modern complimentary medicines).
'Of Thorn-apple I well know that the plant is altogether disused in Physick, and described by authors as highly noxious both to men and to beasts. For all of them unanimously write, that the Thorn-apple disorders the mind causes madness, destroys our ideas and memory and occasions convulsions.' (Anon, 1745).

1746 Henbane fell into disuse and was omitted from the London Pharmacopoeias of 1746 and 1788 and restored in 1809 when it started being used for convulsions.

1747 The *'Jāmi' al-javāmi'-i Muhammad-Shāhī'* was a large pharmacopoeia of at least several volumes by Hakīm Muhammad Hāshim ibn hakīm Muhammad Hādī Qalandar ibn Muzaffar al-Dīn 'Alavī Shīrāzī 'Alavī Khān (d1747 or 1749).

Examination of drugs to prevent adulteration. Apothecaries' Petition to the House of Commons Committee, to Whom the Petition of...Apothecaries of the Cities of London and Westminster...Were Referred. By Sir William Calvert. Bill to revive, explain and amend the Act for the better viewing, searching and examining all drugs, medicines and waters, oil and compositions used in medicines.

Evidence from members from the Society of the Art and Mystery of Apothecaries, alleges that unskilled or dishonest practitioners are dispensing drugs of dubious quality, often comprising incorrect ingredients.

George Key wrote *'A dissertation on the effects of mercury on human bodies, in the cure of the venereal disease'* and gave the following as its adverse effects: *'purging, swelling chaps[135], indurated glands, aching and painful, teeth loose, intumescence[136] of the tongue, head and face swelling to a monstrous size, violent convulsions, dysenteries, contortions of the bowels, jaws oft-times so firmly locked up through contractions of their muscles, destroy the bones of the nose, and sometimes those of the palate.'* (Key, 1747). It would seem in the last two instances that he is mistaking the results of syphilis with those of mercury.

Dr John Steadman, late Surgeon-Major to the regiment of the Royal Grey Dragoons in a letter to Dr John Pringle in whilst in Dutch Brabant.

<u>White Henbane</u>: *'Five men and two women of the regiment took, in error, a brew of leaves of this plant (Hyoscyamus albus): giddiness, staggered as if drunk, incoherent, high delirium, low irregular pulse, slavered, frequently changed colour, eyes looked fiery, legs powerless. One of the women had hands stiff and swelled.'* A Mr William Watson commented that it must have been *Hyoscyamus niger* (Pringle, 1751).

Many non medical people wrote medical guides or tracts for the lay public that couldn't afford proper medical care. A good example was John Wesley who wrote, in addition to his religious works, *'Primitive Physick'*. He read widely contemporary medical

---

[135] chaps = cheeks
[136] intumescence = swelling

literature and consulted an apothecary and a physician before starting to write.

'It is, because they are not safe, but extremely dangerous, that I Have omitted (together with Antimony) the four Herculean medicines, Opium, the Bark, Steel, and most of the preparations of mercury. Herculean Indeed! Far too strong for common men to grapple with. How many fatal effects have these produced, even in the hands of no ordinary Physicians? With regard to four of these, the instances are glaring and undeniable And whereas Quicksilver, the fifth is in its native form as innocent as bread or water.'

His favourite treatment seems to have been electricity. One of his recipes does contain Antimony: 792,Or, after purging take about 15 grains of ceruse of Antimony (Sb_2O_2) in white wine. Some of his remedies seem quite drastic *'Twisting of the guts. Many at the point of death have been cured by taking one, two or three pounds of Quicksilver in water'*. However by not using these drugs he probably caused fewer unnecessary adverse effects than the normal physician.

1748 In the Journal *'Gentleman's Magazine'* for August 1748 a list of quack remedies was given under the pseudonym of 'Publicola'. These were referred to as 'Nostrums', which were defined as medicines with secret ingredients, and 'Empirics', which were defined as medicines which have been shown by experience to have benefits. He lists 202 such potions and gives the type of medicine, its use, its inventor, place of sale and cost. Here is a sample of his list:

Drops; Gleets[137]; Dr Ratcliffe; Vere Street; 3s 6d[138] a bottle.
Elixirs; Fevers; Dr Boerhaave; Denmark Street; 1s 6d a bottle.
Plaisters; Coughs; Helmont; St James' Churchyard; 1s 0d a bottle.
Pills; Cancer; Mr Durham; Holbourn; 10s 6d a box.
In the magazine there were numerous advertisements for similar preparations:
Dr Steer's Oil for Convulsions, 2s 6d the bottle.

---

[137] gleets = purulent urethral discharge
[138] 3/6 = three shillings and sixpence in UK currency and this is worth in 2008 £24.59 based on the Retail Price Index or £260.92 on average earnings (http://www.measuringworth.com/calculators/ppoweruk/result.php?use%5B%5D=CPI&use%5B%5D=NOMINALEARN&year_early=1748&pound71=&shilling71=1&pence71=&amount=0.05&year_source=1748&year_result=2009) Accessed 10th September 2009

Dr Hooper's female pills, 1s 1½d the box.

Henry's Calcined Magnesia, 2s 6d the bottle.

Orskirk Medicine for the bite of a mad dog, 5s 5d the packet.

Daffy's Elixir, 1s 1d the bottle (Jones, 1957).

Some of the inventors bear famous names, but whether these were genuine must seem doubtful. These were extortionate prices and would have been unaffordable by the masses.

1751 The *'Dispensatory of the Royal College of Physicians'*, London, translated into English with remarks, etc. by H Pemberton, MD. No ADRs mentioned.

1752 *'Pharmacopoeia Universalis* or *New Universal English Dispensatory'* by R James MD.

White hellebore: *'caustic or burning force attracted into the nostrils after the manner of snuff excites an invincible sneezing: taken into the stomach it purges upwards and downwards with fever, gripings, sometimes excites convulsions.'*

Hellebore niger: *'Gripings–excites a tenesmus.'*

Henbane: *'Disturbs the reason'* ... *'Even an external application of henbane may procure madness' 'They soon become delirious who take the papaver, mandrake or hyoscyamus inwardly; but their pulse at such time is very slow.'*

Opium: *'Heats very much, which is a sure proof that it dissolves and rarefies the blood and this appears also from its causing an itching in the skin; sometimes sweats…. But the abuse of it is very great and destructive and a hundred times more is used in England than ought to be.'*

Mercury: *'For the miners and others employed about it, though of the strongest constitutions imaginable, seldom remain four years in that state, but are seized with trembles and palsies, and die miserable. By an injudicious use of it, whether outwardly applied, or inwardly taken, the nerves are likewise affected, weakened, corrupted, and contracted. Whence tremblings, spasms, palsies and too great attenuation of the fluids, which often brings on a fatal salivation, ulcers in the mouth and throat, and incurable loosenesses'. 'Those seem to be in great error…. Use sublimate mercury since this, when received into the pores, greatly disposes to violent headaches, hemicranias, and looseness of the teeth.'* (James, 1752).

The German medical periodical *'Rebus in Scientia Naturalis et Medicina Gestis* [Accounts of happenings in natural science and medicines] published in Leipzig containing abstracts of medical books.

1753 *'Treatise on opium, founded upon practical observations'* by George Young, London, 1753, 197pp.

James Lind on scurvy wrote *'Experience shows that the cure of the adventitious scurvy is very simple, viz. a pure dry air, with the use green herbage or a wholesome vegetables, almost of any sort; which for the most part prove effectual'.* (Lind, 1753). It is interesting to note that he first mentions fresh air as a requisite.

1754 Richard Brookes in *'An introduction to physic and surgery'* devoted a chapter to *'The poisonous effects of certain medicaments':*

'Among Medicaments that have poisonous effects, violent emetics, drastic purges, mercurials, and other opiates may be justly reckoned.

Antimonial emetics are the most violent and virulent, especially when given in substances; such as Glass of Antimony, Mercurius Vitae, and Crocus metallorum. These Antimonials given in powder purge upwards and downwards, and often, by their super-purgations, hurry the patient out of the world...

Violent purges have likewise been the cause of grievous diseases, and sometimes death. Among these may be reckoned black and white Hellebore....

Of the Bad Effect of Mercurials

Mercurial medicaments are strong remedies made of quicksilver with the addition of salts, which greatly affect the glands, and by a violent stricture promote the motion of the lympha (lymph), *and being corrosive produce spasms in the nervous parts.*

It is the peculiar property of mercury to affect the fauces with the larynx, tongue, and teeth; for if the joints or other parts are annointed with a mercurial ointment, the tongue and amygdalae (tonsils) *will swell, the fauces wil be full of apthae[139], and saliva will dribble away with a stench, the gums will be flaccid and the*

---

[139] apthae = blister on mucous membrane usually in the mouth

*teeth loose… Quicksilver is innocent and has no drastic effect
alone, but acquires its force and virulence from the addition of
salts…*

Of the Bad Effects of Soporiferous Medicines

*Soporiferous medicines are otherwise called hypnotics, or
anodynes. The strongest are termed narcotics, or stupfactives.
These diminish or destroy the sense and motion of the solid parts.
The most usual and common of these is opium; the stupfactives
are mandragora, henbane, nightshade, strammony, and datura.*

*Too large a dose, or too long an use of opiates or narcotics will
render the pulse languid, depressed, and small, and bring on
a strait and difficult breathing; a sopor and torpor of the head;
a stupor of the senses, and an alienation of the mind. As also a
decreased appetite, costiveness, a weak digestion, and a failure
of strength. However, it is universally allowed they are of great
service in grievous pains and fluxions.'*

He also deals with: Cantharides, *Nux vomica*, gold, copper and
lead (Brookes, 1754).

1755 Boerhaave Herman in '*Materia medica, or the Druggists guide,
and the physician and apothecary's table-book. Being an account
of all drugs*' said of Henbane: '*The black (henbane niger seeds)
are accounted poisonous: but they are not used.*' (see 1735).

1756 '*A mechanical account of poisons in several essays*' by Richard
Mead. 5th edition (1st edition 1702) London: J. Brindley,
Mercury Sublimate: '*violent griping pains, distension of the belly,
vomiting of a slimy frothy matter, sometimes mixed with blood
and stools of the same, an intolerable heat and thirst with cold
sweats, tremblings, convulsions... spasms, contractions, palsies*'.
Compare the wording with that of De Quincy in 1718.

'*The Effects of Semen Hyoscyamui Albi*' by Dr Archibald
Hamilton: '*Lassitude, dryness of throat, swallowing was like to
choke him, gripes in his belly, convulsions, tremors, startings,
eyes open and rolling, insomnia, degree of insensibility after
nearly 25 grs.*' (Hamilton, 1756).

1757 '*I-hsüeh Yüan Liu Lun*' by Hsu Ta-Ch'un. The author in chapter
22 says '*It is difficult to kill a person through [a treatment with]
the wrong drugs*' and goes on to say '*Only drugs with a very hot*

or very dry [nature] kill people in a most violent way. The reason is that hot natured drugs are often toxic. Also their yang nature is urgent and fierce. As soon as they enter the body's viscera and bowels, the blood bubbles up and the influences rise. If a person's yin influences were depleted beforehand, or if it is a hot day, or if the patient has been harmed by summer-heat or [other] heat already, as soon as he takes hot [drugs] the two fires clash, and all types of terrible symptoms will appear at the same time. [The patient's] eyes turn red and his stools are blocked, his tongue loses its moisture and his teeth dry out. His mouth is thirsty and his heart is troubled, his flesh shows cracks and his spirit is disturbed.' (Unschuld, 1998). This is the only instance in which I have found adverse event symptoms have been given in the early Chinese literature. The symptoms are those of the Solanaceae family containing tropane alkaloids, e.g. henbane.

Dr You-Ping Zhu of the Hwa To Centre for Chinese medicine at Groningen University commented '*You are probably right in thinking that classical Chinese herbal texts do not mention specific adverse reactions associated with specific herbs. In TCM, safety is taken into consideration in the overall treatment strategy in relation to patients' specific conditions rather than simply look at specific herbs independent of patients' conditions.*' (personal communication, 2008).

1759 '*Dictionnaire Universel des Drogues Simples*' [A universal dictionary of simple drugs] by Nicolas Lemery, Paris.

Hellebore: '*Ils purgent par haut et par bas*' - they purge both upwards and downwards.

Hyoscyamus: '*Elles sont narcotique, stupéfiant, assoupissant et souvent mortelles aux animals qui en mangent.*' They are narcotic, stupefying, soporific and often mortal to animals who eat it.

Salix (saule marceau): '*The bark, leaves and seeds are astringent and refreshing. One makes a decoction to stop 'les ardeurs de Venus.'* – lust.

Mercury (Hydrargia): '*the head swells, the gums, the tongue and the palate ulcerate, the salivary vessels relax and one feels the pains such as happens if one has put on corrosive sublimate somewhere excoriated, these accidents are accompanied by a copious involuntary salivation*'.

144

François-Marie Arouet de Voltaire, French author, humanist, rationalist, & satirist. (1694–1778).

'Doctors are men who prescribe medicines of which they know little, to cure diseases of which they know less, in human beings of whom they know nothing'. Voltaire also said *'the art of medicine is to amuse the patient while nature cures the disease'*.

In Candide Dr Panglos was *'all covered over with sores, his eyes half dead, the tip of his nose eaten off, his mouth turned to one side, his teeth black, speaking through his throat, tormented with a violent cough, with gums so rotten, that his teeth came near falling out every time he spit'*. A description of the mixture of symptoms and those of mercury.

1760 Dr Anton Storck tried hemlock on a dog and when it remained well, took one grain (65 mgm) of hemlock extract with a cup of tea without ill effect. Subsequently he prescribed it for cancers, ulcers and cataracts.

A controlled study comparing two forms of mercury treatment for syphilis was undertaken in Geneva. Twelve patients were treated by rubbing in a mercurial ointment and 12 with Keyser pills (mercuric oxide and acetic acid) with the result that 23 were cured; two failed to respond to rubbing, one of whom was cured with the pills (Louis-Courvoisier, 2007; Repertoire du Registre CC, 1761).

Leopold Auenbrugger applied the technique of percussion, which he had learnt as a brewer, to the chest and thereby was able to diagnose fluid on the chest and consolidation of the lobes of the lung, but it would not become generally used until the turn of the century.

1761 William Lewis (1708–1781) wrote *'Experimental history of the materia medica'* London, H Baldwin for the author & R Willcock, 1761.

Hellebore Nigra: *'very strongly, though not very violently cathartic.'*

Hellebore alba: *'violently sternatory operating with great violence both upwards and downwards. Has sometimes brought on convulsions and other terrible symptoms. It affects the tongue, produces a strangulation and suffocates with extreme anxiety.'*

<u>Hyoscyamus niger</u>: '*mighty narcotic, violent disoprder of the senses, sometimes fatal.*'

1763 '*An essay on the internal use of thorn-apple, henbane and monkshood*' by Anton Störck, Vienna (1731–1803).

<u>Thorn-apple</u>: '*highly noxious to man and beast*'... *disagreeable taste. Disorders the mind, causes madness, destroys ones ideas and memory and occasions convulsions.*'

<u>Henbane</u>: Most authors forbid the internal use of it. He gave it to dogs–pupils dilated, staggered, trembled, very weak, sight almost gone, vomited three times and stools open 5 times. He treated 13 patients and reported the effects: middling dose–pupils dilated, languor, eyes open, staggered, anxiety in sleep. Case II chilliness and shivering all over the body, with anxiety, a cold sweat, weakness of sight and a sense of beginning fainting fit. Case IV unquenchable thirst and colicky pains.

He conducted animal experiments with some traditional herbs, eventually trying them on himself: hemlock, colchicum, thorn apple, henbane and monkshood (Störck, 1763).

The Reverend Edward Stone wrote in the '*Philosophical Transactions*' that the bark of the willow tree was a successful remedy for the agues. He added '*It seems likewise to have this additional quality, viz. To be a safe medicine; for I never could perceive the least ill effect from it, though it had been always given without any preparation of the patient*'. (Stone, 1763).

'*Essay on the effects of opium as a poison with the cure*'. By John Awsiter.

The general effects of opium are as follows, viz. '*Upon almost immediate taking, the first symptoms are a heat, and weight at the stomach, succeeded by an extravagance of spirits, even to violent laughter, listlessness of the limbs, giddiness, head-ache, loss of memory, dead look of the eyes, imperfect speech, drowsiness, slow and full pulse, short and quick breathing, nausea, and an extreme florid complexion,…. The more violent and extreme effects are itching of skin, madness, vertigoes, vomitings, hiccups, heavy and dead sleeps, unequal pulse, contraction of jaw, convulsions, profuse sweats, universal relaxation, faintings, coldness of the extreme parts and lastly a cold breath, a certain indication of death.'* (Awsiter, 1763).

In 1763 appeared *'The Medical Museum or a repository of cases, experiments, researches, and discoveries; collected at home and abroad whether in: anatomy, botany, medicine, chemistry pharmacy, surgery, physiology, etc'.* By Gentlemen of the Faculty; this consisted of the three volumes with a total of 1,835 pages. The first volume contained 53 separate monographs, e.g. Jones, John, (1645–1709). The mysteries of <u>opium</u> reveal'd by Dr. John Jones ... who:

Gives an account of the name, make, choice, effects, &c. of opium.

Proves all former opinions of its operation to be meer chimera's.

Demonstrates what its true cause is, by which he easily, and mechanically explains all (even its most mysterious) effects. Shows its noxious principle, and how to separate it, thereby rendering it a safe, and noble panacea, whereof. He shews the palliative, and curative use. 1700.

Usual and frequent (tho' not constant) Effects of Opium, used internally in a moderate dose. (Those in 'Side Effects of Drugs' have an *).

'Sleep*, which is so far from being a constant effect of *opium, that it will in me, and many other persons, prevent sleeping, even when otherwise inclin'd to it; causing meat to stay long at stomach; sweat*; deadness of the eyes, as you see in drunkenness; dilatation of the pupil.'* (actually causes constriction) *'itchings in the skin*; much urine; nausea*; swimmings in the head; a kind of dubious state, between sleeping and waking.'*

The rare Effects of Opium, taken in a moderate dose.

'Temporary palsies, as of the bladder*, and sometimes of other parts, tho' (although) *very rarely; faltering of the tongue; looseness of the lower jaw, as in the drowsy, drunkards, &c.; prevention of sweat, in such as sweat too much for want of perspiration; abortion; intumescence of the lips; anxieties and distresses; vomitings* and hiccoughs*; convulsions; syncopes, leipothimies[140] and faintings; death*, tho' very rarely, and that*

---

[140] leipothimie = lipothymy = sensation of being about to faint.

in very weak people; purging; a long stay thereof at stomach sometimes; stoppage of urine*; It sometimes proves dangerous after haemorrhages and large evacuations.'

Thomas Bayes published '*An Essay towards solving a problem in the doctrine of chances'*. This has become the gold standard for the assessment of causality of adverse drug events (Bayes, 1763).

1764 "*Pharmacopoeia Universalis*" or "*A New Universal English Dispensatory*" of 1764, by R. James, M.D., which described not only the therapeutic actions but also the toxic and addictive properties of opium. One effect he describes is that, after taking opium, '*The peristaltic motion of the intestines becomes more languid.'*

1765 Samuel Bard (1742–1821), experimented on himself taking 1½ grains of opium and checked his pulse every half to one hour and found that the rate had dropped from 71 per minute to 57 per minute, starting about an hour after taking the drug and the effect wore off about 7 hours later. He repeated the experiment on himself three times and then on three friends and six patients (Maehle, 1999).

Fabre recommended much circumspection in the use of mercury, because of fear of 'accidents orageux': swelling of the tongue, engorgement of the salivary glands, swelling of the head, dysentery, fever, delerium and convulsions (Fabre, 1765).

'*Ben CaoGang Mu Shi'* [Supplements to compendium of materia medica] by Zhao Xue-Min.

'*Cowpox and Its Ability to Prevent Smallpox'* by Jon Fewster, an apothecary of Thornbury, was submitted to the Medical Society of London, but was not published (FPH RCP, 2000).

1768 William Watson (1717–1787) in '*An account of experiments, instituted with a view of ascertaining the most successful method of inoculating the smallpox'* London: J Nourse. He compared the pretreatment of children inoculated against smallpox. He made three groups as similar as possible and he measured the number of pustules or pocks and compared the means. It was not known at that time how to take into account the small number with very high pock count. The three groups were: mercury, senna plus rose syrup and no pretreatment. One mercury patient had more pocks that the rest of the group together. This is one of the earliest studies using an untreated control group and a quantification of the results. However the largest group only contained 11 patients and it wasn't until much larger groups were used that there was a chance of picking up type 'B' reactions[141] (Boyston, 2008).

1770 The Edinburgh College of Surgeons introduced a diploma for country surgeons (Maehle, 1853).

Van Swieten (1700-1772) had 4,880 registered cases of syphilitic patients treated orally with 0.1% mercuric chloride (corrosive sublimate).

1771 Albrecht Van Haller (1708-1777) published the *'Pharmacopoeia Helvetica'* and wrote on testing new drugs: *'In the first place the remedy is to be tried on the healthy without any foreign substances mixed with it. Having been examined as to its colour and taste, a small dose is taken, and the attention directed to all effects which thereupon occur: such as pulse, the temperature, the respiratory, the excretion. Having thereby adduced their obvious phenomenon is healthy you may pass to experiments upon the sick body.'* (Earles, 1961).

1773 The journal *'Medical and Philosophical Commentaries'* launched in Edinburgh, containing abstracts of books relevant to clinicians. In 1796 it became the *'Annals of Medicine'* and in 1805 it became the *'Edinburgh Medical and Surgical Journal'* and later *'The Edinburgh Medical Journal'*.

1774 De Malon in his book *'Preserver of the blood: or bleeding demonstrated to be always pernicious, and often mortal'* said *'Whereas bleeding destroys one fourth of the sick in general'* (p57) *...'and its martyrdom is much the longest in the rolls of physic'* (p61) *'bleeding is necessary in no kind of disorders, whatever, since we have instances of all sorts of diseases cured without its aid'*. The tide is turning against bleeding.

In the Pharmacopoia Reformata the author 'MS' said *'No new*

---

[141] type 'B' reactions = hypersensitivity or idiosyncratic reaction (Rawlins & Thompson, 1977)

medicine how strongly recommend so be, receive the solemn sanction of the college (Royal College of Physicians, London) *before its real worth be duly enquired into.'* (Earles, 1961).

1776 *'Histoire des plantes vénéuses de la Suisse'* Contenant leur description, leurs mauvais effets sur les hommes et sur les animaux, avec leurs antidotes; rédigée d'après ce qu'on a de mieux sur cette matière, & sur-tout d'après l'Histoire des plantes helvétiques de m. le baron de Haller; mise à la portée de tout le monde, avec le lieu natal de chaque plante pour la France, les figures nécessaires, & plusieurs observations nouvelles. Par Mr. P.R. Vicat ... etc. First Edition, Yverdon, 1776.

['History of the poisonous plants from Switzerland'. Containing their description, their bad effects on men and on animals, with their antidotes; edited after the best of this material, and especially from the History of Swiss plants by Monsieur Le Baron de Haller; placed at the disposal of everybody, with birth place of each plant in France, the necessary diagrams, and several new observations. By Mr. P.R. Vicat...].

Hyoscyamus niger: *'difficulty swallowing, frenetic and stupid, lighty deluded, rather gay, sad dreams, dangerous fever, quarrelsome, furious, violent, loss of all senses, hydrophobia, drunk, vertigo, trouble with vision, double vision, blind, eyes inflamed, can hardly speak, stops speaking, profound sleep, frightening dreams, cramps, convulsions, risus sardonicus, trembling of the limbs, swelling of the limbs, excess diarrhoea, swelling of the lower abdomen, pains in all the body–head, intestines–paralysis takes hold of half of the body, radiant warmth, lived colour, fainting, palpitations, strong irregular pulse, swelling of the vessels–neck, face and limbs, numbness which lasts for months on end.'*

Hyoscyamus blanc: *'Similar, slumber, convulsions.'*

Hellebore niger: *'purgative, excess diarrhoea, hiccups, vomiting, convulsions, inflamed intestines.'*

Papaver somniferum: *'sluggishness of the stomach, intestines, urine and pupils, insensible, respiration difficult, bitterness, nauseous, salivates, sensation of warmth.'*

In his introduction he says 'á propos' the sensory system:

150

'*Je veux parler des sens, soit extérieur soit intérieur de ces gardiens vigilans que la nature á sa sagesse établie pour veiller á le conservation de notre santé et de notre vie.*' 'I want to speak of the senses, either exterior or interior of these vigilant guardians that nature, in its wisdom, established to look after our health and our lives.' This phrase could be applied to Pharmacovigilance.

A French Royal declaration dated 28th April 1777 separated the spicers (grocers) from the apothecaries and forbade grocers and all other persons to make, sell or to retail salts, compounds or preparations for humans in the form of medication under the pain of a fine of 500 pounds or more; reserving the work of the pharmacy for apothecaries.

John Millar (1733–1805) wrote '*Detached cases however numerous and well attested are insufficient to support general conclusions*'. Most adverse reaction reports had been either case reports or case series.

1778 The Société Royale de Médecine became the only competent authority for the authorization for new medicines. This right was abolished during the revolution, but was re-established afterwards.

The first pharmacopoeia published in the United States was compiled for army use and appeared in Philadelphia in 1778.

1779 Wouter van Doeveren, Professor of Medicine at Leiden, (February 8th 1779): In his '*Sermo academicus de remedio morbo, sive de malis, quae hominibus a remedied, sanandi causa adhibitis, saepenumero accidere solent.*' [An academic lecture concerning deadly remedies, or concerning the illnesses which often are accustomed to happen from remedies applied in the interests of cure], warned '*Lest you will not be too easily persuaded to hand out medication which may carry the risk of your adding a second ailment to the first, or through which you may perhaps even invite death or accelerate it*'. Wouter van Doeveren succeeded Herman Boerhaave as professor at Leiden and argued against blood-letting, but he promoted inoculation with cowpox after Leiden had prohibited vaccination with smallpox (Grootheest, 2003).

1780 '*Almanach oder Tschenbuch fuer Scheidekunstler und Apotheker*', [Almanach or Pocket book for chemists and apothecaries] pharmacy journals published.

'Clinical Experiments, Histories, and Dissections' by Francis *Home. Experiment LXXXIV March 16th 1780*
   '*Janet Burn, 21, has been subject, for two months to globus hystericus, fainting fits, frequent vomitings, attended often by haematemesis. After bleeding, cold water used externally and internally, Tincture of Rosar, laxatives, &c. were employed in vain, I ordered extract of hyoscyamus seeds (Henbane). She began with gr.i. four times a day, and came at last to take gr.viii each time. The smallest doses were attended with nausea; the greater doses produced vertigo, and dimness of sight. She continued this medicine for 20 days, but without success in the cure of the haematemesis, or even of the vomiting. Hence, notwithstanding Stork's trials, it neither, appeared to me antispasmodic, nor anti haemorrhagic*' (Home, 1780).

1781 '*Observations on the poisonous vegetables which are indigenous in Great Britain or cultivated for ornaments*' by B Wilmer in the London Journal, volume 1, 1781. Concerning henbane: '*two women became maniacal and were so furious that strict confinement was necessary for several days.*' Two servants had '*uncommon agitation of the mind and were dancing about the room with all the appearance of maniacal persons*'. A shepherd was found staggering about a field like a man intoxicated.

Johannes Rayoux in '*Dissertatis Epistolaris de Cicuta, Strammonionio, Hyoscyamus et Aconito*' [Accounts of the use of hemlock, the thorn apple, henbane and aconite] said of henbane: '*A 40 year old man was seized with a sense of coldness. He was unable to stir and his pulse could hardly be felt. He complained of a painful sensation of heat in his throat and face and his vision was extremely confused. A weakness of sight lasted even a month after his recovery, but he did not lose his understanding and neither was he convulsed. He pronounced his words with difficulty and his memory seemed to have suffered.*' (Rayoux, 1781).

1782 '*A treatise on the medical properties of Mercury*' by John Howard
   Part 1. Salivation

'The devastation made by the sudden and unexpected appearance of the Lues Venereii towards the close of the 15th century called forth the attention of mankind to the wonderful properties of mercury. We shall at once see, that neither increased perspiration, preternatural[142] flow of urine, nor any laxicity of the bowels, short of a dysenteric kind of purging can measure the antivenereal power of mercury with so much certainty as salivation… when the medicine has been so urged as to produce a permanent degree of weakness; to a very considerable degree a general irritability often joined a partial one thus if sloughs have formed behind the dental molar there will some time put on a kind of phagedenic[143] appearance spread towards the uvula.
(Howard, 1782).

1784 *'On the efficacy of opium in the cure of venereal disease'* by F Michaelis: Opium causes diarrhoea and salivation (Michaelis, 1784).

'A description of mercurial lepra' by Dr Moriarty.

1785 *'An account of the foxglove and some of its medical uses'* by William Withering (1741–1799): with practical remarks on dropsy, and other diseases' wrote *'The foxglove, when given in very large and quickly-repeated doses, occasions sickness, vomiting, purging, giddiness, confused vision, objects appearing green or yellow: increased secretion of urine, with frequent motions to part with it, and sometime inability to retain it; slow pulse, even as slow as 35 in a minute, cold sweats, convulsions, syncope and death.'*

'When given in a less violent manner, it produces most of these effects in a lower degree; and it is curious to observe, that the sickness, with a certain dose of the medicine, does not take place for many hours after its exhibition has been discontinued; that the flow of urine will often precede, sometimes accompany, frequently follow the sickness at the distance of some days, and not unfrequently be checked by it. The sickness thus excited, is extremely different from that occasioned by any other medicine; it is peculiarly distressing to the patient; it ceases, it recurs again as violent as before; and thus it will continue for three or four

---

[142] preternatural = beyond normal
[143] phagedenic = pertaining to a progressive and rapidly spreading and sloughing ulceration

days, at distant and more distant intervals.

These sufferings of the patient are generally rewarded by a return of appetite, much greater than what existed before the taking of the medicine.

'But these sufferings are not at all necessary; they are the effects of our inexperience, and would in similar circumstances, more or less attend the exhibition of almost every active and powerful medicines we use.

Perhaps the reader will better understand how it ought to be given, from the following detail of my own improvement, than from precepts peremptorily delivered, and their source veiled in obscurity.

At first I thought it necessary to bring on and continue the sickness, in order to ensure the diuretic effects.

I soon learnt that the nausea being once excited, it was unnecessary to repeat the medicine, as it was certain to recur frequently, at intervals more or less distant. Therefore my patients were ordered to persist until the nausea came on, and then to stop. But it soon appeared that the diuretic effects would often take place first, and sometimes be checked when the sickness or a purging supervened'. Fuchs and Tragus[144] in 1542, pictured the plant, but remarked that it was a violent medicine. Parkinson commended it in 1640. However, This was not the first account of the benefits of digitalis. Withering wrote on the 1st July 1785 whilst Dr Simmons of the Westminster General Dispensatory wrote in the London Medical Journal, Volume 2, on the 11th March 1785 *'An account of the effects of Digitalis Purpura in dropsy' 'Without its seeming to be of much efficacy Digitalis purpura ranks among poisonous plants, and may, if indiscreetly administered produce alarming and even fatal effects',* but went on to say his patient passed 9 pints of urine. A letter from a Dr John Warren in reply said a trial of the virtues of this medicine about six years ago in a patient with anasarca[145], ascites and hydrothorax produced in 36 hours nearly seven gallons of urine and was perfectly cured, but had a great deal of nausea and frequent attempts to vomit.

---

[144] Tragus = Hieronymus Bock
[145] anasarca = generalised massive oedema

Observations on the use of opium in removing symptoms supposed to be owing to morbid irritability (1785) by Alexander Grant, Senior surgeon of His Majesty's Military Hospitals during the late war in North America (1779). He used Opium in cases of syphilis where mercury was not working. *'a tremor, which sometimes came on never obliged me to decrease the dose unless the bowels were disposed to be costive.... Except sometimes a giddiness... pulse decreased to between forty and fifty strokes per minute.... On the second or third day with some headache... with some diarrhoea. Increased secretion of saliva is not uncommon as well as urine'* (Grant, 1785).

First documented medical use of the word 'placebo' which means 'A common place method or medicine' in the 'New Medical Dictionary, and general repository of physick containing an explanation of the terms and a description of the various particulars'. 2nd edition. (Motherby, 1785).

1786 *An experimental inquiry into the properties of opium, and its effects on living subjects: with observations on its history, preparations and uses.* Being the disputation which gained the Harveian Prize for ... 1785 by John Leigh, Edinburgh: C. Elliot, 1786. *'I prevailed on a healthy man to take 15 drops of it in a short space of time and it began to operate and brought on such a vomiting as deterred me from making further experiments of this nature'.* He tried opium in his own eye and it gave him very severe pain lasting for 5 minutes.

Experiment XXV He gave a 30 year old man 2 grains (130 mgm) in alcohol–*'headache, vertigo, drowsiness, unusual heat about his stomach'*...In the same man 3 grains (194 mgm).. *'too much whiskey, warming stomach and heart, loss of appetite, weakness and languor'*... same man 4 grains *'violent sickness of the stomach, confusion in the head, fainted, frightful dreams, increased urine, insatiable thirst...'*.

Experiment XXIX 30 year old man–5 grains (324 mgm): sickness, vertigo, headache, drunkenness, great thirst. The same dose in a 25-year-old woman gave violent convulsions. This dose titration in a volunteer is unusual.

1786 Thomas Fowler (1736-1801) of 'Fowler's Solution' wrote a monograph on Arsenic (1786) and described its adverse effects: nausea, and rarely vomiting, slight griping, increased number of stools, certain swellings especially of the face, loss of appetite, uneasiness and pain in the stomach, diuretic, slight eruption like nettle-rash, sweat, headache and slight tremor. He reported on 320 cases and said that one third had nausea, one third '*open body*' (increased stools) and one third griping. This is one of the first papers giving rough incidences to ADRs. He also gave numbers cured with (27) and without relapse (144), suspended by solution (51), relieved by solution (20) and not relieved by solution (5) out of a total of 247 patients. He referred to his '*mineral solution*' which contained arsenious anhydride in powder form, plus potassium carbonate, 10 grammes of each, plus 30 ml of compound tincture of lavender and distilled water to one litre [Fowler's solution]. (Fowler, 1786). This produced a 1% solution of potassium arsenate (KH_2AsO_3). The ADR he mentions fall short of the ADRs mentioned by Lewin in 1881 who gives much more emphasis to the skin eruptions and also mentions salivation, thirst, the mucous membrane of the mouth, cough, bronchitis and hoarseness, tinnitus, dizziness and anaphrodisia. Twentieth century reports also include cirrhosis of the liver and various cancers. Fowler's ADRs will have been limited by the numbers that he treated, the dosages that he used and the

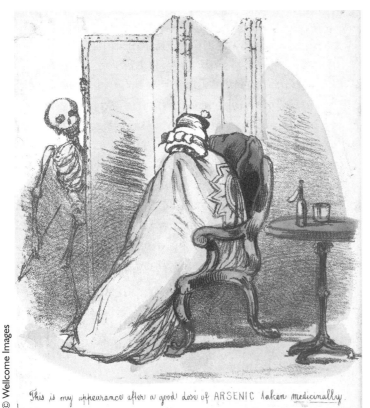

This is my appearance after a good dose of ARSENIC *taken medicinally.*

lack of knowledge of his period. He also wrote medical reports on tobacco, bloodletting, sudorifics and blisterings in defined diseases.

1787 *'An essay, on the operation of mercury, in the human body; in which, the manner how salivation is produced, by that medicine, is attempted to be explained: interspersed with observations on the treatment of the venereal disease'.* By Robert Maywood, M. D. London: Printed for the author, at the Literary-Press, No. 14, Red-Lion-Street, Clerkenwell: and sold by all booksellers. MDCCLXXXVII. *'That languor, inability to perform wonted[146] exercise, loss of appetite, paleness of the countenance and flabbiness of the skin, laxity, paleness and sponginess of the gums, vertigo, profuse sweats on slight exertions, nausea, a quick weak and small pulse, fever, swelling of the lips, pains in the articulations, extreme debility and foetid breath.'* (Maywood, 1787).

<u>Mercury</u>: *'Surely a worse malady cannot seize the vision than large quantities of motion bring on through the whole intestinal canal, which, from a pthisis or ulcerated state becomes incapable of bearing the lightest food without occasioning diarrhoea in which much ichod[147] is commonly discharged, and the patient doesn't constantly suffer from tormenting gripes, or if he escapes this violence, is frequently experiences a pain about the bones in many parts of the body that make his life miserable.'*

1788 The sixth edition of the *London Pharmacopoeia* (1788) paid special attention to the use of chemistry in pharmacy, some 400 years after Paracelsus first advocated it. Significantly, this edition was the first authorized English-language edition. The 10th and last *London Pharmacopoeia* appeared in 1851.

'An account of some experiments with opium in cure of the venereal disease' extracted from the correspondence of the military hospitals of France and communicated to Dr Simmon by Dr JF Croste, First physician to the French army. He treated 30 patients; after giving a purgative he gave one grain of pure opium and increased the dose the next day to two grains and then increased the dose by one grain per day thereafter.

---

[146] wonted = customary
[147] ichod = ichor = a watery foetid discharge from a wound

This gave the following side effects: Sweating, increased urine, itching skin eruption, vomiting, increased stools, pulse quickened, occasional giddiness, hiccoughs, increase in internal heat, a kind of intoxication, disagreeable dreams and colicky pains. Of the 30 patients he rated 18 as cured, 7 as doubtful cures, 4 as not cured and one died from TB (Coste, 1788).

'Practical observations on venereal complaints' by Franz Swediauer, Edinburgh, 1788. Adverse events associated with mercury were: *'salivation, disagreeable smell, painful mouth ulcers, vertigo, trembling of the extremities, chronic violent pains in the articulations, oppression of the breast, fever, headache, griping, total derangement, profuse sweating and diarrhoea.'* (Swediauer, 1788).

Two French Pharmacopoeias were published : *'Les Eléments de pharmacie et de Chimie'* [The elements of pharmacy and chemistry] by Baumé, and *'Le Manuel de Pharmacie'* [The manual of pharmacy] by Demachy.

1789 *'A Treatise of the Materia Medica'*: William Cullen's (1710–1790) *'Substances which excite a kind of fever, as very strong coffee, pepper, aconite, ignatia[148], arsenic, extinguish the types of the fever. I took by way of experiment, twice a day, four drachms of good China. My feet, finger ends, etc., at first became cold; I grew languid and drowsy; then my heart began to palpitate, and my pulse grew hard and small; intolerable anxiety, trembling (but without cold rigor), prostration throughout all my limbs then pulsation in my head, redness of my cheeks, thirst, and, in short, all these symptoms, which are ordinarily characteristic of intermittent fever, made their appearance, one after the other, yet without the peculiar chilly, shivering rigor.'* He was probably the first to use the word 'placebo' in a medical context during a lecture in 1772 (Kerr et al, 2008).

Mercury: *'A small quantity of mercury very suddenly excited a copious salivation and which continued to be very copious for many days.'*

Henbane:.. *'henbane and all other narcotics, may be very hurtful.'*

---

[148] ignatia = This may refer to St Ignatia's bean, which is the seed of *Strychnos ignatis*

Opium: '*In very many of the fevers of this climate, there appears in the beginning of them to be more or less of an inflammatory diathesis in the system; and during this state I hold, and have often seen, the use of opium to be extremely hurtful. It does not then either induce sleep or relieve pain, but aggravates the inflammatory symptoms, and often determines to particular inflammations, which prove afterwards fatal…. Opium is subject to the law of custom by which the force of impressions in which the body is passive becomes weaker by repetition; and that when frequent repetitions are requisite, it is always necessary to increase the dose.*' An example of the development of tolerance.

'*Every body knows that sedatives… particularly opium are employed in restraining excessive evacuations.*' He goes on to say that opium has been much used in dysentery, but that this is wrong since one must make use of frequent use of gentle laxatives. It would be equally evident that opiates must be commonly hurtful. An acknowledgement of its constipating qualities (Cullen, 1789).

1789 '*The New Family Herbal; or, domestic physician*' by William Meyrick, surgeon, Birmingham.

Opium: '*It promotes perspiration and sweat, but checks all other evacuations…An overdose of opium occasions either immoderate mirth or stupidity, redness of the face, swelling of the lips, relaxations of the joints, giddiness of the head, deep sleep, accompanied with turbulent dreams and convulsive starting, cold sweats and frequently death.*'

White Hellebore: '*It operates both upwards and downwards with great violence, and has sometimes brought on convulsions and other alarming symptoms. It has been remarked to affect the upper part of the throat, in a very peculiar manner, causing a kind of strangulation, or suffocation, with extreme pain and anxiety.*'

Henbane: '*Madness, convulsions and death.*'

1790 '*Medical Botany*': by William Woodville containing systematic and general descriptions, with plates of all the medicinal plants, indigenous and exotic, comprehended in the catalogues of the materia medica, as published by the Royal Colleges of

Physicians of London and Edinburgh. London: Printed and sold for the author, by James Phillips ... 1790–1793 Published in three parts and a supplement by the Cumberland physician William Woodville (1752–1805) between 1790 and 1795.

<u>Henbane:</u> *'Dr Patoullat... relates that nine persons, in consequence of having eaten the roots of hyoscyamus, were seized with most alarming symptoms: "some were speechless, and showed no other signs of life than by convulsions, contortions of their limbs and the risus sardonicus; all having their eyes starting out of their heads, and their mouths drawn backwards on both sides; others had all the symptoms alike; however five of them did now and then open their mouths, but it was to utter howlings.... And what is remarkable.. that on their recovery, all objects appeared to them as red as scarlet, for two or three days"...* 'Henbane is poisonous to birds and dogs; but horses, cows, goats and swine it does not affect.'

<u>Hellebore</u>: *'a scruple of the extract brought on violent spasms and convulsions.'* (Woodville, 1790).

1793 *'An inquiry into the nature and properties of Opium wherein its component principles, mode of operation, and use or abuse in particular disease, are experimentally investigated, and the opinions of former authors on these points impartially examined by Samuel Crumpe.'.*

The author experimented on himself and kept very accurate records: *'the pulsation of the head and arteries are first rendered quickly fuller and stronger... large dose - breathing slow stertorous and laborious.*

Forty-five minutes after twelve P.M. my pulse beating 70 in a minute, I took two grains and a half of opium (162 mgm) dissolved in an ounce of water:'

Table 2. Crumpe's experiment

Minutes	5	10	15	20	25	30	35	40	45	50	55	60	75	90
Pulse	70	74	74	76	78	80	72	70	64	64	66	70	70	70

'In twenty minutes perceived a slight warmth, and soon after a degree of moisture on my skin, the fullness of pulse increasing as well as its frequency. In half an hour I found myself, or at least imagined myself, more alert and sprightly than before;

in 40 minutes perceived a pleasing kind of languor gradually increasing; in 90 minutes a dull headache; in two hours time the headache was much increased, and attended with drowsiness and nausea; in two hours and a half every disagreeable symptom was increased, my pulse 70; took a spoonful of vinegar, which somewhat relieved the nausea; in two hours and three quarters found all the above symptoms still increasing, and slight vertigo, and tremors in my hands–pulse the same as before. In three hours and a half the nausea was considerably augmented, the other symptoms as before, and I at length threw up the contents of my stomach. The headache and vertigo were soon relieved; but I continued in a stupid state for the remainder of the day.' (Crumpe, 1793).

1796 Edward Jenner published his work on the vaccination against smallpox (see 1906 AD allergic reactions).

Samuel Hahnemann (1755–1843) wrote his *'Essay on a New Principle for Ascertaining the Curative Powers of Drugs'*. He commented on the effects of several drugs:

<u>Mercury</u>: For syphilis *'no more efficacious remedy could be found'*. It causes trembling, slow, very debilitating fever, thirst, great and rapid emaciation. The treatment for the 'mercurial disease' was opium.

<u>Henbane</u>: *'Possesses the power of producing haemorrhage, especially bleeding of the nose. In large doses it produces: suspicious, quarrelsome, spitefully-calumnious, revengeful, destructive, fearless mania. Also difficulty of moving, and insensibility of the limbs, and apoplectic symptoms… convulsions, want of memory, sleeplessness, dry cough, dryness of the mouth and nose, flow of mucus from the nose, and from the flow of saliva.. convulsions in the facial and ocular muscles… vertigo, and a dull pain in the membranes lying under the skull.'*

<u>Hellebore Album</u>: *'That most incomparable remedy'* It causes: *'inflammation and swelling of the skin of the face, sometimes (from larger doses) the whole body, heat of the whole body, burning in different external parts, cutaneous eruptions, constriction of the gullet, larynx and a sense of suffocation, rigidity of the tongue with tough mucus in the mouth, constriction of the chest, pleuritic symptoms, cramp in the*

calve, an anxious sensation in the stomach, nausea, gripes, and cutting pains here and there in the bowels, great anxiety, vertigo, headache (confusion of the head), violent thirst, tremblings, stammering, convulsions of the eyes, hiccough, sneezing, vomiting, painful, scanty evacuations with tenesmus, local, or (from larger doses) general convulsions, cold sweats, watery diuresis, ptyalism, expectoration, general coldness, marked weakness, fainting, long profound sleep'...

1797 'Mercury stark naked': a series of letters addressed to Dr Beddoes, stripping that poisonous mineral of its medical pretensions by Isaac Swainson. *'Spasms, loss of sight, hearing, taste and smelling; acceleration of the pulse, prostration of strength, giddiness of the head with swooning, bleeding at the nose, increase of salivation, pain and swelling of maxillary glands, brassy taste in the saliva, stubborn costive habits, aching head, throbbing in the temple arteries, eyes hot and reddened, cholic, attended with palsy of a limb or general palsy.* This was followed by an advertisement for Velnos' vegetable syrup. This damnation of mercury seems to be a prelude to his advertising his own remedy (Swainson, 1797). [Velno's Original Vegetable Syrup contained sublimate mercury alongside the more benign ingredients of gum arabic, honey and syrup].

1798 *'Observations and experiments on the broad-leaved willow bark'* by William White. Bath: printed and sold by S. Hazard; sold also by Vernor and Hood, London, 1798. *'I have to say in favour of the willow that except in a single instance (which may be noticed in the case of Collins* [diarrhoea]*) I never found it to disagree with the stomach or bowels...'.*

In short in all cases of ague and intermittent fevers that have come within my practice I have found this bark without a single exception, an infallible remedy. I have never found it to disagree with the stomach, or bowels.' (White, 1798).

'A Compendious Medical Dictionary'. Containing an explanation of the terms in anatomy, physiology, surgery, materia medica, chemistry, and practice. London, by Robert Hooper MD.

Salix: *'Salix, the willow, is recommended to be a good substitute for Peruvian bark and is said to cure intermittent and other diseases requiring tonic and astringent remedies'.*

<u>Hellebore Album</u>: *'It acts very powerfully upon the nervous system, producing great anxiety, tremors, vertigo, syncope, aphonia, interrupted respiration, sinking pulse, convulsions, spasms and death.'*

<u>Hellebore Niger</u>: *'At present it is exhibited principally as an alterative, or, when given in a large dose, as a pugative. It often proves a very powerful emmengogue[149] in plethoric habits, when steel is ineffective or improper... a florid redness frequently appeared on the face, and various cutaneous efflorescences upon the body... in some pleuritic symptoms, with fever supervened... nor were alarming affections of spasms and convulsions unfrequent...many sweated profusely, in some the urine was considerably increased, in others the saliva and mucous discharges;'*

<u>Opium</u>: *'Taken into the stomach in immoderate doses proves a powerful poison producing vertigo, tremors, convulsions, delirium, stupor, stertor and finally fatal apoplexy.'* (Hooper, 1798).

'Mercurial Lepra' by Whitley Stoker.There was a flurry of papers about the skin reactions to mercury about the turn of the century.

1799 A letter to the *'Medical and Physical Journal' (Volume 1, Number 1)* on April 24th 1799 under the pseudonym of Aliquis wrote *'On Quackery, and the most effectual means of checking its dangerous progress'.* He wrote *'If we might venture to offer a few hints on a subject apparently of so much consequence, we would submit to the legislature the propriety of erecting a public board composed of the most eminent physicians for the examination, analyzation and approbation of every medicine before an advertisement should be admitted into any newspaper or any other periodical publication and before it should be vended in any manner whatsoever.... But we are well aware, that the plan we have proposed is extremely imperfect, and the execution of it in its present form would be attended with many difficulties. We can only plead in excuse for offering it, our zeal to remedy an increasing evil, and hope, that our humble attempt may induce*

---

[149] emmengogue = emmenagogue = encourages menstrual flow

some much abler writer to suggest a plan, better calculated to answer the important end for which it is designed'. As Penn has said 'This *plea for legislation had no effect whatsoever and little progress was made until the next century.'* (Penn, 1979).

A letter in the same journal dated June 12th 1799 gave an account of the deleterious effects of the *lolium* or *darnel*. A sack of leafed wheat with an equal quantity of tarling wheat (i.e the refuse seeds which pass the sieve) abounding very much with darnel (perennial rye grass)…were ground and dressed together, and in the evening about ten o'clock, bread was made of a part of it…. *'of this bread, Robert, aged thirteen, eat the next morning… he fell giddy, and had pain of the head during the whole of the first day, with great pain and tightness of the legs especially of the calves of the legs, extending to the ankles, attended with redness and swelling, and itching of the skin, but it did not vomit or purge him until the third day… the pain and inflammation continued to increase, till it terminated in gangrene; sphacelous* (necrosis) *succeeded and he was under the necessity of suffering amputation of both legs.'* This is an early account of a case of ergotism.

A further letter in the same journal 'According to an account given by Dr De Witt, physician in the city of Albany, *the effects of the Datura stramonium, thorn apple, appear to be so extraordinary* (due to the anticholinergic action of the tropane alkaloids), *that well deserve the further notice and investigation of practitioners… found to produce:*

1. Unusual pain and anxiety

2. Convulsive motions

3. Apparent dread or aversion to water or fluids of any kind

4. Vesication on the skin, after the violent symptoms had subsided; and

5. Large and involuntary discharge of urine.' (Witt, 1799).

These two reports emphasize the importance of anecdotal reports of adverse drug effects, which has become the main source of pharmacovigilance data.

Terminology

The oldest written sources are from the Hippocratic era and were therefore written in Greek. The Arabs translated hundreds of the Greek texts from 800–1000 AD and then added their own knowledge and this was imported back to Italy via Salerno in the 12th century. In the first century AD when the Roman empire became powerful the Latin language took over and the Greek texts were translated into Latin. The dominance of Latin in medical literature persisted in England until the end of the 17th century, but continued in Europe into the mid 19th century. Thereafter the national medical language was usually used, but with French,German and English being used for international communication (Wulff, 2004). Probably because of the USA becoming the most powerful country in the world English or American has now become the dominant language for medical communications.

Originally there was no set phrase to refer to what we now call 'Adverse Drug Reactions' (ADR), but the word poison or poisonous was used to describe drugs with adverse effects. Richard Brookes (see above), in 1754, uses the terms *'poisonous effects'* and *'bad effects'*. In 1789 Wouter van Doeveren gave a lecture at Leiden, with the title *'Sermo academicus de Remedio Morbo, sive de malis, quae hominibus a remedies, sanandi causa adhibitis, saepe numero accidere solent'* [Remedio morbo, drug diseases or ailments which often affect people as a result of remedies administered to them for therapeutic purposes] (Grootheest, 2003). An ADR was not usually seen as an entity so they used a perjorative adjective plus a noun such as 'effect', e.g. 'pernicious effects' or 'noxious effects'. Lewin in the 1883 translation of his book *'Die Nebenwirkungen der Arzei mittel'* [Untoward effects of Drugs] said: The greatest variety of names may be found in medical literature for these untoward symptoms following the exhibition of drugs. In Germany they have been and still are known as *'nebenwirkuingen'*, *'physiologische nebenwirkungen or arzneisymptome'* and are also spoken of as the *'special'* or *'accidental'* or *'peculiar'* action of the drug. French authors refer to them as *'inconvenénients'* or *'inconvénients thérapeutique'* or *'accidents'*, *'cas d'accidents'* or *'effets secondaires'*. In England they were occasionally termed *'unpleasant symptoms'*. The first mention that I can find where the phrase *'side effect'* is used was in 1891 (Stern, 1891). Gradually the two words tended to be used together to describe an ADR as an entity, e.g. side effect, and with continual use it became hyphened *'side-effect'*. This term was used by Richard Doll in 1969 but since then it has, more or less, dropped out of use except by the lay public (Doll, 1969). Other terms used have been 'toxic effect', 'side reaction', 'toxic reaction', 'toxic manifestation' and 'collateral effect'. The use of the words 'side' and 'collateral' imply that the effect occurred at the normal therapeutic dose and that it was intrinsic to the drug rather than dependant on individual idiosyncrasy. It is now used by the lay public to refer to all adverse effects of drugs whatever the dose.

In France in 1865 in a book on new medicines the phrase 'accidents léger périodiques' was used (Guibert, 1865). Later 'l'effets secondaire' or 'effet toxique' or 'effet latéral' or 'effet indésirable' succeeded it (Bégaud, 1995). The Italians use the phrases 'effetto collaterale', 'eventi avversi da farmaci' (ADE), 'eventi indisiderati' and 'effetti secondari'.

Botanical nomenclature has always been a problem. A binomial nomenclature was first mooted by Joseph Pitton de Tournefort (1656–1708), although it has been claimed that Joachim Jung did so about 1640 (Morton,1970), but a superior system was suggested by Carl von Linné, but known as Linnaeus (1707–1778) in his book 'Systema naturae' published in Leiden in 1735 (Taylor, 1979)

The typing of ADRs into type 'A' and type 'B' started in 1977 after a paper by Rawlins and Thompson (Rawlins and Thompson, 1977). The term 'adverse event' was suggested for the collection of data in clinical trials in 1965 (Finney, 1965). The phrase 'adverse drug reaction' dates back to 1957, but 'drug reaction' was used in 1934. Both the words 'reaction' and 'effect' imply certainty that something named caused the reaction or effect. Doubt can only be expressed by adding an adjective, e.g. possible, etc. The phrase 'adverse drug event' refers to an association between drug and event, which is not necessarily causal and is therefore used prior to clinical assessment of individual cases or statistical analysis in clinical trials.

Self-experimentation

The first known self-experimenter was Shen Nung in 2500 BC and it is likely that there were many others after him before Storck. This process has continued at an increased rate as more and more drugs become available, but in a more formalised way as in phase I studies. It is common for students, clinical pharmacologists and pharmaceutical industry personnel to volunteer for these self-experiments and receive payment. Any ADRs may be exaggerated, as the volunteers would not have the disease for which the drug was intended, e.g. postural hypotension with an anti-hypertensive. The merit goes to those who took drugs for the first time as their successors now knew the risks. There were three areas where there were many self-experimenters:

Anaesthetics. Here the rapid reversal of the effect meant that there was less risk. The commonest were nitrous oxide, ether and chloroform.

Local anaesthetics. These were usually given subcutaneously and entailed little risk. The commonest was cocaine.

Hallucinogenic drugs. Many of these were taken for non-scientific purposes. Commonest were LSD and mescalin.

Where it has been possible only the first one or two experimenters in these categories are mentioned.

Table 1. Self-experimenters

Date	Physician/scientist	Drug taken	ADRs reported
3500 BC	Shen-nung	Many	Not reported
?1565	Conrad Gesner	Hellebore niger and alba Henbane	
1676	Moyse Charas	Opium	Relaxed, insomnia and itching
1767	Alexander Williams	Camphor	2 G first day no effect, doubled dose on the second day. Convulsions, delirium, foaming at the mouth, raging
		Castor	10-20 G Indigestion
1768	Auenbrugger Joseph	Camphor	2.6 g increased temperature, and pulse rate,
		Nitre (Potassium nitrate)	60 gr diminished pulse, 90 gr giddiness and irregular pulse
1686	Francese Redi	Viper Gall	No effect as it is not poisonous
1701	Richard Mead	Viper venom	Swollen and painful tongue
1727	Isaac Newton	As, Hg, Au, Pb	All these elements were found in his hair after death
1760	Anton Storck	Hemlock (2gr) Aconite Henbane Clematis	No effect
1765	Samuel Bard	Opium	Slowing of the pulse
1793	Samuel Crumpe	Opium	Headache, nausea, drowsiness, tremors, and vertigo
1799	Humphrey Davy	Nitrous oxide	Giddiness, muscle relaxation and tendency to laugh.
1800	SF Hermbstadt	Arsenic (4 G)	Abdominal pain, trembling extremities and cyanosis
1803	Friedrich Wihelm Sertumer	Morphia	Face flushed, nausea, dizzy and stomach pain
1810	Samuel Hahnemann	Many	See his textbooks
1821	Enoch Hale	Castor oil injections	Oily taste, abdominal cramps, headache, and nausea and vomiting

Date	Physician/scientist	Drug taken	ADRs reported
1825	Johann Jorg	17 drugs–hydrocyanic acid (dilute)	?
		Valerian,	Without any discernable action
		Opium,	Light-headedness, inebriation and deep sleep
		Digitalis,	
		Tincture of Iodine	?
		St Ignatius bean	?
			Headaches, abdominal pain and diarrhoea.
1835	Jan Evangelista Purkinje	Ipecac (emetine)	Nausea, salivation, cramps and diarrhoea;
		Belladonna	blurred vision, dry mouth and tachycardia;
		Turpentine	hypnotic effects, euphoria, and stupor;
		Camphor	totally unconscious;
		Digitalis	flickering vision, bradycardia and skipped beats
		Strammonium	
		Opium	
		Henbane	
		Calomel	
1844	Horace Wells	Nitrous Oxide	No painful sensations
1846	WTG Morton	Ether	Numbness of limbs, like a nightmare and the unconscious for 7-8 minutes
1847	Sir JY Simpson	Chloroform	Became unconscious
1848	Erik Jacobson	Disulfuram (Antabuse)	After alcohol–headache, difficulty breathing, vomiting and lowered BP.
1849	Thomas Nunneley	Acetyl Cthloride	Anaesthetic
1855	Cesare Bertagnini	Salicylic acid	Tinnitus and dizziness
1855	Sir Robert Christison	Physostigmine (Calabar bean)	Giddiness, numbness of the limbs, torpidity and faintness
		Oxalic acid,	
		Coniine,	
		Opium,	
		Cannabis,	
		Lead,	
		Strychnine,	
		Arsenic	
1856	John Snow	Amylene	Anaesthesia
1858	AG Field	Nitroglycerine	Nausea, tinnitus, jaw dropped and fullness in the neck
1863	TR Fraser	Eserine eye drops	Contracted pupils

Date	Physician/scientist	Drug taken	ADRs reported
1873	Otto H F Obermaier	Cholera vaccine injection	Died after a few days
1879	Sir Arthur Conan Doyle	Gelsenium (tinct)	Giddiness, severe depression, headache and diarrhoea
		Nitroglycerin	Congestive headache
1880	William S Halsted	Cocaine	Lack of fatigue, but became addicted to it
1884	Ferra Y Clua Jaine	Cholera vaccine	
1886	Il Bardakh	Rabies vaccine	No reaction
1897	Arthur Eichengrun	Aspirin	No ill effects
1899	FC Floeckinger	Acetyl salicylic acid	Headache, tinnitus, flashes of light, increased pulse rate and sweats
1903	Franke	Aspirin	Swallowing difficulties, strangulation, face red, tachycardia of 160 beats per minute, urticaria and sweating.
1902	CF Pirquet	Diphtheria, and scarlet fever and tetanus vaccine	Swollen and painful arm with fever
1914	GR Mines	IV Muscarine	Died due to poisoning
1921	FG Banting	10 units Insulin	No effect
1927	HL Blumgart	Radon	No effect
1930	Chauncey Leake	Furan (wood tar derivative)	Headache and pain on micturition
1933	John A Kolmer	Live attenuated Polio vaccine	No effect
1934	Albert Schweitzer	Yellow fever vaccine (sub/cut)	No effects
1936	LS Goodman	Prostigmine	Difficult breathing, giddiness, weaving movements, fear of death and shock. Required atropine.
1943	Albert Hofman	Lysergic acid diethylamide (LSD)	Restlessness, dizziness, anxiety, dilated pupils and stimulated imagination
		Teonanacatl, Psilocybin	
1944	Scott Smith & Frederick Prescott	D'tubocurarine (Seostim)	Temporarily paralysed
1951	Otto K Hayrhofer	Succinyl choline chloride	Muscle weakness, double vision, ptosis, muscle twitching and paralysis of respiratory muscles.
1951	G Pauletta	Chloramphenicol succinate	No effect
		Chloramphenicol glutarate	Anaphylactic shock and died
195?	JG Hamilton	Isotopes of Na, Cl, Br, I and Plutonium	Developed leukaemia

The main source for this table was: *'Self-experiments: sources for study'* by Arsen P Fiks, edited by P A Buelow. Westport, Conn.: London: Praeger, 2003.

This book contains many other self-experimenters. Some details also from Altman, 1986.

Summary

We now have publication of case series and detailed individual case histories. There are now fuller details of ADRs with doses. Experimentation now plays a part in the study of medicines. Hoffman's response to an epidemic of ergotism is to establish the cause with experiments in animals and this leads to regulatory action. Leigh performs a series of experiments on volunteers to explain the effects of opium. There are more references to figures, e.g. pulse rates, doses and numbers of patients. We have now the whole gamut of pharmacovigilance techniques save for pharmacoepidemiology.

Chapter 7. 19th Century

A lchemy has almost disappeared except for a few fanatics, but
homeopathy replaces it as a pseudo-philosophy . The active principles
are extracted from herbs and synthetic drugs start to make an
appearance.

1800 Humphry Davy anaesthetised humans with nitrous oxide, but it
was 40 years later before it came into general use.

*'A candid inquiry into the education, qualifications, and offices of
a surgeon-apothecary'*: by James Lucas, Bath 1800. *'he may learn
the poisonous efficacy of some preparations..'…'A practitioner,
versed in chemistry, may not only be better apprised of the
noxious effects of some remedies, but be more quick-sighted in
opportunely counteracting their pernicious effects.'* An early
advocate of training in pharmacovigilance.

A study of the relative merits of different treatments for syphilis
was made by John Pearson. He dedicated his book to Thomas
Fowler and in it compared the claims and his experiences of
various herbal and chemical remedies *'to ascertain whether any
other substance than Mercury be a true and certain antidote.'*
(1800). As a surgeon to the London Lock Hospital he had a wide
knowledge of the disease and he tried out, apparently not very
systematically, any likely remedies. He gives the details of thirty
one patients in support of his opinion that guaiac, China root,
sarsaparilla and other treatments recommended as alternatives
were only of value when used in addition to mercury. As to
mercury itself, he states that its effectiveness was demonstrated
in *'not less than twenty thousand cases'* of which he had personal
experience. He was not blind to its disadvantages and looked
forward to further discoveries since *'it were highly desirable to
acquire a medicine equally potent as an antivenereal, and not
possessing certain active properties peculiar to that mineral.'*

This study, based on simple clinical assessment of results, seems to have been highly successful, particularly so since there was at that time little understanding of the pathology of the disease nor were there accurate tests of cure and, as Pearson was aware, symptoms due to syphilis were frequently confused with these of excessive treatment with mercury (Introductory note to: Bull JP (1951).

1801 The first placebo-controlled trial (De Craen et al., 1999) John Haygarth compared the actions of metallic rods known as 'Perkins Tractors', which were supposed to relieve symptoms through electromagnetic influence of the metal, with imitation wooden rods on the same 5 patients and obtained identical results (Haygarth, 1801).

1803 France – The Law 21 Germinal[150] (21st March–18th April) an XI (11 Avril 1803). Only qualified pharmacists could open and practice from a pharmacy, prepare and sell medications (article XXV). Strangely, the law did not lay down any penalty for illegal practise of pharmacy. The law also forbade secret remedies (article XXXII) and there was an obligation to follow only prescriptions given by authorised practitioners (Physicians, surgeons and health officials) (Fouassier, 2003). Article 36 forbade the advertising, distribution, and sale of any secret remedy, but had little effect on the sale of secret remedies (Berman, 1970). 'The government charged the professors of the Schools of Medicine with the members of the School of Pharmacy to edit a 'Codex' or Formulary, containing the medicinal preparations and pharmaceutical preparations that must be held by the pharmacists'. The law was modified in 1805, 1810, 1850 and 1926 (Debue-Barazer, 2003).

1804 *'The Edinburgh new dispensatory'* ... including complete and accurate translations of the ... London pharmacopoeia, published in 1791; Dublin pharmacopoeia, published in 1794; and of the new ed. of the Edinburgh pharmacopoeia, published in 1803. Edited, with extensive alterations and additions by Andrew Duncan, junior.
Tincture Hyoscyamus (Henbane**):** *'causes uneasiness,*

---

[150] germinal = the 7th month of the French revolutionary calendar (March-April)

restlessness and universal irritation. ..Its influence is very much reduced by having alarming effects, intoxication, wild delusions, dilatation of the pupils, convulsions, sweat, eruption of pustules, over the surface...Like other narcotics ...it sometimes gives rise to vertigo, headaches, general uneasiness with particular individuals, it occasions vomiting, colic pains, a copious flow of urine and sometimes purging.'

'White Hellebore: *'violent purging, emetic extreme violence.'* Opium (small dose): *' increases energy of the mind, frequency of the pulse and heat of the body, excites thirst, renders mouth dry and parched, diminishes all the secretions and excretions. Excess dose: headache, vertigo, delirium, convulsions, stertorous breathing, stupor and death.'*

'An essay on a peculiar eruptive disease arising from the exhibition of mercury' by George Alley. Dublin 1804.

'Languor, lassitude, restlessness, cold shiverings, fever, sore throat, white tongue, quick pulse, nausea, headache, thirst, hard dry cough, difficult respiration, anxiety, sense of oppression about the precordium[151], painful tumours, costive, skin hot and itchy.'

1805 Friedrich Wilhelm Adam Sertürner, a German chemist, isolates and describes morphine. He also described the results of experiments in which he and three of his colleagues each orally consumed three half-grain (32 mgm) doses of morphine within approximately 30 minutes. Serturner became alarmed at the response of his friends, and had them drink vinegar, causing a violent emesis.

'The Edinburgh Medical and Surgical Journal' First number. Thomas Spens wrote on January 1st 1805 *'History of three cases of Erythema Mercuriale with observations.'*

1806 *'Essay on Erythema mercuriale, or that eruption which sometimes occurs from the use of mercury'* by John M'Mullin: 'Symptoms copied from Thomas Spens 1804. *'...generally costive. ... On the first or second day rash, papular, distinct elevated like rubella sometimes like intertrigo, In most cases began first on scrotum, inside thighs, forearms, pulse 120-130, cuticle pale continued for 10–14 days, minute blisters, desquamated,*

---

[151] precordium = chest area covering the heart

idiosyncrasy'. He also referred to other similar accounts in 1804.

James Hamilton wrote *'Observations on the utility and administration of purgative medicines in several disease.'* The belief that one should expel evil humours lives on and the diseases that he thought benefitted from purgatives were: chlorosis, chorea (St Vitus's dance), chronic diseases, haematemesis, hysteria, marasmus, scarlatina, tetanus, and typhus (Hamilton, 1806).

1809 Dr Falconer of Bath warns of the dangerous effects of mercury in the 1st Volume *'Transactions of the Medical Society of London'*, May 1809.

In 1809, in Portugal during the Peninsular War at the hospital at Elvas, army surgeon Hamilton and two colleagues made an experiment;

'It had been so arranged, that this number was admitted, alternately, in such a manner that each of us had one third of the whole. The sick were indiscriminately received, and were attended as nearly as possible with the same care and accommodated with the same comforts. One third of the whole were soldiers of the 61st Regiment, the remainder of my own (the 42nd) Regiment. Neither Mr Anderson nor I ever once employed the lancet. He lost two, I four cases; whilst out of the other third [treated with bloodletting by the third surgeon] thirty five patients died.' (Hamilton AL, 1816); (Milne and Chalmers, 2002).

1810 Samuel Hahnemann (1755–1843), the originator of homoeopathy, provided the adverse effects of drugs in healthy persons to support his theory that *'similia similibus curantur'* 'like cures like'. Since they were healthy they were probably victims of accidental poisoning, although one cannot rule out early experiments in clinical pharmacology. The problem with accidental poisoning is the difficulty in establishing which herb was the cause. There is evidence to suggest that some of the symptoms that Hahnemann ascribes to Hyoscyamus were probably due to some other herb. The old mnemonic 'Red as a beet, dry as a bone, blind as a bat, mad as a hatter (or wet hen), and hot as hare' for the adverse effects of henbane or belladonna suggests that the symptoms: contracted pupils, paleness of face, ptyalism, great collection of saliva, cold feet, chilliness and shivering all over for half an hour, long-continued chilliness were due to another herb.

Hyoscyamus Niger: Quoting from 42 'old-school authorities' or sources gives 582 reports of symptoms.

Hellebore Niger: 12 sources and 288 reports of symptoms.

Mercury: 31 sources and 1450 reports of symptoms.

Most of the sources were German and not easily obtainable.

In *'The Organon de l'art de Guérir'* [The system of principles for philosophic or scientific investigations; an instrument for acquiring knowledge of the art of curing] (1824) he says concerning proving drugs that the size of the dose must be such that of normal practice or customary for the prescriber in his recipes (In *'Materia Medica Pura'* he uses the phrase: *'The smallest possible quantity of medicine as potentized development is sufficient for the purpose'* and *'sufficiently strong dose of the medicine,.)..continue use for several days two adequate doses daily of sufficient size to cause or to experience an action from it'...* . He goes on to say that if in the space of some hours there is no action a higher dose must be given , perhaps doubled. If after several hours it wears off the next day a stronger dose should be given. The treatment should continue for several days with progressive doses. The provers were strictly observed for symptoms and watch should be kept for anything that might affect the results, e.g. meals, etc. He pointed out that patients may have idiosyncratic responses. He used about 50 provers from amongst his family and friends, who must have accepted his philosophy - 'Believers'. Despite his efficiency in his experiments we do not know any thing about specific doses causing specific symptoms nor do we know any incidence figures despite the fact that he must have known the number of provers that had taken each drug. As far as I can make out no physical examinations were made of the provers, so that we cannot link symptoms with definite physiological changes. Without any control group the symptoms must be taken as being adverse events rather than adverse reactions.

One cannot accept all the symptoms put forward by Hahnemann as reliable evidence of the adverse effects of the herbs mentioned. (http://www.homoeopathie-online.com/ materia_medica_homoeopathica/).

'*Observations on the Hydargyria or that vesicular disease arising from the exhibition of mercury*' by George Alley, second edition, (see 1804) A very detailed description with coloured pictures of the three stages of the rash: Mitis, Simplex-febrilis and Maligna with accompanying symptoms.

'*The mercurial disease. An enquiry into the history and nature of the disease produced in the human constitution by the use of mercury, with observations on its connection with lues veneria*' by Andrew Matthias, 1810. This book seems to have difficulty in separating the adverse events due to mercury from those of the disease, in that in addition to the usual problems he talks of: mercurial buboes, mercurial chancre, mercurial ulcerated throat and mercurial disease of the periosteum, tendons, cartilage, and joints. He wrote '*I am convinced that in Europe there is no other remedy which has the least effect in subduing the venereal irritation... it has the power of suppressing, but not of curing the venereal action*'. He was the first to recognise that there was a new discipline, which he called: '*The disease of the remedy*', a forerunner of pharmacovigilance (see table at end of the book).

1811 Hahnemann's thesis '*Medical historical dissertation on the Hellebore veterum of the ancients*' gave the uses as: chronic and hemicranial headache, mania, melancholy, dropsy without fever, epilepsy, paralysis, longstanding gout, diseases of joints, inflammation of the liver, chronic jaundice and odd affections of the trachea.

The ADR of *Hellebore album* were: vomiting, suffocation, face swells, tongue protrudes, face excessively red, the voice goes, delerium, hiccough, cramps (calves, hands and muscles of mastication), excess weakness, pulse almost extinct, thirst, syncope, loss of consciouness, loss of vision, stammering, mind deranged, precordial burning, profuse sweat and sneezing. These are fewer than he gives in his provings.

A famous English physician, John Coakley Lettsome, (1744–1815) founded the London Medical Society in 1773 . He was the butt of a poem:

' Whatever patients come to I
I physics, bleeds and sweats 'em
If after that they choose to die
What's that to me, I Lettsom.'

Expelling bad humours still remained a strong philosophy.

1813 *'De l'influence de l'émétique sur l'homme et les animaux'*; mémoire lu à la première classe de l'Institut de France, le 23 août 1813 et suivi du rapport fait à la classe (Lecture given by F Magendie) par MM. Cuvier, Humboldt Pinel et Percy Paris : Crochard, 1813. [The influence of Antimony on man and the animals; dissertation read to the first class at the Institute of France the 23rd August 1813 and followed with an account made to the class].

'Antimony given in large doses: *'enormous evacuations both up and down with atrocious pain, convulsions, dyspnoea, haemorrhage, swelling of the lower abdomen, inflammation, erosion and gangrene of the stomach and the intestines and which finishes by death …Devouring heat and wrenching in the region of the epigastrium, switching from syncope to convulsive agitation followed closely by violent vomiting of frothy yellow matter and sometimes mixed with streaks of blood… frequent fainting fits and painful cramps in the legs.'*

1814 *'Treatise on Gonorrhoea virus and Lues Veneris'* by Benjamin Bell first reported *'eczema mercuriale as well as purgation, nausea and vomiting, increase discharge of urine, some degree of diaphoresis, salivation, foetor, gums red and somewhat tender, salivary glands hard and tender, mouth ulcers, fever, restlessness, anxiety, general debility, very distressful irritable state of the whole system, excites heat over the whole body, quickness of the pulse, coppery taste, pain on chewing, loose teeth, very distressful tumefaction of the tongue and fauces.'*

1815 The Apothecaries Act or An Act for better regulating the practice of apothecaries throughout England and Wales. It was an attempt to separate licensed practitioners from the unlicensed 'quacks'. It was possible to buy an MD from Aberdeen University and St Andrew's University if you had the money and two recommendations. Whereas 'quacks' or 'irregular practitioners' varied from true charlatans to experienced educated men. The problem was that there were too many practitioners for the population and therefore the trained practitioners wished to squash the untrained competitors.

Dr Francis. *'On the effects of mercury in its natural state and on its abuse in certain diseases'*: indigestion, loss of appetite, nausea and vomiting, languor of whole system, convulsions, sanguineous discharge from alimentary canal, haemorrhage from lungs, salivation, extreme weakness, preternatural decay of teeth, loss of sight, memory and voice, and deafness.

1816 France – The Royal Ordonnance of 8th August 1816 ordered the *'Codex Medicamentarius seu* [or] *Pharmacopae Gallica'* and it was published by the Minister of the Interior in 1818 in Latin. It was compulsory for all French pharmacists to have one and to conform to it within six months of its publication. There were many later editions: 1837, 1866, 1884, 1908. 1937.

1819 *'Observations on the use and abuse of mercurial medicines in various diseases'* by James Hamilton.

This monograph on mercury has an extensive section (Section 1) on its ADRs: *'On the effects of mercury'*
'The aching pain which so often follow courses of mercury'
'an inordinate action of the heart and arteries'
'Among other ill effects it tends to produce tremors and paralysis, and not infrequently incurable mania,'
'Erythismus'
'with frightful dreams–impaired or depraved vision –'
'Mental derangement with eventual fatuity,'
'Erythema Mercuriale'
'Death has supervened, apparently in consequence of a very trifling exertion or agitation (see pages 259-262).

A Bill was presented to Parliament (UK) entitled 'A bill for establishing regulations for the sale of poisonous drugs and for better preventing the mischiefs arising from inattention of persons vending the same'. It was opposed by the Chemists and Druggists and was withdrawn.

1820 UK Dangerous Drugs Acts. This was the start of numerous acts and regulations to control dangerous drugs.

In France the task of approving proprietary medications passed to the newly founded Academy of Medicine and its Commission on Secret and New Remedies, with unimpressive results (Berman, 1970).

Quinine was isolated from the bark of the cinchona tree by the French chemists Joseph-Biename Caventou and Pierre-Joseph Pelletier in 1820.

Establishment of the United States Pharmacopoeia (USP), which was first published in 1820 following a convention of medical societies in Washington, DC.

Frederick Accum wrote *'Treatise on Adulteration'* and concluded that in England and Wales *'nine tenths of the most potent drugs and chemical preparations used in pharmacy [were] vended in a sophisticated* [i.e. adulterated] *state.'*

John Ayrton Paris wrote *'Sometimes the unpleasant or perverse operation of a medicine may be obviated by changing the form and its exhibition, the period at which it is taken, or the extent of its dose'* (p121)... *'constitutional peculiarities ,or idiosyncrasy will sometimes render the operation of the mildest medicines poisonous'*. (Paris, 1820).

1821 A Geneva pharmacist, Peschier, isolated hyoscyamine from henbane in impure form.

Francois Magendie, father of experimental pharmacology, published his *'Formulaire'* which discussed the therapeutic use of the newly discovered alkaloids and halogens on the basis of animal experiment (Ackernecht, 1970).

1825 A poem appeared in a Virginia publication warning physicians of the dangers of calomel, mercurous chloride (Hg_2Cl_2):
> 'Since Calomel's become their boast,
> How many patients have they lost?
> How many thousands they make ill,
> Of poison, with their calomel.' (Shryock, 1947).

Richard Carmichael in *'An essay on venereal diseases and the use of mercury in their treatment'* 2nd edition, 1825 gave the various treatments that he used for different manifestations of syphilis:

Astringent washes	Antimonials	Purgatives	Hyoscyamus
Leeches	Blisters	Poultices	Blood letting
Sarsaparilla	Mercury	Local bleeding	Guaicum
Tar ointment	Bath of suphurated Kali	Nitro-muriatic bath	Sulphorous fumigation
Tartarised antimony oint.	Fomentations	Opium	Terebinth
Cicuta	Nitrous acid		

After 1814 many patients were treated without the use of mercury (Carmichael, 1825).

A James Morison (1770–1834) manufactured and sold in their millions Morison's Vegetable Universal pills for all ills, which contained: gamboge, aloes, cream of tartar (potassium hydrogen tartrate) and colocynth. They cost only a shilling a box so it was cheaper than going to the doctor. The pills killed many people due to 'mortification of the bowels'.

'A neighbouring tradesman having learned from his friend, Bottles the chemist, that I had put myself under a regular course of medical treatment loses no time on presenting his card. Bye the bye Mr Sadd is the same gentleman who proposed getting up an anti-Morison demonstration – he says that he considers Morison's pills are a most unjustifiable interference with the vested rights of Undertakers.'

A neighbouring tradesman having learned from his friend Bottles the chemist, that I had put myself under a regular course of medical treatment, loses no time on presenting his card. By the bye Mr Sadd is the same gentleman who proposed getting up an anti-Morison demonstration, – he says that he considers Morisons pills are a most unjustifiable interference with the vested rights of Undertakers.

Another example of the effect of 'secret remedies'.

1826 <u>Salicin</u> (which is converted to salicylic acid in the body) was isolated by Barthlomew Rigatelli. The following year The Institut de France named a commission, which approved the drug, but the medical public were less enthusiastic and by 1865 it was *'un peu abandonée'* in France but thrived in Spain and Portugal (Guibert, 1865).

Benjamin Shaw, a Lancashire mill mechanic, kept a recipe book mentioning several simple mixtures including: *'Take of snake root 15 grammes[152], Cadir (chopped willow bark) 10 grains, sulphur 3 grams, syrup of sugar to mix, and make into a bolus... given in the worst kind of malignant fevers, extended with convulsions and diarrhoea...If plentifully prescribed it requires to be well diluted with small liquor, it will cause a sweat'.* (King, 2001). This kind of mixture where the active salicylate would have been efficacious in fevers combined with seemingly irrelevant herbs might cause adverse interactions. Virginian Snake Root was used for the fever in the Great Plague of 1665, but it is difficult to find if it had any active principle. There were several different snake roots: Virginian, Indian and Chinese.

'Formulaire pour la préparation et l'emploi de plusieurs nouveaux médicaments, tels que la noix vomique, les sels de morphine, l'acide prussique, la strychnine, la veratrine, le sulphate de quinine, la cinchonine, l'émétine, l'iode, l'iodure de mercure, le cyanure de potassium, l'huile de croton tiglium, les sels d'or, les sels de platine, les chlorures de chaux, et de soude, les bicarbonates alcalins, les pastilles digestive de Vichy, l'écorce de la del racine de Grenadier, les préparations de phosphore, etc., etc.' par F. Magendie. Imprint, Paris: Chez Méquignon-Marvis, 1927. [The formula for the preparation and the use of several drugs, such as nux vomica, morphine salts, prussic acid, veratrine, quinine sulphate, cinchona , emetine, iodine, mercuric iodide, potassium cyanide, croton, tiglium oil, gold salts, platinum salts, calcium and sodium chloride, the alkaline bicarbonates, Vichy digestive pastilles, root bark of pomegranite and phosphorus preparations, etc, etc.]

---

[152] gramme (French and English) = gram (customary English usage) = gramma (Greek)

1828 PCA Louis (1787–1872) of the Charité Hospital, Paris, showed that when patients were bled for pneumonia that the longer it was delayed the better the outcome for the patients and he suggested that if no blood was let the outcome might be improved even further (Louis, 1828; Wade, 1970; Morabia, 2006). He was one of the early enthusiasts for group comparisons where the subjects were to be taken *'indiscriminately,* one group for treatment A and a similar sized group for treatment B. With groups of 500 he hoped that they would be similar in all other attributes *'all things being equal'*. He also hoped that the errors in the two groups would compensate each other (Morabia, 2006). This was an important step in the history of pharmacoepidemiology.

Dr Schabel of Tübingen said, *'I have...long discarded hellebore'*.

Friedrich Wohler (1800–1882) synthesised urea, the first synthetic organic chemical and heralded the birth of the present pharmaceutical industry.

1829 Henri Leroux isolated Salicin from White Willow (Leroux, 1830).

1831 Discovery of chloroform.

1832 Henri Gerland synthesised Salicylic acid.

1835 A Swiss chemist, Karl Jacob Löwig, isolated Salicylic acid from *Spiraea ulmaria* (meadowsweet).

The Nuremberg salt test double blind trial compared distilled snow water with ordinary salt in a homeopathic C30-dilution of distilled snow water. There were responses from 50 out of the 54 participants. Only eight persons reported experiencing anything unusual – 5 from the dilution group and 3 from the water group. The conclusion was that the homeopaths claims were *due to fruit of imagination, self-deception and preconceived opinion–if not fraud.* (Stolberg, 2006). Unfortunately this false philosophy has been supported by British royalty.

1838 Raffaele Piria, working in Pisa and Turin, Italy, isolated salicylic acid from willow bark (Pirèa, 1838).

1839 Francois Magendie (1783–1855) presented to the Académie des Sciences and to the Société Philomatique the results of his first experimental work, which he carried out in collaboration with the botanist and physician Alire Raffeneau-Delille (1778–1850). In a series of ingenious experiments on various animals, the two investigators studied the toxic action of several drugs of vegetable origin, particularly of upas, nux vomica, and St.-Ignatius's bean. These experiments mark the beginning of modern pharmacology. For the first time an experimental comparison was made of the similar effects produced by drugs of different botanical origin. Magendie held that the toxic or medicinal action of natural drugs depends on the chemical substances they contain, and it should be possible to obtain these substances in the pure state. He discovered anaphylaxis by giving repeated doses of egg albumen to rabbits (Magendie, 1839).

The Manchu government attempts to prohibit further importation of opium and precipitates the Opium Wars (1839–1842, 1856)'.

1841 Sir Astley Cooper gave the effects of mercury as '*Brassy or smoky taste in the mouth–the gums white and swollen–the teeth unusually sensible to cold air and water-gums ulcerated about the roots of the teeth–the cheeks ulcerated opposite the dentes sapientiæ–the teeth loose and often painful–increased quantity of saliva secreted-bleedings from the gums and cheeks–and exfoliations of the lower jaws. Chilliness–sensation of cold water running down the back–pulse quickened–increased secretion of urine–loss of appetite–restlessness–sweating–purging often–tenesmus, vomiting, irritation in the skin–pains in the joints.*' *(Cooper, 1841).*

1842 Ether was used for the first time as an anaesthetic by Crawford Long in the US.

1845 '*A Treatise on Poisons*', by Robert Christison, 4th edition,
   <u>Black Hellebore</u>: '*Vomiting, delirium, convulsions, burning pain in stomach and throat, cramps of the hands and cold sweat.*'
   <u>White Hellebore</u>: '*Pain in belly, swelling of the tongue, soreness of the mouth, giddiness, dyspnoea, weakness, stiffness of hands, blindness, dilatation of the pupil, faintness, convulsive breathing and a small pulse.*'

1846 The inunction of 1ʒ of mercurial ointment produced severe symptoms of mercury poisoning in a patient with Bright's[153] disease and the recognition that poor renal function resulted in increased blood levels of renally excreted drugs (Harrison, 1846).

1847 First use of chloroform by James Simpson in Edinburgh and first death due to chloroform (Thomas, 1974).

1848 The first American national law, The Drug Importation Act, came in 1848 during the Mexican War. It banned the importation of adulterated drugs because the United States had become a dumping ground for counterfeit, contaminated, diluted, and decomposed drug materials. American troops in Mexico had suffered from spurious medication for malaria. To demonstrate to Congress what exactly the problem was, the Select Committee catalogued a long list of common adulterations in imported drugs:

1. The 'blue mass pill', for example, which contained 33½ percent mercury when pure, was imported and sold with only 7½ percent mercury. The rest of the pill was made up of 27 percent clay, 16 percent water, 34 percent 'soluble saccharine matters,' 12 percent 'insoluble organic matter,' and trace percentages of colouring and sand.

2. Sulphate of quinine, derived from Peruvian bark, was adulterated by being combined with chalk, plaster of Paris, and the salts of willow bark.

3. Imports of scammony, (The active principle is the glucoside scammionin or jalapin), $C_{34}H_{11}O_6$. Scammony is inert until it has passed into the duodenum where it is converted into a powerful purgative). *'It contained generally only about one-half the active principle of the genuine article.'* The rest was *'a worthless vegetable extract commingled with clay.'* It was also an anthelmintic.

   The Act did not apply to US produced adulterated drugs, so it was only a partial success. A Spurious Solution to a Genuine Problem: (Walch, 2002). This bill did not prevent the rapid growth of the patent medicines industry.

   Dr Sibson pointed out that in four cases chloroform caused

---

[153] Bright's disease = acute glomerulonephritis

death by paralysis of the heart; In all the four cases it is manifest that the immediate cause of the instantaneous death lay in the heart' (London Medical Gazette vol xiii, 1848 p 100).

'Zhi Wu Shi Tu Kao' [Atlas of medicinal plants] by Wu Qi-Jun.

1851 The Arsenic Act. The retail sale of arsenic was restricted and the purchaser had to be known to the seller and records had to be kept. Up to this time more than a third of poisonings were due to arsenic (Royal Pharmaceutical Society of Great Britain (RPSGB), Theme E, sheet 1).

1853 Charles Gerhardt, professor of chemistry at Montpellier University, synthesized acetylsalicylic acid.

1854 Invention of the hypodermic syringe by Doctor Alexander Wood of Edinburgh (Wood, 1855).

1855 Cesare Bertagnini in 1855 published a detailed description of the classic adverse events associated with a salicylic acid overdose, which he studied by deliberately ingesting excessive doses, about 6 grammes in two days. The first day there were no problems, but on the second day there was: a continuous noise in the ears and a kind of dizziness. He said that his superior, Professor Piria, had taken salicin but the effect of a large dose was so disconcerting that he did not do any more research. (Bertagnini, 1855).

The UK House of Commons Select Committee on Adulteration of Food, Drinks and Drugs discussed adulteration of chloroform, opium, scammony, etc.

1857 Claude Bernard wrote *'Leçons sur les effets des substances toxique et médicamenteuses'*. [Lessons on the effects of toxic and medical substances] in which he dealt with sulfocyanine de potassium (KCNS), oxide de carbone (CO) and curare. He tried the latter on rabbits, frogs and dogs, but said that it was innocuous by mouth (Bernard, 1857). Claude Bernard and Francois Magendie made great advances in the science of clinical pharmacology. Apparently early in his life he took a job with a pharmacist who had a 'Theriac Jar' and when ever a drug fell into disuse it was added to the 'Theriac jar'. The latter retained its therapeutic properties despite its ever changing contents (Richet, 1919).

*'Notwithstanding the extreme subtlety of the aether, it is
perfectly innocent and safe to take, as it contains nothing that
is acrimonious or corrosive; so that it may be given even to the
youngest children without hesitation. It neither purges nor
vomits; nor does it increase any of the sensible evacuations, except
that of urine, and sometimes that of sweat, if taken when in bed';
To apply it externally, you must procure a bit of linen rag, of
such a dimension as to be conveniently covered by the palm of the
hand; moisten this rag with a little of the aether as it lies upon
your palm, and instantly apply it to the part affected, pressing
it very close, so as to prevent the escape of its fumes, for two or
three minutes. The general dose for a grown person is a common
tea spoonful; and the best vehicle to take it in is a draught of
cold water. If it be only stirred, in the water with the spoon,
and the mixture drank immediately it strikes the nostrils by its
volatility,'* (http://www.gutenberg.net). Title: An Account of the
Extraordinary Medicinal Fluid, called Aether. (Matthew Turner;
Crockett, 1857).

1858 John Snow pointed out in *'Chloroform and other anaesthetics'*
that 'in recorded cases of fatal inhalation of chloroform none
of them have taken place in a gradual manner, but that in all
cases the fatal symptoms, if not the actual death, have come
on very suddenly.'…. *'Occasional sequelae of the inhalation of
Chloroform: sickness, faintness, depression (more in the feeble
and disabled), hysteria, death coming on very suddenly.'*

'The Dispensatory of the United States of America' by George
Wood and Frankilin Bache, 11th edition 1858, 1st edition 1833.

Opium: *'headache, nausea and vomiting, tremor, secretions
diminished, peristalsis lessened, stertorous respiration, dark
suffused countenance, slow labouring pulse, cold extremities,
restlessness, delirium, and itching.'*

Henbane: *'sense of heat in the throat, sleep, vertigo, pain in
the head, dilated pupils, occasionally diaphoresis, or diuresis,
pustular eruption, often laxative. Overdose–disordered vision,
loss of speech, difficult deglutition, delirium, intoxication, stupor,
some times tonic spasms, convulsions, paralysis, pain in bowels,
diarrhoea, feebleness of pulse, petechiae, and death.'*

Hellebore Niger: *'vomiting, hypercatharsis, vertigo, cramps, convulsions, and death.'*

Hellebore Album: *'vomiting, hypercatharsis with bloody stools, general prostration, and sneezing.'*

Hellebore Viridis: *'vomiting, faintness, somnolence, vertigo, headache, dimness of vision, dilated pupils, and bradycardia.'*

The different species seem to produce different symptoms, but this is not borne out by subsequent books.

Mercury: *'small frequent pulse, anxiety about the praecordia, pale, nervous agitation, debility, eruption, salivation, coppery taste, sore gums, foetor, and tongue swelling.'*

This was the first dispensatory that dealt with adverse effects of the drugs.

1860 First clinical description of mercurialism in hatters was published in the transactions of the Medical Society of New Jersey in 1860. The exposed workers complained of *'the shakes', tremor, gastrointestinal disturbances, sore mouth, psychic disturbances such as irritability, timidity, irascibility and difficulty in getting along with people, headaches, drowsiness, insomnia, weakness, loss of coordination, slurred speech, loosening of teeth, memory loss, depression, irritability and anxiety.'* (O'Carroll et al., 1995).

'On the injurious effects of mercury in the treatment of disease' by S O Habershon, 1860: *'salivation, taste, breath, gums, diarrhoea, nutrition impaired, effusions into cavities, vomiting, cough, coma, convulsions, mercurial fever, tremor, dry skin, loss of memory, sleeplessness, delirium, mercurial cachexia, deficient in red cells, pulse irritable, palpitations, swelling ankles, anasarca, erythema and death.'* At the end of the book is an advertisement for his own recipe, so not all these books are for enlightenment but some were to sell their own products.

Kolbe and Lautemann made synthetic salicylic acid from phenol.

1861 Holmes OW. *'Currents and countercurrents in medical science with other addresses and essays.'* Boston: Ticknor and Fields. *'I firmly believe that if the whole materia medica, as now used, could be sunk to the bottom of the sea, it would be all the better for mankind,– and all the worse for the fishes.'*

1862 *Des éruptions médicamenteuses pathogénétiques'* [Pathogenic drug-induced skin rashes]. Paris, Thesis by Leon Guérard. 1862. 55 pages.

'The diagnosis of drug eruptions is generally easy; one is alerted by the sudden appearance of the illness, its sharp and rapid progress, the site, the form and arrangement of the rash, etc.' This thesis covers: resins (balsams), belladonna, arsenic, mercury, iodides, antimony, opium, morphine, iron, cod liver oil, silver nitrate and quinine sulphate.

Erythema due to <u>belladonna</u>/<u>henbane</u> or strammonium apple: minimal dose–*a diffuse reddening, especially on the face and neck. Lack of fever and dilated pupils confirm the diagnosis. Rapid onset within the first few hours, and lasts for only a few hours'.*

<u>Hydrargyrie</u>/<u>mercurial</u> eczema: Apparently rare in France as compared with England. Uses the scheme put forward by Alley (see 1804) and he gives a full description of the three phases.

<u>Opium and morphine</u>: *'pseudo-exanthemata, either erythematous or papular, secondary to the sweating and itching.'*

This seems to be the first collection of ADRs referring to a group of drugs rather than to a single drug.

1863 Johan Adolf von Baeyer, a twenty-nine-year-old assistant of Friedrich August Kekule (the discoverer of the molecular structure of benzene) in Ghent, synthesizes barbituric acid, the first barbiturate. It is said that he named it after St Barbara since he discovered it on her saint's day – 4th December 1863 (Cozanitis, 2004).

The forerunner of salvarsen, Atoxyl was discovered by Béchamp A.

1864 The Royal Medical and Chirurgical Society (now the Royal Society of Medicine) published a *'Report of the Scientific Committee on the uses and the physiological, therapeutical and toxical effects of chloroform, as well as into the best mode of administering it, and of obviating any ill consequences resulting from its administration'.* The inquiry was sparked by 123 fatalities following its administration. They found that chloroform depressed the action of the heart and frequently killed by producing syncope[154] (Royal Medical and Chirurugical Society, 1864; Thomas, 1974).

---

[154] syncope = in this context it meant cessation of the heart beat, but normally it refers to a faint.

1868 UK Pharmacy Act set up a register of people qualified to sell, dispense and compound poisons. The Pharmaceutical Society was granted powers to deem a substance a poison and to decide which substances should be available for sale, and who should be allowed to become either an authorised chemist or druggist and who should be a listed agricultural or horticultural supplier (RPSGB).

1869 *'The old vegetable neurotics[155]: hemlock, opium, belladonna and henbane; their physiological action and therapeutical use alone and in combination; being the Gulstone Lectures of 1868 extended and including a complete examination of the active constituents of opium.'* by John Harley

Henbane: Use–Cardiac and pulmonary asthma, neuralgia, nephritis and enuresis.

Dose: 1/40 gr dryness of the mouth, reduces pulse 80 to 60 beats or 50 to 45 beats not less than 40 beats.

1/16–1/12 gr 'sedative, little heat, somnolence, cheeks occasionally a little flushed, membranes eye slightly injected, pupils slightly dilated and pleasing delirium with illusions of the sight'.

1/8 gr Giddiness, pulse raised by 12 beats, slightly twitchy.

1872 The German Imperial Order attempted to regulate drug quality by restricting the sale of pharmaceuticals to recognised apothecaries (Abraham, 1995).

1874 *'Des éruptions provoquées par l'ingestion des médicaments'* [Rashes provoked by the intake of medication], Thèse pour le Doctorat en Médicine, 59 pages, by Jean Berenguier. Paris, (Berenguier, 1874). The medicines covered were: bromides, balsams (copahu, cubèbe, térébenthine or turpentine), belladonna, chloral, mercury, arsenic and iodides, but he also mentioned rashes caused by opium, quinine sulphate, antimony tartrate, antimony trisulphide, hypophosphites, copper sulphate, digitalis, iron, sulphur, henbane, datura and valerian. This was before the discovery of allergy in 1907 and the only hint of type B reactions was in the phrase: *'One must take account of a special aptitude, of an individual predisposition that one*

---

[155] neurotics = medicines that act upon the nervous system

cannot call into question'. He mentions some predisposing factors: youth, femininity, weak, lymphatic (pale flabby or sluggish) and scrofulous (tuberculous) patients. He describes the rashes covering the sites of predilection, detailed accounts of the objective and subjective symptoms with case histories, but without any histopathology.

The Japanese clarified their principles of dispensing with the 'Medical Service Order' of 1874.

1875 UK Sale of Food and Drugs Act, but despite this many counties failed to test drug samples and less than one third of cases where adulteration was proved were prosecuted (Abraham, 1995).

The Canadian passed the Inland Revenue Act , which despite its name, aimed at preventing the adulteration of food, drinks and drugs. This act was tightened up in 1884 with the Adulteration Act and fixed official standards for drug composition. Secret remedies were tackled by the 1909 Proprietary or Patent Medicines Act. Biologics were included in the 1927 Food and Drugs Act. The 1953 Food and Drugs Act controlled the conditions of manufacture and remains current. (snippits-and-slappits.blogspot.com/2009_07_01_archive.html) Accessed 21st July 2009.

1876 At the post-mortem of a TB patient who had taken 12 grammes of salicylic acid (forerunner of Aspirin) Goltdammer found several gastric ulcers (Goltdammer, 1876). Salicylic acid caused buzzing in the ears, (tinnitus), difficulty in hearing (Bertagini, 1855), urticaria (Leube, 1879), oedema of both eyelids (Heinlein, 1878) and petechiae (Freudenberg, 1878) and albuminuria... inflammation of the parenchyma of the kidneys (Balz, 1877). 'Forewarned is forearmed' all these occurred later with Aspirin (Lewin, 1881).

Stricker (Stricker, 1876) and MacLagan (MacLagan, 1876) found that salicylic acid was useful in the treatment of rheumatic fever. At this time the Hottentots of South Africa were using a decoction of willow-tops for rheumatic and other fevers (Volmink, 2005). During the period 1876–1880 there was much discussion as to the relative worths of salicin and sodium salicylate in the treatment of acute rheumatism.

1877 The British Medical Association set up in Manchester a committee to investigate the sudden deaths with chloroform. This was the first time that a committee had been set up to solve an adverse event problem.

1879 The individual predisposition to injurious effects of certain drugs may be hereditary (King,1879).

From 1879 to 1905 at least 190 bills related to US federal control of foods and drugs were proposed but none were passed (Abraham, 1995).

The employment of black hellebore is nearly obsolete but the drug is still imported from Germany and sold for use in domestic animals (Flückner & Hanbury, 1879).

1880 The BMA committee, known as the Glasgow Committee, on chloroform deaths concluded that chloroform was hazardous because it depressed respiration and had a deleterious effect on the heart–The McKendrick Report. They had carried out many investigations in animals (rabbits and dogs) and had analysed reports of fatal accidents in patients. This produced a backlash in that the Hyderabad Commission on chloroform in 1889 reported that chloroform was safe, but that any deaths were due to asphyxia and not to cardiac arrest. A second Hyderabad Report in 1890 said that chloroform was *'as safe as whisky and water'*. They had carried out the experiments on over 1,000 animals (dogs and monkeys). The truth is that chloroform sensitises the myocardium to catecholamines, which may induce a variety of cardiac arrhythmias including fatal ventricular fibrillation (Wade, 1970).

Van Harlington referring to skin ADRs said *'I endeavoured to collect and collate cases arranging them into groupings under the heading of each drug the various lesions of the skin which have been attributed to its influence.'* These drugs included: arsenic, belladonna, chloral, iodine, mercury, morphine, quinine and salicylates (Laughlin & Jackson, 1986).

1881 Louis Lewin published *'Nebenwirkungen der Arzneimittel: Pharmakologisch–Klinisch Handbuch'* [The Incidental Effects of Drugs: A Pharmacological and Clinical Hand-book]. (1882)

W. Wood. There are 783 pages and drugs are dealt with in turn after a 38-page introduction. This would seem to be the first collection of ADRs from all body systems.

Lewin recognised 'type A' and 'type B' ADR but did not use those terms *'There has been some hesitation in regarding these 'nebenwirkungen (adverse events)' as poisonous effects. And very properly so, for we are not justified in regarding one or more symptoms as the effects of a poison, simply because they may not occur in 999 cases and yet appear in the thousandth. In addition to this it may be noted that the majority of these unwanted effects do not, in any particular, correspond with the symptoms induced by a poisonous dose of the drug, and that we cannot, at will, effect these untoward symptoms and especially such as manifest themselves in cutaneous eruptions.'* As Paracelsus implied 'poison' being a question of dose means that it refers to a 'type A' event.

Quinine: Vépan mentions a lady who took 1½ grains (97 mgm) *'and afterward 2 1/2 grains (162 mgm) of quinine for neuralgia, two days afterward her entire body was covered by purpuric spots, which disappeared in the course of nine days but to reappear after the administration of the drug was resumed'.* Lewin says that in this case the severity of the eruption was in proportion to the size of the dose, and during its existence there was bleeding of the gums (Vépan, 1865); he adds that Gauchet also noticed an eruption of this kind in a lady who had previously expectorated blood after taking quinine. The petechiae were profusely spread over the entire body; it disappeared after the suspension of the drug' (Gauchet, 1871).

Opium: *'Brochin reported* (Brochin, 1877) *a case in which the 'idiosyncrasy' against morphine was so great that 1/25 of a grain (2.6 mgm) of the drug administered hypodermically caused irregularity of the respiration, momentary suspension of the heart-beat and profound narcosis, intense mental confusion, vertigo, headache, convulsions, buzzing and ringing in the ears, tinnitus, confusion, dimness of vision, disturbances of hearing, unconsciousness, twitching, tremor, temporary paralysis, dry throat, nausea and vomiting, anorexia, profuse diaphoresis, face turgid and reddened, hot to touch, pruritus opii, skin eruption, stupor, and colicky pains.'* (Gould & Pyle, 1997).

<u>White Hellebore</u>: *'sneezing if in contact with the nasal mucous membrane, similarly the conjunctiva, sense of pricking and increased heat, restlessness, anxiety, petechial or vesicular eruption, lowers pulse rate, blood pressure, temperature, and frequency of respiration, dryness of the mouth, difficult deglutition, nausea and vomiting, choking, salivation, colicky pains, diarrhoea, may be tinged with blood, vertigo, dimness of vision, trembling, collapse, pustular eruption on face, and cerebral symptoms.'*

<u>Henbane</u> (Hyoscin): *'irritability, vomiting, intoxication, speech difficult, swallowing impossible, delirium, laborious respiration, pupils dilated, clonic convulsions, hyoscine from amorphous hyoscyamine gives—feeling of oppression, benumbed sensation, pressure over the eyes, thirst, dryness of throat, nausea, trembling, sensation of heat, laboured respiration, dizziness, numbness, intoxication, and staggering gait.'*

<u>Mercury</u>: *'eczema mercuriale, gangrene, salivation (30–40%), offensive odour, gingivitis, metallic taste, loose teeth, insomnia, tongue swelling, headache, fever, anorexia, weakness, stomatitis, disturbed nutrition, gastro-enteritis, stomach burning, diarrhoea with blood, debility, frightful dreams, emesis, gastric and abdominal pains, albuminuria, glycosuria, peripheral anaesthesia, hyperaesthesia, erethism (bad temper, irritability, diffidence, bashfulness, facial pallor, asthmatic respiration, irregular heart's action, debility), dizziness, vertigo, and tremor.'*

Whereas Withering in 1785 gave as the ADRs of Digitalis: *'sickness, vomiting, purging, giddiness, confused vision, objects appearing green or yellow, increased secretion of urine, with frequent motions to part with it, and sometime inability to retain it; slow pulse, even as slow as 35 in a minute, cold sweats, convulsions, syncope and death'* Lewin adds *headache, dryness in the throat, choking, buzzing in the ears, muscæ volitantes, amblyopia or diplopia, sleepiness, a fall in temperature and an 'erysipelatous affection'*. However, none of these are mentioned in the 14th edition of 'Side Effects of Drugs' 2000 other than *'flickering sensation'*, which may represent muscæ volitantes[156]. Lewin did mention a papular eruption with positive rechallenge,

---

[156] muscae volitantes = flying flies = spots before the eyes

which is also mentioned in SED with other dermatological effects. It seems likely that Lewin incorporated single uncorroborated reports of events.

1881 Japanese pharmacopoeia. The first version was published in 1881 and is revised at least every 10 years.

1882 *'A peculiar idiosyncrasy (induction of pyrexia) as to mercury'* by Simeon Snell. Patient took ʒi liq. Hydrarg. Perchlor. And after the third dose felt ill and the drug was stopped and six weeks later it was repeated and next day they had a temperature of 104° vomited and had a headache, there was a positive dechallenge, three weeks later was given Iron citrate and Hydrarg. cum Cret. twice daily and next day had a temperature of 101.6°.

Advertisement

Gowland's Lotion. The formula sanctioned by the medical profession is to take of Jordan almonds (blanched), 1 ounce; bitter almonds, 2 to 3 drachms; distilled water, 1/2 pint; form them into an emulsion. To the strained emulsion, with agitation, gradually add of bichloride of mercury (in coarse powder), 15 grains previously dissolved in distilled water, 1/2 pint. After which further add enough water to make the whole measure exactly 1 pint. Then put it in bottles. This is used as a cosmetic by wetting the skin with it, and gently wiping off with a dry cloth. It is also employed as a wash for obstinate eruptions and minor glandular swellings and indurations. This noxious preparation was first marketed in 1792.

1883 First clinical use of the sphygmomanometer (Basch et al, 1883).

1819–1892 *'I love doctors and hate their medicine'* Walt Whitman.

1884 Carl Koller anaesthetised the cornea with cocaine. Coca previously had been chewed in leaf form in South America for its stimulant properties (Spillane 1995).

1885 In an article by Prince A Morrow entitled *'The Aetiology and Pathogenesis of Drug Eruptions'* the author explores the different current views and concludes that 'idiosyncrasy' is based upon a recognition of their neurotic character'. He gives as predisposing causes: the relative fineness and sensitiveness of the skin of women and children, especially blond children;

heredity, nervous irritability, hysteria, spinal injuries, and other neuroses, eczema and idiosyncrasy (Morrow, 1885).

1887 Discovery of phenacetin (acetophenetidin).

First electrocardiogram recorded in man (Waller, 1887).

Dr Broadbent *'I have seen deaths in acute rheumatism of a kind quite new and strange to me, after prolonged administration of salicylate of soda every four and six hours'*. (Broadbent, 1887).

1888 Paul Ehrlich first described aplastic anaemia, although this name was not used until 1904 (Young, 1996; Erhlich, 1888).

1890 Multiple forms of mercury compounds given to infants and children such as laxatives, teething powders, antihelminthics, nappy (diaper) rash creams and the first organic mercurial antiseptic mercurochrome led to a condition known as acrodynia or pink disease. Although described as early as 1890, the role of mercury was not confirmed until 1948. (See pages 205, 266 and 320).

1891 The first use of passive immunisation when a young boy with diphtheria was cured by an injection of diphtheria antitoxin (Singer & Underwood, 1962). Pirquet and Schich discovered serum sickness caused by diphtheria antitoxin in 1905 (Pirquet & Scich, 1905).

1893 The first recognition of hypertension as a disease entity 'Une maladie d'hypertension arterielle' (Huchard, 1893). A 'hard pulse' had been noted from the early days of Chinese medicine and in 1760 Schaarsschmidt and Nicolai treated 'spastic constrictions of the blood circulation with nitrate salts'. (Backer, 1944). And then after Hale's discovery clinicians started to associate high blood pressure with different disorders. Treatment with Sodium thiocyanate was the first treatment of 'hypertension' in 1900 (Esunge, 1991).

1894 Introduction of anti-diphtheria serum.

The Therapeutic Committee of the British Medical Association set up an inquiry regarding the importance of ill-effects following the use of antipyrin, antifebrin, and phenacetin. The aim *'was to ascertain the 'impression' which any ill-effects, met with had made on the mind of the observer; in particular whether that impression was of such a kind as to prevent him using the drugs as frequently as he would otherwise have done'.* They approached the 34 BMA branches and invited them to furnish a limited list of names of members to whom an inquiry might usefully be addressed. Each doctor was told *'There seems to be an impression that the effects are of such a character and frequency as materially to limit the usefulness of these drugs'.* They were then asked the following questions:

The amount of experience you have had in the use of these drugs, whether as an antipyretic or analgesic agent.

The doses you habitually give.

The nature of any ill-effects you have observed.

Their comparative frequency.

Your opinion as to their comparative importance. Do they materially limit the usefulness of the drugs?

Twenty seven branches responded. The results showed that the ill-effects were strikingly infrequent and that placing them in the order their freedom from ill-effects: phenacetin, antipyrin and antifebrin. It is easy today to criticize the methodology used, but this was one of the earliest attempts to find the ill-effects of a series of drugs.

Biases: answer suggested, arbitrary choice of doctors, memory dependent, dependent on doctors' diagnoses of ADRs. More of an opinion poll than a scientific investigation (see 1909) (Leech & Hunter, 1894).

1895 Buss introduced sodium salicylate (Buss, 1895).

Heinrich Koebner (1838–1904) published a study on quinine eruptions.

The first study of a drug interaction: Adrenal extract caused ventricular fibrillation in a dog anaesthetised with chloroform (Oliver & Schaefer, 1895), Lewin had mentioned that the English Chloroform Committee had remarked that persons under the influence of emotion, whether it be fear, fright or care were peculiarly liable to succumb to the action of chloroform. He also said that chronic alcoholics had abnormal reaction to chloroform needing larger quantities than the normal person and also showing a high degree of excitation. He uses the phrase

' thus inebriates, through a combination of the action of these two agents are more liable to unpleasant untoward symptoms'. An appreciation of a drug interaction.

1896 Scipione Riva-Rocci developed the mercury sphygmomanometer, but like most new inventions its use only spread gradually over the next 20 years.

1898 *'King's American Dispensatory'* by HW Felter & JU Lloyd. Pub. Ohio Valley Co.

Opium: *'nausea, emesis, restlessness, startling, disagreeable visions, delirium, anxiety, unpleasant prickling sensation on the surface of the body or a troublesome itching occasionally accompanied by a slight eruption, giddiness, languid pulse, sickness at the stomach, cephalgia, tremblings, want of appetite, mucous secretions become suspended, constipation is induced, cutaneous secretion is increased, retention of urine, diminution of the frequency of the pulse, slow stertorous respiration, flaccidity of the extremities, coma, first livid or turgid afterward pale features, livid lips, excessively contracted pupils, coldness of the limbs, profuse cold perspiration, convulsions may precede death.'*

Hyoscyamus (Henbane): *'dryness of the mouth, flushing of the face, pupillary dilatation, quickened cardiac and respiratory action, illusions, hallucinations, loss of memory, deranged vision, giddiness, fullness of the pulse, flushing of the face, weight in head, headache, loss of muscular control, tremulousness, mental confusion, incoherence of speech, somnolence, furious delirium, unconsciousness, coma, cold sweat, convulsions, nausea and vomiting, intestinal pain, and purging.'*

White hellebore: *'sore mouth, swelling of the tongue, gastric heat and burning, severe vomiting, profuse diarrhoea, vertigo, tremors of the extremities, feeble pulse, loss of voice, dilatation of the pupils, spasms of the ocular muscles, blindness, cold sweating, mental disturbance, stupor, convulsions, and severe coryza when snuffed up through the nostrils.'*

Green Hellebore: *'nausea and vomiting, watery diarrhoea, slow pulse, dilatation of the pupils, cold sweats, failure of sight, coma, sneezing, muscular weakness, reduced temperature, slow shallow or stertorous breathing, sleepiness, dizziness, faintness, increased kidney, lung and liver secretion, and fatal.'* Again one wonders whether these are true differences between the different types of hellebore.

Salicylic Acid: *'tinnitus, deafness, pain in forehead, manual tremors, excess debility, hurried respiration, lesions of the kidneys, tingling in the extremities, delirium, amaurosis, dimness of vision, ptosis, strabismus, asphyxia, nausea and vomiting, pyrosis, diarrhoea, angina, redness of face, burning mouth, and increased saliva.'*

Diacetylmorphine (heroin) was synthesized in Germany. It was widely lauded as a *'safe preparation free from addiction-forming properties'.*

First US National Pure Food and Drug Congress. Anxiety about the adulteration of foods had been growing since the 1848 bill and the drug regulations came in on the back of the food regulations.

Johannes Andreas Fibiger performed the first randomised controlled trial comparing patients with diphtheria who were randomised according to their day of hospital admission to either standard treatment or standard treatment plus serum treatment. Serum sickness affected approximately 60 % of the serum treated patients (Hróbjartsson et al., 1998).

1899 Acetyl salicylic acid marketed as 'Aspirin' by Farbenfabriken vormals Friedrich Bayer & Co. The sodium salt of aspirin and sodium salicylate were tested on normal rabbits and on cold-blooded animals, which *'showed clearly that aspirin is less poisonous than salicylic acid'.* The clinician, Floeckinger, even went so far as to take two large doses of aspirin himself: first 75 grains (4.86 G) and then another 60 grains (3.9 G). After the first dose he found himself *'without toxic effects, except violent headache and tinnitus'* which lasted for 16 hours, until it subsided following profuse sweats. After the second dose, Floeckinger experienced *'increased pulse, reduced temperature, and flashes of light before the eyes.'.* Nonetheless, Floeckinger concludes his article as follows:
'It presents several advantages over salicylic acid. It does not irritate the stomach. There is no cardiac depression. In ordinary doses there is no tinnitus or headache...and [it] is best prescribed in wafers or sachets for acute and chronic rheumatism,

polyarthritis, and pleurisy...but it is ineffective in neuralgias and pleurodynia.' (British Medical Journal, December 9, 1899; p. 96.) It was marketed at a dose of 625 mgm four hourly.

Original reservations about the effects of Aspirin (ASA) on the heart prevented its widespread use; however, persistent provision of ASA to local physicians returned nothing but praise and optimistic results.

Witthauer said *'..it can be given without deranging the stomach... ringing in the ears is hardly ever observed with aspirin... Its taste is much less unpleasant than salicylate of sodium.'*

Wohlgemuth described a case of a 21 year old with fever and swelling of hand and knee. Given 3G Aspirin daily in dilute alcoholic solution the pain was at once relieved. After a few days the patient complained of pain in the stomach, this immediately subsided when the medicine was stopped. There was no loss of appetite or tinnitus. *'The pain in the stomach was no doubt due to the alcohol'*; the patient at the first disliked the strong smell of alcohol in the medicine. In the further experiment aspirin was given in the form of powder in a dose of 1.0 G. No pain in the stomach was noticed when the drug was given in this form (Wohlgemuth, 1899; Wohlgemuth, BMJ, 1899).

July 22nd 1899. The Bayer Company stated *'..not dissolving appreciably in water but easily in alcohol. It disappears, however, in weak potash solutions, the addition of acid to this alkaline solution leading to the reappearance of a crystalline substance. This fact is of clinical importance, since aspirin would pass through the stomach unchanged until it reached the alkaline digestive juices in which it would be decomposed and the salicylic acid would be appropriated. On this account the irritation in the stomach caused in some cases by salicylic acid and its salts is prevented. Further, it is said that owing to aspirin decomposing gradually the singing in the ears sometimes produced by ordinary salicylates is to some extent avoided. Aspirin is almost free from taste but is slightly acid; it is not sweet like the salicylates'*. The suggested dose was 15 grains (972 mgm).

Placebo

Placebo-controlled studies allow the establishment of the common ADR pattern of new drugs prior to marketing. Ethically, placebo treated patients should be kept to a minimum, but from the point of view of establishing the factors responsible for the ADR pattern as well as those factors affecting efficacy large numbers are important. The adverse events occurring whilst on placebo are grouped together in the analysis and allow one to define the adverse events due to the drug, but these 'placebo' adverse events consist at least three different elements:

1. Adverse events that have occurred because the patient believes that they may be on an active drug. These are the true 'placebo effects'.
2. Those adverse events, which are due to the underlying disease(s) or new diseases (diseases in this context includes the minor symptoms of everyday life).
3. Adverse events due to unidentified parallel interventions, e.g. 'white coat hypertension.

It has been suggested that where there is also an untreated group one is able to define more accurately those adverse events due to the giving of placebo by subtracting those of the untreated group from those on placebo. (Ernst & Resch, 1995), The adverse events occurring whilst on placebo have been called: Nocebo (Kitchener et al, 1996) or 'Placebo-induced side effects' (Schindel, 1968), 'Nonspecific medication side effects and Nocebo phenomena' (Barsky et al, 2002), Introduction of the term 'nocebo' meaning the patient's expectations producing adverse effects from placebo, from 'nocere' meaning 'to harm' (H̶a̶h̶n̶e̶m̶a̶n̶,̶ ̶1̶8̶1̶0̶ Kennedy, 1961).

From what has been said above many of the adverse events are not true 'effects' of placebo or nocebo.

Secret Remedies

Since the begining of time medicines had been sold without any description of their contents. In 1731 the French King's physician authorized remedies that had been prepared in advance for the cure of certain illnesses after taking the advice of a committee representing the physicians, surgeons and apothecaries. In 1778 The Société Royale de Medicine was charged with examining new drugs giving Royal Warrants authorising their sale and distribution and this legalised the secret remedies. On 8th August 1793 all the licensed academies and societies were su*f*pressed and as a result the secret remedies multiplied (Kassel, 2002) The French law of 1803

200

specifically banned secret remedies and they were definded as 'those of which the formula is kept secret by their inventors'. Only those drugs that were mentioned in the 'Codex' and those preparations magistral[157] could be provided by pharmacists. The pharmacists probably felt aggrieved by this especially as the charlatans continued to flout the law. The law was modified on 14th June 1805 those that had previously been on the market were allowed to stay. As well as those that had been approved by the medical authorities as long as they were useful and new. On 18th August 1810 this was again modified to put a commission in place to examine the medicines to judge whether they were innocuous efficacious. The 3rd May 1850 saw yet a further change The French Academy of Medicine had to confirm that they conformed with four demands:

They were mentioned in the 'Codex'.

They were prescribed by a doctor.

Had been published by the Government.

That they had the approval of the Academy of Medicine and the latter had published details in their bulletin.

If these conditions were not met then they were labeled 'secret remedies'. However, it was only when there was a disaster that the law was invoked. By 1926 there were so many 'secret remedies' that something further had to done, so a decree on 13th July 1926 said that as long as they were labelled on the bottles, boxes, packets or packaging with the name and dose of each drug as well as the name and address of the pharmacist then they were legal. This left two problems: It was not possible to patent medicines in France, so anybody could copy the formula and secondly since the drug now had the name of its contents on the outside anybody could read them and guess the patient's disease, e.g. mercury meant they had syphillis. The industry synthetised more and more drugs and they were able to patent their mode of manufacture. The pharmacists could now benefit by selling these new drugs made by the industry (Debue-Barazer, 2003).

In Britain the BMA published two books: The first of 195 pages in 1909 entitled '*Secret Remedies What they cost and what they contain*' and the second in 1912 '*More Secret Remedies*'. These books listed all the medicines and the results of chemical analysis and pricing of their constituents. Needless to say most of the ingredients were in low doses, often without efficacy and worth only pence. The Pharmacy and Medicines Act 1941 made the disclosure of the active ingredients obligatory.

---

[157] magistral = medicines prescribed by a physician

Adverse Reaction Committees

From c2500 BC Emperors and Kings were making decrees about the use of drugs and ordering the compilation of pharmacopoeias. Then eminent physicians such as Hippocrates (370 BC) and Galen (60 AD) were advising on the adverse effects of drugs. This was followed by professional bodies making regulations for their members as to the use of drugs, e.g. in 1271 the faculty of Paris forbade the prescribing of medicines except by qualified physicians and in 1566 the faculty forbade the use of antimony. The RSM 1864 report and the McKendrick 1880 report on chloroform were, however, the first occasions when professional bodies set up committees to assess a specific ADR problem.

Health Insurance schemes

The end of the nineteenth century saw the realisation that a form of National insurance against the vissitudes of life would spread the burden more equally. Various mutual benefit clubs had started in the 18th century. One for seamen who had to pay sixpence a month towards the seamen's hospitals for decayed seamen, their widows and children was ordained by an Act of Parliament in 1696. The benefit clubs paid doctors out of weekly contributions made by members. The club managers usually paid the doctors on the basis of an amount per member, i.e. a capitation fee. The first National Insurance scheme was in Germany and was started by Bismark in 1883. The British scheme started in 1911 by the National Insurance Act of 1908. Where drugs were paid for by a scheme there was strict supervision to make sure money wasn't wasted by giving expensive medicines. This meant that more people were able to benfit from drugs and that there was enough supervision to prevent the prescribing of quack medicines.

Interactions

I have found no mention of any interaction between herbs other than the reference in 220 AD that toxicity can be reduced by adding another herb. In 1667 George Castle says 'The mixing of things which are harmless sometimes produces a poison'; but this refers more to chemical interactions. The lack of references to interactions may be because there were few herbs with active principles and, therefore, few interactions. There are some herbs that contain more than one active principle and there is the possibility that these interact and it has been suggested that two of the digoxin glycosides, digitoxin and verodoxin, interact so that the action of digitoxin is enhanced, but I can find no evidence to support this. This situation has been called 'The SEES[157] theory' (Sutrisno, 1978). It must, however, have been obvious that herbs with similar properties should not be combined, e.g. belladonna, henbane and mandrake, which all contain tropane alkaloids, i.e. pharmacodynamic interactions should have been recognised. Pharmacokinetic interactions would have been more difficult to appreciate and may have been even rarer. St John's Wort is known to affect CYP 1A2[158], 2C9 and 3A4 and thereby increases the metabolism of digoxin so that on stopping the St John's Wort the concentration of digoxin rises and may cause an ADR. The stopping of the St John's Wort may have occurred long after the starting of the digoxin so that the ADR would not appear to have been caused by the digoxin. It was not until the explosion in synthetic drugs in the late 19th century that were powerful active principles to interact. The first mention of the interaction between salicylates and sodium bicarbonate was in 1944 and with aspirin in 1949. There is no mention of drug interactions in Medline before 1964. An adverse event caused by an interaction will occur after the second drug or substance has been started and may reverse on stopping the second drug leading to the opinion that the second drug is the sole cause of the ADR. However, if the second drug increased the blood level of the first drug the adverse event will have the characteristics of an ADR to the first drug not the second drug. Any factor in the causality of an ADR may be considered as interacting with the drug.

Summary

There are still many papers/books/letters on the mercurial treatment of syphilis. The symptoms of the ADRs of most our marker drugs are now well established. The laws and regulations start dealing with dangerous drugs, but still continue to check the quality of drugs. The first publications that devote themselves to the adverse effects of more than one drug concentrate on the skin, which is easy to describe although the vocabulary has always been arbitrary. About mid-century there is the beginning of new synthetic drug industry which will fuel a new powerful pharmaceutical industry. Clinical trials use placebos, double-blinding and randomisation, but little attempt is made to collect ADRs systematically.

---

[157] SEES = Side effects Eliminating Substances or Secondary Effective Eliminating Substances
[158] CYP = isoenzymes of cytochrome P450

Chapter 8. 20th century

*S*ynthetic drugs start to displace herbals medicines. Allergic
reactions become recognised and pharmacology becomes a powerful
force in medicine.

1901 On October 26th 1901, a five-year-old girl in St. Louis, USA, was
admitted into hospital with diphtheria and was given antitoxin,
two days later she died in the city hospital from tetanus. The
admitting physician stated that she had most likely presented
at the hospital nine days earlier with spinal meningitis, but was
given the diphtheria anti-toxin prophylactically. The municipal
health officials investigated the case and found that the horse
from which the anti-toxin had been taken had produced over
30 quarts of diphtheria antitoxin in his career, but had been
destroyed after contracting tetanus. Investigators concluded
that instead of destroying all of the horse's contaminated serum,
two officials had allowed some of it to be distributed resulting
in the deaths of twelve more children throughout St. Louis.
(Roberts 1996). Also in the autumn of 1901, nine children in
Camden, New Jersey, died from tainted smallpox vaccine and
nine children in New Jersey died from contaminated smallpox
vaccine, setting the stage for the adoption of rigorous standards
for the emerging biological products industry.

A pamphlet produced by Bayer says *'The innocuity of Aspirin is
absolute. No action on the stomach or the digestive tract'.*

1902 The Biological Control Act passed in the US to ensure purity and
safety of serums, vaccines and similar products used to prevent
or treat diseases in humans. This required that biological drugs
be licensed and produced in licensed facilities and production
supervised by a qualified scientist. The Act was prompted by
The Medical Society of the District of Columbia following these
deaths (see above). The Hygienic Laboratory, forerunner of the

National Institutes of Health, was authorised to conduct regular inspections of the establishments and to sample products on the open market for purity and potency testing (FDA, 2006).

Barbital was first synthesized in 1902 by German chemists Emil Fischer and Joseph von Mering. They published their discovery in 1903 and it was marketed in 1904 by the Bayer company as Veronal. By 1913 it was implicated in fatal accidents and suicides. By 1950 barbiturates were established as 'true' drugs of addiction, but they were known to cause habituation from 1941 (Medawar, 1992). In 1979 the Committee on Review of Medicines (CRM) said they should be reserved for severe cases of intractable insommnia.

Hirschberg describes anaphylaxis due to aspirin (Hirschberg, 1902).

Charles Richet, in 1902, injected a dog with a dose of poison derived from the tentacles of the actiniae and with no harmful effect whatever. Twenty-two days later he reinjected the dog with exactly the same dose, expecting to reach larger doses later and a condition of prophylaxis to the poison. To his surprise, hardly had he finished the injection when the animal became extremely ill and died in thirty-five minutes. This being the exact opposite of prophylaxis he called it 'anaphylaxis' (Coke, 1921). Richet described an experiment whereby a watery extract of various tissues from an Egyptiam mummy over 3,000 years old was made and injected into guinea-pigs, and a month later it was found that these animals had been made anaphylactic by means of human albumins (Richet, 1910).

1903 Acrodynia (Pink Disease) The first known case was presented at the Cassel Congress, in 1903 although possible cases had been reported in Australia as early as the 1880s. The report reads: *'The disease is observed in girls aged 18 months to three and a half years. It is characterized by sadness, anxiety, and eventually a progressive loss of language, with psychiatric symptoms (hallucinations, coprophagy, delirium during sleep, etc). In addition, there are sweats and their consequences: viscous, humid skin, swollen, red and cold hands and feet. The patients feel cold and permanently irritated. They complain of being itchy,* *lose their hair primarily at the temples, but sometimes to the point of complete baldness. Almost certainly infection of the nail cuticles and abscesses follow. Internal organs are not affected.'* An association between mercury and Pink disease (infantile acrodynia) was suggested by the work of Warkany and Hubbard (1948, 1951), Fanconi et al (1947) and Fanconi and Botsztejn (1948). In 38 of 41 investigated cases Warkany and Hubbard found an abnormal quantity of mercury excreted in the urine. Then in 1945 a severely affected child was admitted to hospital in Cincinnati, Ohio, under the care of Dr Josef Warkany. The disease was rare in Cincinnati and Warkany's interest was aroused. He had a hunch that heavy metal poisoning might be implicated, so he asked his laboratory to measure the levels of the common, industrial heavy metals in the child's urine. The results were all negative. But one element-mercury-had not been measured, as there was no adequate test for it at the time. By luck, Warkany discovered that in Cincinnati there was a young chemist, Mr Donald Hubbard, who had recently developed a sensitive method for measuring urinary mercury, so for the sake of completeness he asked Hubbard to do the measurement on his patient. The result was strongly positive (Thiele, 2006). Mercury in the urine doesn't prove causality, just an association; it could be due to protopathic bias where early fever due to a virus infection could be mistaken for teething (fever, flushed cheeks, peevish, disturbed sleep, lower jaw moved from side to side) hence the giving of a mercury (calomel) containing teething powder (Thomson, Steele & Reid, 1896). (http://www.users.bigpond.com/difarnsworth/pink53.htm (2 of 5) Accessed[05/28/2000 1:43:49 AM].

In 1947 there was the recognition that mercury in teething and worming powders caused Pink disease (Black, 1990). However in a standard textbook on children's diseases 1954 said *'Common disease of unknown aetiology' giving four theories of causality – vitamin deficiency, neurotrophic virus infection, chronic mercury poisoning and salt-deficiency'*. By 1953 mercury had been banned from teething powders in parts of Australia. Since the 1950s the disease has disappeared and this seems the strongest evidence that the cause was mercury in teething powders. (The causes of Pink disease by Diane Farnsworth) (http://www.pinkdisease.org/causePD.htm).

1905 A patient with severe rheumatism was given 15 gr. Aspirin and after 2 days there was violent palpitations, difficult respiration, extreme weakness, approaching unconsciousness and the voiding of green urine. There was a positive rechallenge (Barnett, 1905). There was little published in the Lancet between 1900 and 1910 on the ADRs of Aspirin, but one noted originally in a French paper was an account of unpleasant symptoms caused by the new synthetic substance aspirin: some cases of gastric pain, vomiting, giddiness, painful oedema of the eyelids and the lips extending at times to the head and to the mucous membranes of the pharynx. A single case of a scarlatinform rash was also reported plus a case of epistaxis (Notes, Lancet, 1905).

Aspirin-induced fixed drug eruption with a positive rechallenge was reported (Freund, 1905).

Aspirin goes on sale in the UK on 30th October 1905.

The American Medical Association organised 'The Council on Pharmacy and Chemistry', which evaluated new drugs and re-evaluated old drugs.

Pirquet and Scich gave the first detailed description of serum sickness (fever, lymphadenopathy, cutaneous eruptions and arthralgias) caused by diphtheria antitoxin in 1905 (Pirquet & Scich, 1905). They defined it as *'specific acquired reactivity which follows initial response to foreign protein'*.

1906 The Pure Food and Drugs Act (USA) concerned labelling and prohibited interstate commerce in adulterated food and drugs. This had been prompted by the popular press protesting against *'filthy conditions in Chicago's packing plants'* and *'nostrums laden with arsenic and other harmful ingredients, the unfounded cures for cancer, TB, syphilis, narcotic addiction and a host of other serious as well as self-limited disease'*. (FDA, 2006). Drugs had either to abide by standards of purity and quality set forth in the US Pharmacopoeia and the National Formulary, or meet individual standards chosen by their manufacturers and stated on their labels. Proprietary drug manufacturers and business lobbies kept the food bill from becoming law earlier (Young, 1981).

Clemens Von Pirquet coined the term 'allergy' (Pirquet, 1906).

1907 Synthesis of arsphenamine (Salvarsan) in Germany by Alfred Bertheim (Williams, 2009).

1908 Sulfanilamide synthesized.

Toxic effects of Aspirin: After 10 gr. Aspirin + Exalgin 1½ gr. thirty minutes later lips, throat and nose swell, speech impaired, pupils unduly dilated, pulse 110, bulli on the nape of neck, violent sneezing and lacrimation (Ewing-Hunter, 1908).

The UK Pharmacy and Poison Act. Revised schedule of poisons and listed sellers of non-medical poisons. Purchasers of opiates had to be known by the seller and an entry made in the Poisons Register (RPSGB).

Paul Ehrlich and his co-worker Sahachiro Hata found that the 606th compound that they tried was effective against syphilis and they named it Salvarsan (compound 606). This was arsphenamine (i.e. made from arsenic). It was used in more than 20,000 patients prior to marketing compared with the median number in 1987–89 of 1528 with 95% confidence limits of 1194–1748 and a range from 43 to 15,962 (Williams, 2009; Rawlins & Jefferys, 1993). It was marketed in 1910 and Neosalvarsen was marketed in 1912. The price of a single injection of Salvarsen in 1911 was 10 shillings (2008 value by the retail price index was £37.95 or $ 70.38; by average earnings £198 or $368). This meant that only the rich could have afforded it, whilst the poor would have had ung. hydrarg./ liq. arsenicalis or sodium aresenate.

The US Department of Agriculture (Bureau of Chemistry) undertook a survey of US physicians to ascertain their views on 'The harmful effects of acetanilide, antipyrin and phenacetin'. The purpose of the study was to 'collect information relative to the poisonous nature of acetanilide, antifpyrin and Phenacetin'. They wrote to the physicians throughout the US and asked the following questions:
1. To what extent do you use these drugs in your practice?

2. What dose do you ordinarily preseribe for adults?
3. Do you prescribe them more or less frequently than formerly? Why?
4. What is your opinion with regard to the relative safety of these three drugs?
5. Have you observed instances of acute or chronic poisoning or cyanosis caused by these drugs? How many of each?
6. In what form was the drug administered?
7. About what dates did the poisoning occur?
8. Were the patients adults or children?
9. For what ailment was the drug taken?
10. Was it ordered by a physician?
11. Was it used internally or externally?
12. Quantity taken?
13. Give brief history of cases observed by you, omitting details.
14. Have you observed any cases of habitual use of any of these drugs or of any preparations containing them?
15. In what form was the drug taken?
16. Were there any ill effects? Give brief description.
17. Were there any protracted ill effects?
18. Give a brief clinical history of each case.

Nine hundred and twenty-five letters were sent out and there were 400 replies (Total number of doctors in the US at the time – 125,000). Quote: *'Granting that the 525 physicians who did not reply had no cases to report.'* They, therefore, calculated that there were 925 patients with 814 cases of poisoning, which included 28 deaths ascribed to the drugs and and 136 cases of habitual use. They gave the results of an extensive worldwide literature search. The results were similar to those of the BMA survey (see 1894). The use of all three drugs was diminishing at the time of this survey. These biases were similar to those with the BMA survey (Kebler et al., 1909). Acetanilid (antifebrin) was removed from the Japanese market in 1971 due to its propensity to cause aplastic anaemia. Antipyrin (phenazone) was removed from the market in Argentina in 1981, Malaysia in 1986 and also in Bahrain.

In a lecture on Salvarsen in 1910 Wihlem Wechselmann said *'Is the eventual risk of the drug in an acceptable balance with the size of its [beneficial] effects'?* (Wechselmann, 1910). This probably the earliest correct version of the cost/benefit ratio.

1911 Founding of the Drug Commission of the German Medical Association as a panel of the German Society of Internal Medicine. Its main objective: '*...if it is possible that the congress could independently take action to set a boundary to the escalating mischief regarding to production and particularly marketing of new drugs which becomes more and more intolerable'.*

The UK National Insurance Act 1911 provide medical treatment and attendance, including provision of proper and sufficient medicines. The bill was strongly opposed by the BMA due to inadequate money for the doctors.

The UK Select Committee Report on Patent Medicines recommended the creation of a Medicines Commission, that all medicines should be registered for an annual fee and that the qualifications for being on the register should be that of quality, safety and efficacy. These were not enacted because of the outbreak of the First World War (Select Committee on Patent Medicines, London: HMSO [Her Majesty's Stationary Office]).

1913 The Medical Research Council (MRC) was set-up with funding by the government under the 1911 National Insurance Act.

1915 '*The Committee* (MRC) *venture to urge that members of the medical profession would be performing a service of national importance, in the present emergency, by keeping accurate records of cases in which the new preparations are used, and by placing such records at the disposal of the committee for their private information and guidance. Particular stress must be laid upon the desirability of recording in every case, the name of the preparation used and the serial number applied by the manufacturer to the particular batch employed together with such details as to dosage, the precautions taken to ensure purity of the water used and finally the results of the administration, both as regards therapeutic efficacy and the presence or absence of special incidental symptoms.'* (BMJ Editorial, 1915). The first public request for spontaneous reporting of 'incidental symptoms'.

First experimental evidence of cancer by chemicals reported when repeated applications of coal tar to the ears of rabbits resulted in skin cancer (Yamagiwa & Ichikawa, 1915).

Otto Seifert wrote '*Die Nebenwirkungen der modenen arzneimittel [The side effects of modern drugs]*. This was followed by a supplement in 1922. There are eighteen chapters in 278 pages and the book covers all groups of drugs. Each drug has a section on its use followed by a list of its side-effects, which are well referenced. Of the drugs dealt with in part 3 of this book he mentions: antipyrine, aspirin, phenacetin, amidopyrine, phenobarbitone, phenolphthalein, cincophen, piperazine, bismuth subgallate and phenformin (Seifert, 1915).

1916 First placebo-controlled clinical trial (Delay and Pichol, 1973).

In a standard UK medical textbook, '*Wheeler's Handbook of Medicine*', there is no mention of 'adverse reactions' or 'side effects'. Common mild adverse effects are rarely mentioned; the only ones mentioned being for quinine (singing in the ears) and for salicylates (tinnitus, air-hunger, delirium, vomiting and acetonuria). Important drug adverse effects are mentioned as 'intoxications' so for causes of jaundice we have chemical poisons: phosphorus, toluene-diamin, mercury, arsenic, chloroform and ether. For secondary anaemia: poisoning - we have lead, mercury and arsenic. For toxic purpura there is quinine, antipyrin, copaiba, mercury, etc. Albuminuria may be caused by arsenic and excess morphia. Causes of peripheral neuritis include; alcohol, arsenic and bisulphide of carbon.

Aplastic anaemia is under 'pernicious anaemia' as a '*few cases with no bone marrow reaction*' and, of course, there is no mention of Vitamin B_{12}. There is no mention of agranulocytosis. The ordinary treatment of syphilis is Hutchinson's pill (Hydrarg. c. Cretâ gr. i and Pulv. Ipecac.Co. gr. i one or two thrice daily), but if treatment is more urgent inunction of blue ointment (4G daily) or hypodermic injection of corrosive sublimate gr ⅛ or calomel gr. i-ii injected intramuscularly once a week, but there is no mention of adverse reactions. Under another heading Salvarsen and Neosalvarsen are mentioned as giving good results. Drug treatment for miliary TB is 'purely symptomatic' and for ordinary pulmonary TB Tuberculin is recommended, but serum treatment was not successful. Great emphasis is given to vaccine treatment for tetanus, anthrax, actinomycosis, Malta fever, septicaemia, erysipelas; and anti-sera, which was used for typhoid, diphtheria, scarlet fever, erysipelas, lobar pneumonia, anthrax, dysentery, plague, croup, and acute endocarditis. Treatment for rheumatic fever is salicylate of sodium or Salicin gr.xx every two hours and only if salicylates disagree other salicyl compounds, e.g. aspirin, may be used. 'Tonics' play a large part in treatment, especially arsenic, iron and strychnine. Although Galen's humours have lost most of their influence, emesis, purging and venesection still play a part in some diseases:

Emesis: in collapse of the lung and bronchopneumonia.

Purges: in hepatic engorgement, high blood pressure, chronic bronchitis with cardiac dilatation, chronic haemoptysis, acute and chronic Bright's disease, mumps, glandular fever, yellow fever, gout, acute tonsillitis, worms, hepatic cirrhosis, infantile paralysis, simple meningitis, cerebral haemorrhage, Meniere's disease, migraine and Trichina spiralis infestation.

Venesection: in chronic bronchitis with cardiac dilatation, lobar pneumonia, meningeal haemorrhage, simple meningitis and cerebral haemorrhage. (Jack, 1916).

James McDonagh, referring to Salavarsan, said *'There is no drug, which has not at some time or another given rise to toxic symptoms, so differently constituted in each human frame'.* (Williams, 2009). He seems to have been against the use of Salvarsan and in favour of mercury treatment.

Prior to the introduction of Kharsivan, the English version of Salvarsan, the UK Board of Trade tested it and published an official report on the 'Toxicolgy of Salvarsan' (1st April 1916). Animal toxicology had been performed on white mice, white rats and rabbits. The clinical details were given of the adverse effects and the individual reports of deaths, but no statistics were given. (Wilcox & Webster, 1916). There was no mention of any specific liver problems.

An army captain reported (29th April 1916) on the effects of 600 injections of Kharsivan. He stated that 72% of patients had no adverse reactions. This important information on new drugs is rarely given even today. He also gave percentages for the adverse effects: headache in 17%; rigor in 5%; vomiting in 7%: diarrhoea in 10%; transient albuminuria in 0.3%; Herxheimer's[160] reaction in 2.3%, etc. There were no reports of liver problems. This is the first report that I have found that gives good statistics on ADRs and which gave that information to prescribers (Lucey, 1916).

There was an outbreak of acute yellow atrophy in patients who had been given neoarsphenamine benzoate for syphilis at a military hospital near Cambridge. The same problem had occurred in Germany and there had been two official reports in 1914 and 1917. The Medical Research Committee appointed a 'Special Committee on the manufacture, biological testing and clinical administration of Salvarsan and its substitutes', which reported in 1922 that the most probable cause was the toxicity of the organo-arsenical compounds. *'The Committee hope that a plain statement of the rare fatalities and other untoward effects known to occur after the use of arsenbenzol preparations may encourage the communication to the Ministry of Health of details concerning such accidents, for it is only in the light of such information that investigation and measures with regard to their prevention can be successfully undertaken.'* Shah says that this was the forerunner to monitoring of adverse reactions (Shah, 2001). However, in retrospect, it was probably viral hepatitis. The Committees report in 1922 said that after a course of Salvarsan there was, in practically every instance, 'evidence of hepatic insufficiency' demonstrated by two tests: the laevulose toleration test (discovered the previous year) and the estimation of lipase (more a test of the pancreatic function than liver function). There were few positive tests after a course of six injections, but after three months all tests were positive only to become negative at six months. The report doesn't come to a conclusion as to the exact cause of the acute yellow atrophy (Salvarsan Committee, 1922). In 1902 there were no liver function tests mentioned (Hutchinson & Rainy, 1902), but in the same book eleven editions later in 1951 the

[160] Herxheimer's reaction = transient immunologic reaction commonly seen after treatment of syphilis and attributed to the release of endotoxin like substances from dying microorganisms.

laevulose test has been replaced by the galactose tolerance test measuring carbohydrate metabolism and there are tests for protein metabolism: Takata-Ara test, colloidal gold reaction, cephalin-cholesterol flocculation test, the thymol tubidity test and plasma prothrombin. There were two tests of excretion and detoxification: the bromo-sulphone-phthalein test and the hippuric acid test. There was only one enzyme test–alkaline phosphatase (Hutchinson & Hunter, 1951).

A similar outbreak in Dublin in soldiers treated with neoarsphenamine concluded that malaria had been transmitted via the apparatus for the neoarsphenamine injection. The former outbreak might have had the same mechanism (Wade, 1970).

1919 William Osler (1849–1919) *'We doctors have always been simple trusting folk. Did we not believe Galen implicitly for 1500 years and Hippocrates more than 2000 years.'*

1920 UK Dangerous Drugs Act. These drugs: cocaine, morphine and opium could be sold only to a physician's prescription and import, export and manufacture of raw opium, cocaine, heroin and morphine was prohibited except under licence (RPSGB).

Insulin discovered.

MRC Salvarsen Report. In addition to the problem of acute yellow atrophy there were problems with encephalitis haemorrhagica, which occurred within 2–3 days after a injection, and exfoliative dermatitis. A course of treatment was usually followed by a period of hepatic insufficiency, which was thought to be due to the drug (Salvarsan Committee, 1922).

Widal describes asthma, rhinitis and urticaria with aspirin (Widal et al., 1922) 9th February 1921 after 100 mgm aspirin there was an immediate hemoclastic crisis with a fall in leucocytes, general erythema, spasmodic coryza, an attack of asthma, and after 4 hours there were repeated attacks of spasmodic coryza and continuing asthma while the urticaria began to subside. There was a positive rechallenge. This became to be known as the 'Widal syndrome'.

1924 Haber's law (Zur Geschichte des Gaskrieges) [On the history of gas warfare] says that the incidence and/or severity of a toxic

Dear Reader,

Several reviewers have said that this is a history book; but most history books that I have read are continuous narratives reflecting the opinions of the authors. There is frequently little primary evidence and usually there are no references, but rather a bibliography, which consists of secondary sources. I have based the book on the structure of a scientific paper with the aim, methods and limitations in the preface whilst the remainder of the book forms the results and conclusion sections. I hope that there is sufficient information for the readers to form their own opinions and to support my own conclusions.

The cut-off date of 1960 was determined partly by the great change in attitude and regulations concerning the adverse effects of drug after the thalidomide disaster, partly because extending it to the present time would have more than doubled the size of the book and partly because it would be better written by others.

I apologise that my inadequate proof-reading has meant that there are many errors. I have corrected most of these and added extra references. In Part 3 the 'drug lifespan' are unreliable because varying criteria were used and similarly with the withdrawal times so that the graph (figure 9) on page 379 is inaccurate. However, when the latter is corrected the graph remains substantially the same.

The further one goes back in time the more inaccurate are the dates and they are not reliable before about 1500.

The transliteration of Chinese and Arabic has been difficult as over the years different systems have been used. Wherever possible the Chinese system has been Pinyin, but the Arabic format is the same as in the references used.

Perforce the book is about the adverse effects of drugs and there is little reference to efficacy, but this is not to deny that the efficacy of modern drugs has saved many millions of lives including my own.

Myles Stephen.

reaction depends on the total exposure, i.e. exposure to the drug x duration of exposure. This law is applied in carcinogenicity testing (Haber, 1924).

1925 Therapeutic Substances Act (USA) regulated the manufacture and sale of substances requiring biological testing.

Therapeutic Substances Act (UK) regulating manufacture, but not sale of antitoxins, and sera, vaccines, posterior pituitary preparations, insulin and arsenicals.

1926 Insulin was produced.

A French decree (July 13th 1926) resolved the problem of secret remedies (Berman,1970).

1927 Thyroxine synthesized.

Fleming discovered penicillin.

W Trevan created the a marker for toxicity: LD$_{50}$ mgm/kilo body weight, the median lethal dose.

In a discussion on blood-letting, at the RSM in 1927, it was said that within the last decade it came to be discarded in hospital practice, but persisted in private practice. In 1927 it was still being used for a variety of conditions:
   Right-sided heart failure (over distended heart, one of the
      criteria being 'lividity').
   Uraemic states following scarlatinal nephritis.
   Apoplectiform seizures
   Status epilepticus
   Heat stroke
   Asphyxia by non-irritant gases.
   Acute alcoholic poisoning.
   Polycythaemia
   High blood pressure
   Pain caused by aneurysms
   Mushroom poisoning
   Gunshot wounds to the chest. (Spencer et al, 1927).
   These have now been whittled down to 1, 2 and 8, i.e. where there is iron-overload, pulmonary oedema secondary to renal failure, cor pulmonale. So we have seen over more than 800

years the erosion of the mythical use of blood-letting and the establishment of the logical reasons for removing blood.

1928 Norwegian legislation developed regulations relating to drug safety and efficacy (Abraham, 1995).

Formation of the Food, Drug and Insecticide Administration (later the Food and Drug Administration).

Chauncey Leake suggested that the evaluation of new drugs should entail study of the toxicity of the different members of the series and that this required a large number of animals and much patience. He was astonished how unreliable and meagre toxicity figures were for even standardized preparations. The minimal lethal dose, (killing three out of five) depended on many factors among which were:
   (a) Species
   (b) Condition of animal
   (c) Solvent and concentration
   (d) Mode and rate of administration.
He went on to say that these variables took considerable experience to control in order to arrive at sound estimates.

He also advocated that before venturing to clinical trials one should submit the selected substances to study in regard to their action on normal human beings (Phase I studies).

'Many drug firms make the mistake of believing that their chemists can furnish trustworthy pharmacological opinion. Indeed some eminent chemists impatient with careful pharmacologic technique, have ventured to estimate for themselves the clinical possibilities of their own synthetics... There is no short cut from the chemical laboratory to the clinic except one that passes too close to the morgue.' (Leake, 1929).

Sir William Willcox referring to the dangers of new medicines said: *'Recently many new drugs, a large proportion of them of foreign manufacture, had been placed on the market, and their virtues were highly extolled by the manufacturers and the vendors. Attention was rarely called, however, to the toxic and other harmful effects which were liable to follow their use. He thought it most unfortunate that the makers of drugs did not more fully take the medical profession into their confidence.*

Certainly the medical practitioner would feel more confidence in a new drug brought to his notice if all the possible sources of danger were carefully indicated.' (Willcox, 1928).

1930 Isolation of digoxin from Digitalis lanata (Smith, 1930).

In the Lubeck Municipal Hospital 249 infants were given oral doses of BCG[161] between late February and Mid-April 1930. By June 67 infants had died and 80 were critically ill. Eventually approximately 75 died. The BCG had been contaminated with tuberculosis bacilli.

1931 Sir William Willcox gave a warning as to the control of drugs:
'The great variety of drugs in common use which might act as liver poisons and produce dangerous toxic jaundice showed how necessary it was that, before they were placed on the market, these drugs should be submitted to careful toxicological and therapeutic tests on the human subject as well as on animals. The medical profession should be fully informed, not only of the therapeutic properties of new drugs, but also of the dangers which might arise from idiosyncrasy or overdosage. At present doctors were insufficiently informed of the dangers resulting from the new drugs introduced into the country in increasing amount. The present system of scheduling poisons was quite inadequate to keep pace with the rapid developments of the chemical manufacturing industries, which were daily launching new and imperfectly tried complex organic drugs on the market'... The system of control and sale of drugs possessing powerful toxic properties was most imperfect and unsatisfactory, exposing the people of this country to great danger from the taking of new drugs advertised as possessing wonderful curative properties, without any mention of their toxic effects. (Willcox, 1931).

Notices appeared in 'The Telegraph' on the 31st July:
'The Medical Research Committee (UK) announce that they have appointed a Therapeutic Trials Committee, as follows, to advise and assist them in arranging for properly controlled trials of new products that seem likely on experimental grounds to have value in the treatment of diseases.' They examined 59 drugs between 1931 and 1939. The instigators of the Committee were the Association of

---

[161] BCG = Bacillus Calmette-Guérin vaccine with efficacy of 70–80% against TB

British Chemical Manufacturers who had made representations to the Medical Research Council for an official scheme for the clinical testing of new remedies which in laboratory tests had given promise of therapeutic value'. (Green, 1944).

The UK Therapeutic Substances Act came into force on 25th July 1931.

1932 There were several popular US books written about the dangers in foods and drugs: *'100,000,000 Guinea pigs, dangers in everyday foods, drugs and cosmetics'.* Written in cheap journalese with chapter headings such as: The quack and the dead; little white lies; to make the best of a bad law, etc. These books helped to put pressure on the FDA. Many similar books have been published since then on both sides of the Atlantic.

Gerhard Domagk (1895–1964) discovered the sulphonamides in December 1932.

1933 July 15th dinitrophenol found to cause weight reduction, but caused severe skin rashes, agranulocytosis, jaundice, and fatal hyperthermia. This product was not covered by the 1906 law, because it was a diet potion. (see under regulatory responses).

A group consisting of FDA officials, USDA (United States Department of Agriculture) staff and private lawyers drafted a bill to expand government authority to inspect manufacturers and require firms to carry out premarketing food and safety tests. The bill languished in the House Commerce Committee for the next five years (Cavers, 1939).

Madison and Squier suggested that amidopyrine and other drugs containing a benzene ring might be a cause of agranulocytosis. The OTC (Over The Counter) sale of amidopyrine was prohibited in the UK in 1936 and in the US in 1938, but it remains on European markets (Wade, 1970). (see under regulatory responses).

The UK Pharmacy and Poisons Act. It contained a Fourth Schedule which listed poisons, which could only be sold to the public in accordance with a prescription written by a doctor, dentist or veterinary surgeon (RPSGB).

1934 Swedish drug law required manufacturers to demonstrate the safety and efficacy of their products prior to approval. Germany and the UK had no pre-market safety and efficacy regulations in place until after Thalidomide. The Norwegian and Swedish law requiring drug safety before marketing did not prevent them from authorising Thalidomide.

Ciba Geigy started marketing clioquinol in 1934 for amoebic dysentery. The company marketed it in Japan in 1953. By 1970, 10,000 Japanese citizens suffered from the adverse reaction of subacute-myelo-optico-neuropathy (SMON). See 'Marker drugs'. *Part III*

1935 First use of prontosil red (sulfamidochrysoidine), the first commercially available antibacterial with a relatively broad effect. Discovered in 1932 by Bayer chemists, Josef Klarer and Fritz Mietzsch (Turk 1994). Prontosil is metabolized to sulfanilimide (para-aminobenzenrlsulfonamide), a much simpler, colourless molecule, redefining Prontosil as a prodrug (Loudon, 2008).

April 1935. dinitrophenol caused an epidemic of sclerosing cataracts leading to blindness. September. Forced off the market by the FDA in 1935 (Hecht 1987). (see under regulatory responses).

Cortisone and ergometrine isolated.

1935 Carlo Levi qualified as a doctor in 1923 but gave up medicine in 1927 to write and paint. He also became involved in anti-fascist politics. In 1935 he was sent into internal exile in 'the God-forsaken country' of Lucania in the foot of Italy. Here he witnessed the extreme poverty of the peasants who, unable to pay the few incompetent doctors or the unqualified pharmacists for anti-malarial treatment 'quinine' to protect themselves from the endemic disease, died or were crippled by ill-health. They turned to the local witches for incantations and potions. One of their favourite magic amulets carried the word ABRACADABRA. Their poverty protected them from adverse drug reactions. There must have been many similar situations in the developed world at that time and, of course, it must have been normal in the underdeveloped world (Levi, 1945).

1937 September – Elixir Sulfanilamide containing 72% diethylene glycol (DEG) given to 353 patients during the period of a week. On 2nd October 1937 a JAMA editorial warned against its use because of the increasing number of ADRs including dermatitis, photosensitivity, granulocytopenia and haemolytic anaemia (JAMA Editorial, 1937). Days later six patients died from renal failure. There were 105 deaths including 34 children due to renal failure caused by the diethylene glycol (DEG)(Geiling and Cannon 1938; (Wax, 1995). In 1969, in South Africa, 7 children died of renal failure (vacuolar nephropathy) due to DEG. In 1986 there were 14 deaths in Bombay. In 1990 47 children died similarly in Nigeria (Wax 1995). In 1995 there were 51 deaths due to DEG (Hamif et al., 1995). In Haiti 88 children died as a result of paracetamol syrup being contaminated with 14.4% DEG (O'Brien et al., 1998). In 1998 a cough syrup containing DEG implicated in 33 deaths in India (WHO Bulletin 2001). And so it goes on.

The classical study of Sulphonamide for the treatment of puerperal fever by the Therapeutics Trials Committee of the MRC in 1937 included 106 patients with fever and a positive culture of haemolytic streptococcus Group A. They used historical controls from the same hospital and under the same physician, who had been treated with 'Red Prontosil' and 'Prontosil Soluble' in the previous year (1936) and patients from the years 1931–35, who had mostly received no treatment. The death rate in this study was 8% compared with 22.8% in the controls (1931–1935) and 4.7% in the controls treated with the Prontosils. Under toxic effects:

Drug fever: it was difficult to differentiate between the disease and drug effects.

Cyanosis with met- or sulph-haemoglobin–more than 50% (58 patients).

Nervous system: depression, headache, dizziness, blurred vision, 'spots before the eyes' and parathesia of peripheral nerves have occasionally been observed.

Mental disturbances: hysterical type–two.

Joint pains: in a few cases.

Transient skin eruptions: also seen occasionally.

Jaundice: slight in two patients.

Urine: two cases with casts and three with albuminuria (Colebrook & Purdie, 1937).

Perhaps the dramatic saving of life with the sulphonamide compared with no treatment overshadowed concerns for minor adverse effects, but is characteristic of this period that little was done to investigate and enumerate ADRs.

The Swedish authorities published the Lex Maria, which assigned the duty of a local authority to notify the National Board of Health and Welfare (NBHW) and the police of every serious patient injury or the risk of serious injury caused by medical treatment. This was precipitated by the deaths of four patients in the previous year, who had been given mercuric oxycyanide instead of a local anaesthetic at the Maria hospital Stockholm (Ödergård & Löfroth, 1991).

1938 Another study of a sulphonamide, this time M&B 693[162], in the treatment of pneumonia used as controls patients admitted under other physicians receiving the usual standard treatment. These two groups admitted patients on alternate days. The results in a 100 patients gave a death rate as 8% in the M&B 693 group compared with 27% in the control group. Toxic effects: cyanosis appeared in about a quarter of the patients. Frequent white cell counts were made but no cases of agranulocytosis were found. The attention to adverse effects of the drug was even sparser than in the Sulphonamide study of 1937.

Federal Food, Drug and Cosmetics Act (USA) 1938. The DEG epidemic occurred whilst the act was under consideration, so it was not a case of cause and effect, but no doubt gave an added stimulus. It required that firms had to prove to the FDA that any new drug was safe before it could be marketed. It did not specify what kinds of tests had to be performed, but that *the investigations…which are submitted… do not include adequate tests by all methods reasonably applicable to show whether or not such drug is safe for use under the conditions prescribed, recommended, or suggested in the proposed labelling thereof… he shall … issue an order refusing to permit the application to become effective*. The phrase 'new drug' was defined as '*a drug*

---

[162] M&B 693 = The new chemical 693, a sulphonamide, discovered by May and Baker laboratories

which is not generally recognised, by experts qualified to evaluate the safety of drugs as safe when used as directed by its labelling' .There were some exemptions to the act: vaccines, serums, toxins, antitoxins and most blood products which are licensed under the Biologic Control Law. Likewise five antibiotics were later exempt: penicillin, streptomycin, aureomycin, chloramphenicol and bacitracin and their derivatives (Smith, 1956).

Legislation tends to prevent the industry earning money and therefore has been resisted. The changes in the law do not always answer the situation and, in these cases, require amendments. The 1938 law was amended in 1951 with the Durham-Humphrey Amendment because the 1938 law was vague as to what and who was responsible for identifying prescription versus non-prescription drugs - dictated which drugs needed prescription drug labelling. It was on the basis of this act that Dr Frances Kelsey refused to approve Thalidomide.

An FDA Commissioner, GP Larrick, said of the 1938 law:

1. *'The producer of a new drug did not have to establish that his drug would be effective, as well as safe, for its intended uses'* (Without knowing the effectiveness of a drug no cost-benefit judgement can be made).

2. *'We were forced to work against deadlines of 60 and 180 days to prevent the automatic approval of the new drug'* (In 1940 there was only one medical officer working on new drugs which increased to two in 1950) (Larrick, 1965).

3. *'There was no provision requiring regular record keeping and reporting of clinical and other experiences with new drugs.'*

4. *'We could not remove a new drug from the market unless we could prove that it was unsafe; it was not enough to show that new developments had drawn the question of its safety sharply into issue.'*

5. *'There were inadequate controls over the distribution and use of investigational drugs, as the thalidomide episode showed.'* [Richardson-Merrell distributed 2,528,412 thalidomide tablets to 1,267 physicians for some 20, 000 patients in the USA (Sjöstrom & Nilsson, 1972). Over 2,151 patients were given them in clinical trials. There were at least 7 cases of phocomelia (Mellin & Katzenstein, 1962)].

6. *'Prescription drug advertising, at an estimated expenditure of a quarter-of a- billion dollars per year - $1,000 for each physician in the United States–was virtually unregulated.'*
7. *'Trade names were being used without proper relationship to generic names, with resulting confusion to the profession.'*
8. *'The quality of "old drugs" was not assured, as it was with the "new drugs." Only five of the classes of antibiotic drugs used to treat life-threatening infections were subject to routine batch testing and certification by our laboratories.'*
9. *'And factory inspection authority was so limited as to seriously handicap our operations.' (Larrick, 1965).*

Geiling and Cannon proposed that the necessary information for drugs to be supplied by pharmaceutical companies in their New Drug Applications (NDA):

Chemical composition.

Acute toxicity studies in two species

Chronic toxicity studies with different doses in different species.

Observation of the animals.

Pathologic examination of animals.

Studies in animals with experimental lesions.

Studies on the absorption and elimination of the chemical.

Study of interactions.

Knowledge of idiosyncrasies and untoward reactions (Geiling & Cannon, 1938).

These postulates governed toxicological work for the following decades. Some of the drug disasters that followed were because of neglect of these principles (Hodel & Bass, 1992).

The Food and Drugs Act (UK) made it illegal to sell a drug labelled in a misleading way or to publish an advertisement which did so (RPSGB).

1939 An improved standard for measuring the safety margin for drugs was proposed, based on the determination of the dose-effect relationship. The 'standard safety margin' was defined as the zone between the surely effective dose and the lowest lethal dose (Foster, 1939).

1941 First patient treated with penicillin (Ellis 1997).

The major French law of 11th September 1941 on pharmacy

stipulated in article No.1: the preparation of medicines intended for use in human medicine are reserved to pharmacists.

The UK Pharmacy and Medicines Act legislated against 'secret remedies' making the disclosure of the active drugs compulsory. *'Not derived primarily from a concern to protect consumers' interests, but rather from the conflicts of interest within the drug trade with respect to tax exemptions and related privileges.'* (Abraham, 1995).

The Winthrop Chemical Co. despatched 12 shipments of sulfathiazole, which contained no sulfathiazole, but were filled with phenobarbital. Eighty-two people died. The same tabletting machine had been used for both drugs.

1943 February: Nazi government banned all new drugs except those granted special approval by Defence Ministers (Stop-Verornung). This ban continued on into the 1950s (Abraham & Smith, 2003).

The Drafting of the French Pharmacopoeia was placed under the jurisdiction of a National Pharmacopoeia Commission under the authority of the Minister of Public Health.

The Japanese 'Pharmaceutical Affairs Law' was introduced to implement regulations necessary for ensuring the quality, effectiveness, and safety of drugs and medical devices.

Streptomycin discovered by Dr Selman Waksman's team from Rutgers University (see under marker drugs).

1946 The UK Medical Research Council set up the first formal randomised control trial (see under marker drugs).

1948 First modern randomised clinical trial of streptomycin/placebo by the Medical Research Council (MRC). This reported damage to the inner ear, circumoral numbness, nausea and vomiting, albuminuria and urinary casts, raised blood urea, pruritus, urticarial rash, eosinophilia and yellow vision. However, the toxic effects had been reported previously by the Veteran's Administration study (MRC, 1948)(see analysis of marker drugs).

Introduction of chloramphenicol. In 1950 it was found to cause bone marrow aplasia in between 1 in 58,000 and 1 in 75,000 patients (Rich 1950), but the pathogenesis has not been fully elucidated. It was removed from the French market in 1987 but remains on other markets for very restricted use. It led to the establishment of a blood dyscrasia registry in 1952. (see under regulatory responses).

Vitamin B12 isolated.

Tetracyclines discovered

1949 Henbane still mentioned in The British Pharmaceutical Codex, London, The Pharmaceutical Press, 1949, p. 425.

The Mayo Clinic in Rochester, Minnesota set up a Committee on Safety of Therapeutic Agents. Staff members who wished to administer a new substance or therapeutic agent to human subjects were required to register the material with the committee and provide them with all the relevant information. If safety and efficacy could not be proved, the committee would recommend that the use of the agent be discontinued (Nelson, 1997).

1950 German Drug Commission of the Federal Chamber of Physicians was established and issued warnings concerning thorium containing preparations. (see regulatory responses).

1951 '*Schadelijke nevenwerkingen van Geneesmiddelelen* ' [Harmful side effects of some medicines] (192 pages) published in the Netherlands by L Meyler.

UK Dangerous Drugs Act controlled vegetable narcotics, such as *Cannabis sativa* (cannabis) and opium, and a few chemically related synthetic substances.

1952 English version of Meyler's book '*Side Effects of Drugs*' was published. Only 268 pages compared with 14th edition, 1876 pages.

The American Medical Association Council on Pharmacy and Chemistry established the first official registry of adverse drug effects to collect cases of drug-induced blood dyscrasias (Strom, 2000), which became the Registry on Adverse Drug Reactions in 1961.

Dr George Discombe said '*I believe that there is a need for a small standing committee of clinical and forensic pathologists, whose terms of reference should be: "To collect evidence on the production of injurious effects by drugs administered for therapeutic purposes; to deduce from this, and any other evidence available, whether the therapeutic value of any such drug is great enough to warrant its continued use; and to submit representations and recommendations to the Poisons Board on the regulations for the manufacture, sale, advertising, packaging, labelling, or prescription of drugs which have been shown to produce injurious effects*'. (Discombe, 1952).

1953 Renal damage by phenacetin suspected. Chronic use of phenacetin is known to lead to renal papilary necrosis and is implicated in analgesic nephropathy (see under regulatory responses).

Publication of '*Maladies Médicamenteuses d'ordre thérapeutique et accidentel*' [Drug-induced diseases of a therapeutic and accidental nature] by C. Albahary. This book of 751 pages was written two months after Meyler's Side Effects of Drugs. Sodium salicylate figures largely in the French version. It is in narrative form and covers the investigations required and treatment and is obviously aimed at the clinician.

Intravenous *Veratrum viride* was found to be a potent vasodepressor lowering the blood pressure and slowing the pulse. The side effects were: *tingling, a coolness or numbness of the lips, face, tongue and trunk... sensation of warmth usually about the mouth, forehead and chest...perspiration...slight nausea, vomiting, hiccough... sensation of substernal pressure*'. (Elek, 1953).

1954 'Stalinon' An organic compound of tin, diethyltin di-iodide + vitamin K, in a 15 mg/capsule, linoleic acid (100 mg/capsule), which went on the market in 1953 and was used in the treatment of anthrax, furunculosis, osteomyelitis and acne had impurities, ethyl triiodide, triethyltin iodide and tetraethyltin. Of the (estimated) 1000 persons that had taken the drug, there were 102 deaths of a total of about 210 cases of cerebral oedema. Of all the affected people only 10 completely recovered.

Triethyltin iodide is believed to be the primary cause of this poisoning The formation of a cerebral oedema after organotin intoxication had already been seen with mice and monkeys (BMl, 1958; WHO, 1980) (http://openchemist.net/chemistry/show.php?id=analytical&story=env001).

The Stalinon case, resulted in new legislation governing marketing licences and the issue of quality control of medicines in France in 1958-59: the judicial enquiry and subsequent court case in 1958 concluded that the manufacturers (Février) were liable for having put on the market a product of insufficient quality. The Chief Executive, Ms Feuillet, was sent to prison for two years and fined. Apart from the legal penalties, the French State also amended the legislation governing the issuance of marketing licences, enacting the Ordinance of 4th February 1959, which set new requirements for marketing licences, which included the duty to provide details of all clinical trial reports (Bonah, 2007).

Chemie Grünenthal synthesized Thalidomide (alpha-[N-phthalimido] glutarimide) and tested it in mice, dogs, rats, guinea pigs and rabbits (Mellin & Katzenstein, 1962). It had not been tested in pregnant animals, but the same effect was found in mice, rats, hamsters, rabbits, macaques, marmosets, baboons and rhesus monkeys. An LD_{50} (median lethal dose) was never established since there was no apparent toxicty even in high doses (Burley, 1988) (see under regulatory responses).

A year after the *'Maladies Médicamenteuses'* G. Duchesanay produced *'Le Risque Thérapeutique, prevention et traitment des accidents'* (The therapeutic risk, prevention and treatment of adverse reactions). This is again very clinical and covers contraindications and treatment. It deals with methyl salicylate, sodium salicylate and Aspirin.

1955 *'Reactions with Drug Therapy'* by Harry L. Alexander, WB Saunders Company 1955. Despite its general title it only concerns type 'B' reactions, which reflects the authors position as editor of the 'Journal of Allergy'. The 301 pages give considerable details of animal studies as well as human.

In the US there was a nation-wide campaign of poliomyelitis

vaccination using vaccine made by Cutter laboratories. In the next two months 260 cases were reported in vaccinees and their contacts. Two batches of the formaldehyde inactivated Salk type Cutter vaccine were found to contain living virus (Wade, 1970).

The Council on Pharmacy and Chemistry of the American Medical Association produced '*New program of operation for evaluation of drugs*'. It said ' *Pharmaceutical firms are encouraged to cooperate with the Council by forwarding complete data or reports (published and unpublished) of all laboratory and clinical investigations relating to the safety and usefulness of new drugs in order that evaluation reports may be made to the profession at the earliest possible date*'. All this data was made available to a number of recognised experts whose views were given to the Council, who would then consider all the evidence and then write a mongraph, which would be published in *JAMA* after the pharmaceutical company had offered any criticism of the monograph to the Council (Stormont, 1955).

The FDA form (FD 356) for an NDA[163] contained the following statement: '*An application may be incomplete or may be refused unless it includes full reports of adequate tests by all methods reasonably applicable to show whether or not the drug is safe for use as suggested in the proposed labeling*'…*Reports of all clinical tests by experts, qualified by scientific training and experience to evaluate the safety of drugs, should be attached and ordinarily should include detailed information pertaining to each individual treated, including age, sex, conditions treated, dosage, frequency of administration, duration of administration of the drug, results of clinical and laboratory exaninations made, and a full statement of any adverse effects and therapeutic results observed*'. The last clause was used as a primary regulatory strategy to refuse marketing to drugs about which medical officers had scepticism, including Thalidomide (Waxman, 2003).

1956 During clinical trials of Thalidomide (Chemie Grünenthal) Dr Piacenza described a case of polyneuritis, which he had traced to the drug. Although the manufacturers became aware that this was the case in October 1959, they suppressed the information,

---

[163] NDA = New Drug Application (USA)

and later admitted that a neuropathy could occur, but described it as 'reversible' in spite of evidence to the contrary (Sjöström and Nilsson, 1972). The first case of Thalidomide phocomyelia was born on Christmas Day (Lenz, 2000).

The UK Therapeutic Substances Act 1956 this was only concerned with standard of strength, quality and purity of the same substances as in the 1925 act.

1957 1st October Chemie Grünenthal put Contergan (Thalidomide) on West German market as a sedative and mild hypnotic.

1958 Thalidomide on UK market as 'Distaval' on 14th April 1958.

The Drug Commission of the German Medical Association (DCGMA) requested all doctors to report adverse drug reactions to the Commission (www.akdac.de).

1959 The French State amended the legislation governing the issue of marketing licences, enacting the Ordinance of 4th February 1959. Article L.511 Code of Public Health, which set new requirements for marketing licences. The list of data to be submitted for issuance of the licence underwent considerable change; henceforth, applicants must file detailed written analysis and verification of both the raw materials and the finished product, documents that must be corroborated by an expert's report. The manufacturing facilities must be inspected, and reports of clinical trials must be provided.

Senator Kefauver started investigations which three years later led in 1962 to the emasculated Kefauver-Harris Amendment of the 1938 Food, Drug and Cosmetic Act (Abraham & Lawton Smith, 2003).

The Early Clinical Drug Evaluation Unit Program was set up in the USA, because less than 1% of new compounds reached the market (Prien, 1995).

The first benzodiazepine, Librium, or chlordiazepoxide, was introduced in the US and into Britain a year later. The CRM acknowledged that patients could be dependant on benzodiazepines in 1980. In 1988 the Committee of Safety of Medicines (CSM) advised against long-term use of

benzodiazepines because of dependence (Medawar, 1992).
It took many years before the dangers of barbiturates and
benzodiazepines were acknowledged by the regulatory
authorities and this was partly due to their rigorous defence by
the industry.

The ABPI advocated the creation of an 'independent' voluntary
trust to vet new drugs (Hancher, 1990).

November 1959 A UK Working Party was set up to *'review the
legislative provisions which relate to the control of medicinal
substances and to recommend what changes should be made
to rationalise and simplify the law with a view to ultimate
amendment and consolidation'.* The work of this group was
overtaken by events as the Thalidomide story evolved. At the
same time another group, the Interdepartmental Committee
on Drug Addiction recommended 'that *drugs having an effect
on the central nervous system and liable to produce physical
or psychiatric deterioration should be confined to supply on
prescription, subject to the advice of an independent expert body'.*

During 1959 The UK Poisons Board warned of the probability of
hazard to the health of the public from widespread use of potent
medicines for self-medication.

31st December. Dr A Leslie Florence published a letter in
the BMJ 'Is thalidomide to blame?' describing peripheral
neuropathy. He had seen four patients, who had taken
thalidomide, with parathesia of the hands and feet, coldness
of the extremities and nocturnal cramps in leg muscles. By
February 1961 Chemie Grünenthal had more than 400 cases
(Sjöstrom & Nilsson, 1972).

1960 10th November 1960 Dr Frances Kelsey wrote to William
S. Merrell Co. concerning the material on the clinical trials:
*'it fails to report the clinical studies in full detail. The report
should include detailed information relating to each individual
treated, including age, sex, conditions treated, dosage, frequency
of administration of the drug, results of clinical and laboratory
examinations, and a full statement of any adverse effects and
therapeutic results observed.*

Many of the cases reported in the application are in summary form without the necessary details included. In addition, the application is inadequate under section 505 (b) (1) of the act in that insufficient cases have been studied. Many of the 3,156 cited cases are in foreign literature reports and in many instances the reports do not represent detailed studies to determine the safety of the drug. The application should contain more cases in which detailed studies have been done.

The application is further inadequate and incomplete under section 506 (b) (1) of the act in that the chronic toxicity data are incomplete and therefore, no evaluation can be made of the safety of the drug when used for a prolonged period of time'. (Sjöstrom and Nilsson, 1972).

1961 December 16th 1961 Dr WG Mc Bride's letter was published in the Lancet announcing his observation '*that the incidence of multiple severe abnormalities in babies delivered of women who were given the drug thalidomide ('Distaval') during pregnancy as an anti-emetic or as a sedative, to be almost 20%'*. The Distiller's Company in Liverpool had received the news on November 21st 1961. Dr Widukind Lenz from Germany saw a suspected case for the first time on November 11th 1961 and informed the company on November 16th 1961. This changed the whole world of drug safety.

[Dr Mcbride was discredited 20 years later in the Benedectin case when he stated the Benedectin *"is not safe and that it caused birth defects'*. Bendectin - A combined preparation of doxylamine, dicyclomine and pyridoxine was marketed in the US for nausea of pregnancy under the name of Bendectin and in the UK two years later as Debendox. The long shadow of thalidomide claimed it as a victim when it was alleged to cause congenital abnormalities. Nine cohort studies and case-control studies failed to show a causal relationship, but in spite of this the drug had to be withdrawn from the market in 1983 (MacMahon, 1981; Orme, 1985). Finally a legal action found for the company and no damages were ever awarded to the 1100 plaintiffs] (Masheter, 1985).

The plaintiff's case was that there was a relative risk of 1.49 and confidence limits of 0.17 to 3. They did not offer a single study that did not include a confidence interval including 1.0 (Christoffel & Teret, 1991). Another assessment of these studies showed a relative risk of 0.89 with confidence intervals of 0.76 to 1.04 (MacMahon, 1981).

Dr Kelsey said at an open public scientific workshop on *'Thalidomide: potential benefits and risk'* on September 9th-10th 1997: *'I joined the Food and Drug Administration as a medical officer in August of 1960. I spent the first months going around various areas of the Food and Drug Administration getting familiar or getting introduced to the type of work that was done there. On September 1st, I reported to the Bureau of Medicine as a reviewing medical officer. The thalidomide application was filed shortly after September the 8th. Although it was usual to give applications around more or less in rotation, since I was new, they selected an easy one for me…. Now, I should explain, however, that the applications really were quite a bit different from what they are today. A lot of them were for fairly ordinary drugs, minor molecular modifications of long-used drugs, or a new mixture of old drugs. It was rare that a really new and exciting drug came in, and it was in those applications that the best clinical and animal studies were performed. In general, at the time, drug testing was not considered a very scholarly pursuit by most people. Many of the studies in support of new drugs were written really more as promotions than as scientific studies. The ground rules in those days were that after an application had been submitted and filed with the agency, the agency had 60 days in which to decide that the drug was safe for the proposed use or uses. There was no requirement for efficacy, and this of course was one reason why the applications were so much smaller. In fact, the thalidomide application was four volumes in size, as I recall. That was about standard. I think I remember one that was 11, and one that was one or perhaps two. Now, although I guess they're mostly computerized, it's a matter of 100 or 200 volumes.The applications were reviewed, as they are now, by a chemist, and a pharmacologist, and a medical officer. The chemists were in the same little prefab building that we were in on the Mall between 7th and Independence, where the Museum of Science and Industry now is. The pharmacologists were in another bureau altogether, in the Department of Agriculture. The medical officer really had the choice. They could do the pharmacology themselves or they could ask for a consult from the pharmacologist. I chose the latter course. We had, as I said, 60 days. If we hadn't communicated with the company before that, they could have automatically assumed that it was okay, and marketed it. So very close tabs was always kept on the date. We did get our letter out on November the 10th, although I said the application was received on the 8th, or some little time before it got logged in. I think the official date of acknowledgement was September the 15th. So we got our letter out on the 10th of November. In this, we declared that the application was incomplete and inadequate, and could not be filed. Then we gave the reasons for our decision. We all had fairly serious questions. The pharmacologist felt that the chronic toxicity studies had not run for a sufficient length of time. He also felt that there were inadequate absorption and excretion data. The chemist found all sorts of problems or shortcomings with the manufacturing controls. She had concerns about the asymmetrical carbon atom, and wondered what was known about the D[164] and the L forms, and in what proportion they were present, and so on. She, fortunately, had been educated in German, and a lot of this application consisted of German reprints with an English translation. She of course could read the original German, and did find at least one error in the translation. I, who know no German, or just enough to pass a Ph.D. exam in it, was very impressed by this. I had some problems. The data to submit safety was very sketchy and anecdotal. The claims were quite fulsome, you might say, almost. It was of course perfectly non-toxic. It lacked hangover effect. It was non-habituating, or addicting, and so on. But one by one, these claims sort of were modified somewhat. I was particularly – and all of us were – concerned about the fact that you seem to be able to give enormous amounts, both to animals and humans, without any effect of perhaps drowsiness or sedation. In fact, one of the claims or one of the mentions in the brochure included several cases in which persons had tried to commit suicide, and been unable to do*

---

[164] D and L forms = Two substances can have the same chemical composition, because of different optical activity. The dextro (D) form twists polarised light to the right whilst the levo (L) form does so to the left.

so. You've probably heard a later comment that, had thalidomide been on the market, Marilyn Monroe would be alive today. Well, pretty soon it was acknowledged that, like all other drugs of its class, there was indeed some hangover effect, but we were concerned about this non-absorption. We felt there might be conditions of the non-toxicity, which we felt was surely due to non-absorption, and we thought there might be conditions, illness or another drug or something like that, that might change this so much more would be absorbed, and toxic effects might appear. We did not know, for some years later, that a solution of liquid form of the drug had been marketed in Germany, particularly for use in children. When the British company thought they would market a similar one, their pharmacologist was horrified to find out how very toxic this compound was. I can still remember his anguish when he described experiments he had done. It was a micronized preparation in a sweet solution. Despite his findings, however, it was marketed for a while in Britain. As I understand it, the preparation was taken off the market because of some toxicity in humans, but we didn't know this. The application was resubmitted again on January the 17th, which meant that by mid-March we would have to give them another opinion. We were continually concerned about the lack of data on metabolism, excretion, absorption, and this curious lack of toxicity. Then, at the end of February – the 23rd, I think it was, actually – we picked up a number – it was actually the December 30th number – of the British Medical Journal, which contained Florence's article posing the question, did thalidomide cause peripheral neuritis? This was a little late in getting to us, because the mail was on strike. It was actually a shipping strike, I think, and we did not get our British and other foreign publications by airmail in those days. However, this did come in time. When we questioned the company about it, they said they had just seen that, too. They were sort of surprised, and were going over to Europe to find out more, and would let us know when they came back. Now, what we didn't know, again, was the German company had been questioned about peripheral neuritis as early as the winter of December of 1959, before our application was even submitted. The same person that asked them about it this time gave a paper – I believe it was in May of 1960 – describing a number of cases of peripheral neuritis, some of which seemed pretty severe. The British actually answered the first report by saying that they were aware of it, and had put some reference to it in the material that they distributed with the drug. Our company was not obliged to submit foreign supporting material or material of that type at that time, so we were not aware of this side effect. They had independently discovered it about May of 1960, and there is good evidence that the German and the British company had a sort of gentleman's agreement to keep the matter rather quiet until the American company had a chance to get the drug on the market. So we were inclined to believe that the American company had not heard of this earlier. The company did report to us on their trip to Europe. They said that indeed there did seem to be some cases that neither in Germany nor in England were it considered of great moment, and that both companies felt a little note on the labelling would suffice. There were even questions early on whether the drug should continue on an over-the-counter status, as it was in some parts of Germany, and other parts of the world. It was a little time later that the over-the-counter drug status was changed, and the drug became prescription-only. But it's difficult to exaggerate how popular this drug was at this time. I think it was the third largest-selling drug in Europe. As I mentioned, it was considered so safe that it was over-the-counter in many areas. We were concerned about the peripheral neuritis, even if the companies did not seem to be. We sought some outside consultations with neurologists, Dr. John Tower at NIH and Dr. Webb Haymaker in the Army Walter Reed Hospital. They both felt the same. They felt that peripheral neuritis could be serious, painful, and often irreversible. The risk of developing this would not be justified in a drug that was used simply as a hypnotic and sedative, since there were other drugs on the market for this purpose. We continued to feel it might be a serious matter. One of the questions we raised at this time was what would happen if the mother took it through pregnancy, and this drug was taken for quite long periods of time, what would be the effect of the drug on the child? This was not a shot in the dark, because at that time the Food and Drug

*Administration and the American Academy of Paediatrics had
been concerned about the effects of drugs when taken during
pregnancy, and were in the midst of preparing guidelines for the
testing of such drugs. There had been a number on the market
that had been shown to have disastrous effects – aminopyrine,
chloramphenicol, to name a few. I'd had a little experience some
years previously when I worked on the anti-malarial drug project
during World War II. We were given a little time for research,
and we were interested in the metabolism of the effective anti-
malarials, quinine and Atabrine. We established that the quinine
was very rapidly metabolised by the liver of the rabbit, but we
found that the foetal liver had no such activity, and it did not
appear till shortly after birth. This, of course, was the same
situation that causes the chloramphenicol problems. The baby
simply doesn't have the enzymes to protect itself against the
chloramphenicol as the adult did. The answer always was, if it
had had an ill effect, surely it would have been known by now.
That, of course, is a common excuse about any adverse effect. But,
interestingly enough, it had. A German in Bonn, Germany, a
paediatrician and a geneticist, had been struck by the increase of
phocomelia cases in their hospital. They felt it must be due to
some recently introduced substance, and they wrote around to a
number of other hospitals in Germany. Most of them reported the
same thing, that they had had an increase in this very unusual
adverse effect. They then thought they would find out the
experience of other countries where thalidomide had been used.
Most of them had indeed seen this increase. They were thrown
off, ironically, because they were under the impression that the
drug was released in the United States. The promotional
material said it was widely used in North America, and it had of
course been marketed in Canada. They wrote to three centres in
the U.S. where statistics were kept on birth defects. There wasn't
really any indication of an increase. This is, sadly enough, what
put them off the scent. It wasn't until November of 1961 that Lenz
discovered the association. Now, the first report of phocomelia
was announced at the end of November of 1961. The company
immediately phoned us, and told us the news, and said they
didn't really believe it, but as a precaution they would put a halt*

to clinical studies going on in this country. But they did want to continue some that they had just started on its possible usefulness in cancer. That seemed no great problem to us, the benefit/risk ratio being entirely different. In March, early March of 1962, they told us they were withdrawing the application immediately, as they believed there may be some truth to this association. There were some weird differences in wording of their two communications that led us to think it might have been more widely used in this country than we had gathered from the new drug application, so we asked for a complete list of the doctors they had sent the drug to, and were very surprised to find that actually over 1,000 doctors had been given the drug. Most of these were recruited after the application had been submitted in September, in the expectation that it would be rapidly approved. They were told, in essence, "Don't really worry about recording the results. We just want you to try it out, and see if you want to use it in your patients." We then visited, or had the company visit, every one of these doctors, and pick up what remaining stocks they had -- and there were indeed quite a lot -- and find out if they had had any phocomelic or abnormal births amongst the patients they had given the drug to. In all, we found about 10 or 11 cases that we thought might be due to the trials in this country. There were an additional seven patients or subjects where it was clear that the drug had been gotten from a foreign source. Now, the thalidomide tragedy in Europe actually didn't cause a great stir at the time in this country because there really were, except for those few, no victims. The one person who was concerned was Dr. Helen Taussig, who was the professor of cardiology at the Johns Hopkins Hospital. She had heard about the outbreak from an ex-resident of hers who was now in Germany, and he had urged her to come across and see some of the victims, many of whom had cardiac defects. Before going, she had contacted another ex-resident who was working at the Food and Drug Administration, and when she got back she invited both him, Dr. John Nestor, and myself to hear the results. They were essentially published later in the JAMA after she gave a talk to the American Academy of Physicians. It caused a great increase in the science of teratology, or means of testing drugs for

237

adverse effects in pregnancy. So those were some of the immediate good effects. I would say, however, that thalidomide never faded away. I mentioned that we permitted certain trials in cancer to proceed. Some years later, when an application was submitted for leprosy, we felt that was a reasonable use, since there was great need for such a drug in this distressing disease, and the patients would be under pretty good control'.

She also spoke before the House committee, but it really wasn't until mid-July when the article in the Post came out, authored by Morton Mintz, that the country realized the enormity of the problem. Almost immediately, the long-awaited Kefauver-Harris bill was passed in October. This not only required proof of safety, but also proof of efficacy. It also included a last-minute addition that patient consent must be obtained from all subjects in the clinical trials in the future. Meanwhile, FDA had hastened to strengthen the investigational drug requirements, and essentially published early in July, what was finalized in early March, with the addition of this efficacy and consent requirements. So these were the two immediate effects of thalidomide, the strengthening of the law and the regulations, both offering greater protection both to subjects of trials and to the public getting drugs later.

It also stimulated other countries to bring new laws. Many of them had laws such as we did back in 1930, before 1930, when a manufacturer could simply put a drug on the market if he felt it was safe when used as labelled. The onus was on the government to remove them. But many of them introduced laws similar to our 1962 ones, and one of the great forward steps has been the harmonization, the efforts being made to bring the requirements of Japan, the European countries, and the United States into harmony. This of course will add to more rapid marketing of good and safe drugs, and protection against unsafe ones. It also increased greatly the efforts to monitor birth defects. (Provided by the US Food and Drug Administration)

Louis Pasteur gave the inaugural lecture as professor and dean of the faculty of science, University of Lille, Douai, France on December 7, 1854: *'In the fields of observation chance favours only those minds which are prepared.'* Dr Kelsey's mind was prepared.

Preludes to the Thalidomide disaster

Following the Thalidomide disaster most countries hurried to enact laws to try to prevent any recurrence of a similar disaster and at the same time to reduce the risks from new drugs. One must acknowledge the earlier attempts to do the latter:

Ancient Greece: Hippocrates aphorism: *'Drugs may be administered to pregnant women from the fourth to the seventh month of gestation'.* Had this advice been followed the thalidomide phocomelia would not have occurred. The damage caused by thalidomide was between the 34th and 50th day of gestation (Lenz, 1992).

UK: The aborted recommendation for the creation of a Medicines Commission in 1914; the ABPI avocation of the creation of an 'independent' voluntary trust to vet new drugs in 1959 and the commissioning of a UK Working Party in November 1959 to 'review the legislative provisions which relate to the control of medicinal substances'.

France: The Ordinance of 4th February 1959. Article L.511 Code of Public Health in response to the Stalinon disaster.

Sweden: Swedish and Norwegian drug laws in 1934 and 1928 respectively, which required manufacturers to demonstrate the safety and efficacy of their products prior to approval, but they still approved Thalidomide.

USA: Chauncey Leake in 1929: 'The rational introduction of new drugs requires the close cooperation of chemists, pharmacologists and clinicians. Reliable pharmacologic study is necessary in the development of new drugs to estimate

Toxicity

Type and mode of action.

Worthiness of application to human beings.

Reasonable replacement of existing drugs.

'Clinical evaluation should be made under controlled conditions in research hospitals. Physicians should not use new drugs in daily practice until favourable reports from such sources have been published in reputable journals'. (Leake, 1929).

Germany: The Drug Commission of the German Medical Association (DCGMA) requesting in 1958 that all doctors should report adverse drug reactions to the Commission.

All these efforts were to no avail and although the Bundesverfassungsger icht's (Federal Constitutional Court) final position leaves no doubt that most of the charges brought against Chemie Grünenthal by the prosecution were considered to have been legally substantiated and the company paid 114 million marks in a settlement, the court and prosecutors thought that it was not in the general interest to pursue the trial (Sjöstrom & Nilsson, 1972). Dr Roy Goulding, who was a consultant Clinical Toxicologist at Guy's Hospital and a senior Medical Officer at the UK Ministry of Health, said *'Its all very well to say we should have tested it more thoroughly, but we had no means at all for testing for teratogenicity at that time and it took a long while to get any such procedure'* (Goulding, 1997). The Grünenthal website states' *The Grand Criminal Court of the Landgericht Aachen,... Having reviewed all the charges, the court closed the proceedings with a judgement of minor fault'.* http://www.contergan.grunenthal.info/ctg/en_EN/pdf/ctg_en_en_ctg_brosch. pdf) Accessed 22nd July 2009.

Allergic reactions

2640 BC The first mention of a possible case of anaphylaxis was in 2640 BC when Pharaoh Menes died after a wasp sting.

49 BC Carus in 49 BC spoke of *'what is food to one to some becomes fierce poison'* is the first reference to idiosyncrasy.

1586 Marcello Donati described angio-oedema in a patient after eating eggs (Juhlin, 2000).

1740 Synonyms for urticaria were: Uredo (Plinius), Knidosis (Hypocrates) and Zedler used by Urbiano in 1740.

1780 Charles Webster in 1780 referred to *'urticaria medicamentis vix unquam indiget'* [There have almost always been remedies for nettlerash] (Webster, 1780).

1800 Cullen quotes Heberden as saying that urticaria may be caused by wild valerian root (still used as a mild tranquillizer in 2009), eating of fish not sufficiently dressed, mussels, shrimps and even honey, and the kernels of fruits (Cullen, 1800). Dr Lancelot Aery used similar words in a pamphlet dated 1774. He also added Occ. Vel Chel. Cancer, which may refer to allergy to an eye ointment (Aery, 1774).

1839 Magendie produced anaphylaxis in dogs when he gave them repeated albumen injections (Magendie, 1839).

1852 Miale called it *'idiopathic idiosyncrasy'*. (Miale, 1852).

1870 Engelmann described a case of mercurial eczema who had *swelling of the face… itching*, which suggests angioedema (Engelmann, 1870).

1878 Heilein referred to sodium salicylate causing *'oedema of both eyelids, intolerable itching and diffusely scattered wheals'* .(Heinlein, 1878) The latter being urticaria.

1880 Virchow mentions *'mystery of individuality'* and *' it is the individual peculiarities which the tissues of certain persons evince in regard to medicines'.* (Virchow, 1880).

1883 Lewin refers to symptoms, which are not poisonous effects, simply because they may not occur in 999 cases and yet appear in the thousandth' and he called them *'that natural peculiarity of each individual'.* (Lewin, 1883).

1885 Morrow in 1885 referred to some rashes as idiosyncrasy, which he defined as *'abnormal susceptibility to external impressions which is manifest in certain individuals, a condition which has been regarded as inexplicable as it is mysterious, as an ultimate fact, unknown and unknowable'.* He later refers to *'erythematous and urticarial eruptions of arsenic, belladonna, bromide of potassium, chloral, copaiba, digitalis, hyoscyamus, opium, morphia, quinine, strammonium, salicylic acid, etc., as angio-neurotic phenomena, caused by the specific action of the drugs in question upon the vaso-motor system'.* (Morrow, 1885).

1903 Serum sickness was first described (Hamburger, 1903).

1905 CF Von Pirquet and B Schick described serum sickness on giving diphtheria antiserum from horses to man and coined the word 'allergy' (Pirquet & Schick, 1905).

1912 In an article entitled 'Hypersensitivity' in 1912 it says that anaphylaxis appears to be confined to proteins, and vegetables, e.g. serum, milk and bacterial cells, but there is no mention of drugs (Goodall, 1912).

1914 There were cases of anaphylaxis to various drugs including morphine (Silvestri, 1914) .

1915 Another possible case of anaphylaxis to morphine (Scott, 1915).

1914–1915   There was a case of anaphylaxis with mercury which occurred 'some years' before 1917 (Robertson & Fleming, 1918) and this case is the earliest concerning a drug in man that I have found.

1924   Sir Thomas Lewis suggested that some vascular skin reactions may be caused by the liberation of the 'H-substance' (Lewis & Grant, 1924).

1932   In 1932 it was shown that anaphylaxis was associated with histamine release (Dragstedt & Gebauer-Fuelnegg, 1932).

Several sources have said that Case IV in Jenner's book published in 1798 had details of anaphylaxis (Jenner, Edward. An inquiry into the causes and effects of the variolæ vaccinæ, a disease discovered in some of the western counties of England, ... and known by the name of the cow pox. By Edward Jenner, M.D., F.R.S.&c. London, 1798. Eighteenth Century Collections Online. Gale Group). One possible reference to an allergic reaction was on page 43 *'I have inoculated Pead and Barge, two of the boys whom you lately infected with the cow-pox. On the second day the incisions were inflamed and there was a pale inflammatory stain around them. On the third day these appearances were still increasing and their arms itched considerably. On the fourth day the inflammation was evidently subsiding, and on the sixth day it was scarcely perceptible. No symptom of indisposition followed'.* This is not a description of anaphylaxis, but is suggestive of urticaria. Another article (Baxby, 1985) refers to a footnote of his fourth case: Mary Barge as being a case of anaphylaxis. Let the reader judge for themselves:

'Case IV. Mary Barge, of Woodford, in this parish, was inoculated with variolous matter in the year 1791. An Efflorescence of a palish red colour soon appeared about the parts where the matter was inserted, and spread itself rather extensively, but died away in a few days without producing any variolous symptoms. She has since been repeatedly employed as a nurse to small-pox patients, without experiencing any ill consequences. This woman had the cow-pox when she lived in the service of a farmer in this parish thirty-one years before.

'It is reasonable that variolous matter, when the system is disposed to reject it, should excite inflammation on the part

to which it is applied more speedily that when it produces the Small Pox. Indeed it becomes almost a criterion by which we can determine whether the infection will be received or not. It seems as if a change, which endures through life, had been produced in the action, or disposition to action, in the vessels of the skin; and it is remarkable too, that whether this change has been effected by the small-pox, or the cow-pox, that the disposition to sudden cuticular inflammation is the same on the application of variolous matter'.

Poison

The use of this term may not be helpful, since as Paracelsus has said, it is a question of dose. There are five different circumstances:

Where there is a single active principle in a specific species of a herb and it is responsible both for its efficacy and its adverse effect (i.e. a true side effect) and where the amount of the active principle is reasonably constant so that an accurate dose can be given, then the word 'poison' would be inappropriate.

Again where the single active principle in a specific species of a herb is responsible both for its efficacy and its adverse effect, but where an accurate dose cannot be assured, then the term may be appropriate, e.g. if a single farmer always grows the same species of herb and farms in a constant manner, e.g. harvesting and storing the herb in an identical manner over time, then the active principle is likely to have a narrow range and an accurate dose would be possible. However a wholesaler collecting herbs of different species of the same herb from many countries would be likely to have very wide limits for the active principle and be unable to guarantee an accurate dose. A consumer may consider the first sample of the herb to be non-poisonous and the second poisonous.

The third possibility is that there is more than one active principle in a herb and that the active principle responsible for its efficacy is not the same one that is responsible for its adverse effect. Under these circumstances the ratio between the two active principles may vary from species to species and crop to crop so that although an accurate dose may be found for the active principle responsible for efficacy the dose for the second active principle may be very variable and under these circumstances the herb may be considered as a poison.

Where there were several herbs with different active principles but had similar actions, the one with the best benefit/risk ratio may have been called a medicine whereas the one with worst benefit/risk ratio may have been called a poison.

Where there is a narrow therapeutic ratio individual variations in response may mean that a large number experience adverse events and may consider themselves poisoned.

The term was probably used very loosely by the early writers expressing their lack of knowledge of the herb or expertise in using the herb correctly and at the same time wishing to err on the safe side. The Anglo-Saxon word for poison was 'bane' hence 'henbane', but now means 'cause of trouble'.

Demise of Drugs

The life expectancy of humans has increased steadily with acceleration from the 1950s whilst the life expectancy of drugs has been the reverse with a slow decrease accelerating since the 1950s. The factors involved are probably:

The discovery of the active principle of herbs making the herb redundant, e.g. opium → morphia, henbane → hyoscyamine.

The discovery of better drugs for the same purpose, e.g. arsenic for syphilis → penicillin.

The manufacture of the drug is no longer profitable.

A worsening of the cost/benefit ratio due to the discovery of a new serious ADR, e.g. thalidomide.

A change in medical philosophy, e.g. realisation that purging was not beneficial to the patient - hellebore.

The corollary to this is that there are factors, which prolong the life of a drug, such as:

a. The development of a salt of the original drug, e.g. $Hg \rightarrow Hg_2Cl_2 \rightarrow$ Merthiolate/mersalyl.

b. The discovery of a niche market, e.g. thalidomide for leprosy.

c. The discovery of a new application, e.g. aspirin for prevention of diseases. In the Massachusetts General hospital there was steep decline in use of several drugs from 1820 until 1880.

Calomel 1820 - 58 %; 1880 - 5%

Tartar emetic 1820 – 21%; 1880 – 0%

Ipecacuanha 1820 – 12%; 1880 – 0%

And also in procedures: Venesection 1820 – 46%; 1880 – 10%; cupping 1820 – 9%; 1880 – 0%; leeching 1820 – 12%; 1880 – 0% [approximate figures from a graph] (Warner, 1990).

Persistence of drugs

As explained above some drugs continue to be used for very specific purposes despite having ADRs that should otherwise exclude their use. Again this is seen with venesection which has persisted for the removal of a specific blood constituent such as: primary haemochromatosis (ferritin), polycythaemia (haemoglobin) and porphyria cutanea tarda (ferritin). Of the 50 drugs dealt with in this chapter the following are still used for specific indications:

Thalidomide – leprosy and other skin diseases, multiple myeloma and myelodysplastic syndromes.

Mercury (Thiomersal) – vaccine antiseptic.

Antimony – leishmaniasis (pentavalent antimonials).

Arsenic – trypanosomiasis (trivalent arsenic) and dermatitis herpetiformis (Fowler's solution).

Bismuth – peptic ulceration (tripotassium dicitrato bismuthate).

Urethane – animal anaesthetic.

Phenobarbitone – epilepsy.

Oxyphenisatin – enema.

Stilboestrol – hormonal-dependant cancer.

Chloramphenicol – eye ointment.

Panaceas

Named after the daughter of Aesculapius and similar to the Greek word 'panakeia' with 'pan' meaning 'all' and 'akos' cure, a universal remedy, which cannot exist. The panacea in 1916, seems to have been potassium iodide as it was used for: syphilis, yaws, gonorrhoea, leprosy, gout, chronic rheumatism, rheumatoid arthritis, hepatic cirrhosis, amyloid liver, pericarditis, myocardial disease, arterio-sclerosis, aneurism of the thoracic aorta, acute bronchitis, asthma, disseminated sclerosis and goitre. Most of the known active drugs were used for diseases other than their main indication. e.g. chloroform for angina pectoris, hydrophobia, laryngitis stridulosa, asthma, epilepsy and infantile convulsions. Other panaceas were: bleeding, mercury, antimony, quinine, gold and digitalis (Ackerknecht, 1973). Since the drugs had no benefit to the patient, unless thay had the one specific disease which it might heal, any adverse effects were not balanced by the chance of benefit.

The strength of the evidence that an adverse event was caused by a drug

The evidence varies from the weak case reports (1) to the strong randomised clinical trial (5).

1. Case reports.

   These are reports of single patients, which may produce hypotheses;

but rarely give sufficient information to be able to exclude alternative causes. However on rare occasions they can show that a drug did cause the event in that particular patient, e.g. a well-documented positive rechallenge, but even these can be misleading (Stephens, 1983). They can give no idea of the frequency of the reaction. Horace in 23 BC said that after taking Hellebore ' *I've lost the pleasure of imagination',* but gives no information as to how he drew this conclusion. Later in 1596 Paracelsus tried mercury on a persistent case of syphilis and came to the conclusion that this had cured the patient. Self-experimenters often produced strong evidence by taking a drug and then taking objective measures subsequently, e.g. Samuel Crumpe in 1793 with opium. Single case reports, especially as part of spontaneous reporting to regulatory bodies, have been the most successful means of creating hypotheses (Venning IV,1983), but these have rarely been validated (Loke et al., 2006).

2. Large uncontrolled prospective cohorts.

These have been used by pharmaceutical companies as part of Phase IV studies. They almost never discover new ADRs. They played no part in the period covered by this book.

3. Case series.

These are patients who have been exposed to a drug and the adverse events that they have suffered have been reported by the prescriber. They can give some idea of frequency. Again they rarely have sufficient information to be able to exclude alternative causes. Since neither a case report nor a case series have a control group other than historic controls they cannot exclude bias.

When Xenophon in 354 BC said that hyoscyamus drives those who take it mad he was, no doubt, referring to his experience of what had happened to the patients he had treated. An excellent example of a case series was that performed by Samuel Bard in 1765 using opium and making regular recordings of the pulse. He repeated the experiment on himself three times giving a double positive rechallenge. Most of the publications mentioned in this book must have been based on case series of the authors, perhaps with evidence from previous authors. Case series have discovered most of new important ADRs, described in this book e.g. thalidomide, streptomycin and aspirin.

4. Case-control studies.

These are a collection of similar adverse events where one has retrospectively compared antecedent exposures with a similar group without the adverse event. The technique wasn't suggested until 1955 (Neyman, 1955). One can stretch one's imagination to see early stirrings of case-control studies; perhaps those cases of accidental poisoning where the offending herb was not known until enquiry after the event, with the event itself being so unusual as not to occur without having taken some poison. However, although these may have the essential quality of being a retrospective judgement they would not have had a formal control group, e.g. Stedman in 1751 reported a group from his regiment who had taken leaves of a plant afterwards recognised as *Hyoscyamus niger*.

5. Cohort studies.

   These are prospective or retrospective studies of groups of patients who have and have not had an exposure to a drug. In 1061 two patients ran a race one having had ginseng and the other not. At the end of the race their shortness of breath was compared. A cohort of two patients would have been insufficient to draw conclusions, which could have been extrapolated, to other patients. It wasn't until 1662 that Helmont chose cohorts of 200 or 500 patients and divided them into two groups that there were sufficient numbers to provide a controlled study.

6. Controlled clinical trials (unrandomised) Originally when physicians treated a series of patients with a new drug they would have put the results into context by reference to their past experience. Later they would have compared the results with a previous group of patients treated by other means but documented in the same way. Colebrook's study (see 1948) used this method but he realised that comparing treatment with Sulphonamide and previous treatments for *Haemolytic streptococcal* infections might be confounded by the possibility that the virulence of the streptococcus might have declined in the interim, so for the later studies he used concurrent controls allocating treatment in rotation.

7. Randomised controlled clinical trials.

   These are prospective studies where the investigator allocates the treatment by means of randomisation and the MRC trial of streptomycin is a classic example. The use of the word 'caused' means in the context of adverse drug reactions that it was final factor in the production of the event, although this is open to discussion.

The collection of adverse events during a clinical trial for both the active group and a placebo group reveals how false the 'adverse reactions' frequency found in a cohort study without a control group can be. In a low dose aspirin trial, with 22, 071 patients, comparing 325 mgm Aspirin on alternate days with placebo the figure for gastrointestinal discomfort was 26.1% on Aspirin and 25.6% on placebo and for bleeding problems 27.0% for the aspirin group and 20.4% for the placebo group. This difference was statistically significant (Physicians' Health Study Research Group, 1989; Amery, 1994). How many patients had a bleeding problem because of aspirin? If one used the figure obtained from the aspirin group alone the incidence would be approximately four times higher than the incidence when the placebo group was considered in the analysis. A sub-group of clinical trials: large simple randomised controlled studies are useful for detection excess mortality due to the drug, e.g. Clofibrate v placebo (Committee of Principal Investigators, 1980), Salmeterol v Salbutamol (Castle et al., 1993). Randomised controlled clinical trials played very little part in the period covered in this book. These are useful for determing common ADRs, but rarely have sufficient numbers to detect very rare, but important ADRs.

Books on the side-effects and abuse of drugs

The first book dedicated only to side-effects and covering several drugs was Guérard's thesis (55 pages) in 1862 followed by a fellow countryman's thesis, Berenguer (59 pages) in 1874, covering dermatological effects for 12 and 7 drugs respectively. This presaged the first major book covering all major drugs and all types of reactions: Lewin's *The incidental effects of drugs : A pharmaceutical and Clinical Handbook'* (216 pages) published in German in 1881 with an English translation in 1883. This book covered 105 medications. All of these books discussed drug reactions in general and tried to explain them. Their authors were handicapped in their explanations by ignorance of allergic mechanisms, which were not known until Pirquet's paper in 1907. There followed a gap of 34 years before the next book on the side effects of modern drugs *(Die Nebenwirkungen der Modernen Arzneimittel)* was written by Otto Seifert in 1915. Leonard Meyler's first edition of 'Side-effect of drugs' (192 pages) in Dutch appeared in 1951 with an English edition a year later (268 pages). There were subsequent volumes at two - four yearly intervals, but in 1977 a *'Side-effects of Drugs Annual'* was introduced. The latest 15th edition (2007) in 6 volumes dealing with about 1,550 drugs with 4007 pages indicates the vast expansion that has taken place over the last 50 years. Meyler's books are the final expression of the total output of Pharmacovigilance. Two months after Meyler published his first English edition another French book was published '*Maladies Médicamenteuses d'ordre Thérapeutique et Accidentel*' by Claude Albahary (751 pages). This book was written for clinicians with considerable detail on the chemical properties and physiology as well as details of the clinical history with many references. It is 38 times the size of Meyler's first edition. In 1954 G. Duchesanay wrote '*Le Risque Thérapeutique, prevention et traitment des accidents*' (600 pages). The following year '*Reactions with Drug Therapy*' by an American, Harry L. Alexander, was published but this only dealt with allergic reactions.

French dermatologists seem to have been the first of the specialists to take an interest in drug reactions, perhaps because the early treatment of syphilis–the French disease - with mercury produced numerous skin reactions and that the whole of the condition was obvious to both patient and physician from its first manifestation. There has always been a French predominance in the clinical aspects of adverse drug reactions whilst the English-speaking world has been foremost in pharmacoepidemiology. The first book on adverse drug reactions in Polish was written by Professor Jan Venulet and was published in 1964 by Panstowy Zaklad Wydawnictw Lekarskich. Its title was '*Powiklania w leczeniu farmakologicznym*'.

Nearly all the writers from Hippocrates onwards crictize their predecessors and their contemporaries for using the wrong dose, formulation or using them for the wrong diseases. Ackerknecht names Asklepiades, Galen, Paracelsus, Fernelius, van Helmont, Sydenham, Boerhave and Gaub as those who have complained about the misuse or abuse of treatments. He goes on to say that at the beginning of the 18th century the first monographs on iatrogenic diseases appear in Halle in Germany:

1. 1726 GE Stahl '*Examination of badly cured and spoiled diseases*' in which he condemns cathartics, emetics, sudorifics and especially opium which he says produces hectic fevers, dropsy, cachexia, colics and gout. Mercury for epilepsy is a very harmful treatment with gold a swindle and Peruvian bark extremely dangerous. Spas, astringents and iron medication are misused.

2. 1728 GE Weiss '*Doctors as the cause of disease*' mentioning the detrimental effects of bleeding and antimony.

3. 1736 Frederich Hoffmann wrote three pamphlets: '*Unwise medication as a cause of many diseases and death*'; '*On the misuse and the damage arising from the application of the mild medicaments*': '*Ordinary errors in the application of local remedies in practice*'.

4. A series of dissertations in Latin from Halle all dealing with iatrogenic disease: Zweifel in 1701, Curtius in1714, Langguth in 1739, Kühnein 1763, Zeys in 1772, Schlenther in 1777, J Ch WJunker in 1791 and J Ch Reil in 1799.
5. 1788 J Lenhardt '*Medicaments without mask*'.
6. 1802 Curt Sprengel '*Handbook of Pathology*'.
7. 1775 Thomas Withers of Edinburgh wrote '*Observations on the misuse of medicaments*' where he criticizes the abuse of bleeding, emetics, purging, sudorifics, stimulants, mercury, opium, tea, coffee, and bark. He mentions only these two drugs.

Regulations and laws

There are several themes running through the legislation:

The adulteration of drugs and the striving for their purity.

The protection of the pharmacists' monopoly for providing medicines and the protection of the physician's and surgeons monopoly for care of the patient.

The appointment of committees to judge whether a drug should be allowed on the market.

The first two themes have been fairly constant over a long period whilst the third was a product of the 20th century.

There was a growing crescendo of concern, which was overtaken by the Thalidomide disaster.

Summary

The arrival of Aspirin with a very strong sales programme meant that its ADRs would be discovered early due to its widespread usage. It had been preceded by other salicylates, which were also effective and could have competed with Aspirin. The 1894 BMA Survey and the 1908 U.S. Survey of acetanilide, antipyrin and Phenacetin were the forerunners of Prescription Event Monitoring.The rapid increase in synthetic drugs: phenacetin, benzodiazepines, barbiturates, arsphenamine, insulin, thyroxine, penicillin, dinitrophenol, amidopyrine, clioquinol, prontosil, antibiotics, etc; meant that loopholes in the drug-testing programme were soon discovered and various attempts were made to deal with these, but in the end the Thalidomide debacle over shadowed all the other problems. Several laws were iniated to deal with failures, but other influences counteracted any major advances.

Part 2: Analysis of the Marker Drugs

Analysis of the dates when the ADRs were first reported and their descriptions should throw light on the pharmacovigilance processes over time. We need then to compare the ADRs of our six marker drugs found before 1960 with those known today to discover whether the true ADRs were discovered, presuming that those known today give an accurate picture of the real ADRs. The earliest writers mention only symptoms and it isn't until the 1850- 60s that in the UK the physicians started physical examinations beyond taking the pulse and looking at the urine (Newman, 1958). The French were earlier and a manual of pathology was written in 1827 outlining a full physical examination (Martinet, 1827).

Many of the more advanced examinations required instruments, thermometers (1714), stethoscope (1819) sphygmomanometer (1902), etc. (see page 66) which were only developed after the 18th century. The patho-physiological mechanisms had to wait until laboratory investigations were sufficiently advanced.

Chapter 9. Hellebore

Indications: pneumonia, fevers, chronic and hemicranial headache, mania, melancholy, dropsy without fever, epilepsy, paralysis, longstanding gout, diseases of joints, inflammation of the liver, chronic jaundice, odd affections of the trachea (Hahnemann, 1810), diuretic, warts, skin disease, drains black bile, eases toothache and improves the eyesight. It also was used for killing mice (Lev & Amar, 2008).

Table 3. Adverse reactions to Hellebore

Abbreviations: V=Viride, A=Album, N=Niger. H=Hahnemann's provings

Hellebore Adverse Events	Reports prior to 1852	Dispensatory of the USA 1858	Lewin 1881	King's American Dispensatory 1898	SE of Drugs 1952	ADR 2007
Salivation	H		A		V	AVN
Vertigo	1791, H	VN	A	A		x
Stupor	H			AV		N
Thirst	873A, H		A	N		N
Mouth and throat tingling/burning	873A, 1845A, H		A burning	N A (Sore mouth)	V Elek	V burning
Loss of voice	1798A, H			A		
Swelling of tongue/ throat	873A,1845A, H			A		N
Tremor	873A, 1798A			A		
Hiccup	1662, 1776N, H					
Vomiting	400 BC, 199, 783A, 1586NA, 1640A, 1651, 1657, 1662, 1694, 1752A, H 1776N, 1789A, 1845N,	AVN	A	AVN	V Elek	AVN
Diarrhoea (c blood)	585 BC, 1662, 1694, 1752A 1772N, 1789A, 1804A, H	A (c blood) N	A (c blood)	AVN (c blood)	V	VN

Hellebore Adverse Events	Reports prior to 1852	Dispensatory of the USA 1858	Lewin 1881	King's American Dispensatory 1898	SE of Drugs 1952	ADR 2007
Abdominal pain	1662, 1718, 1733,1752A, 1772N, 1790, 1845AN, H	N	A	N		N A
Gastric erosion	873A,			A (gastric heat)		A
Restlessness/anxiety	H	1789A	A			
Delirium	78, 783A,1662, 1640, 1845N, H (fits of madness)		A	N A (mental disturbance)		N
Muscular weakness	1662, 1817A, 1845A, H	A		AV		
Convulsions	370 BC, 1491, 1551, 1619, 1651A, 1662, 1752, 1776A, 1789A, 1790, 1798A, 1845A, H	N	A	AN		VN
Collapse ?hypotension			A			
Danger of suffocation	1586A, 1662, 1694, 1789A, H			V (stertorous breathing)		N
Bradycardia	873A, 199, H	V	A	VN	V Elek	AVN
Hypotension	1845 faintness, 1798 syncope, H	V	A	V	V Elek	AVN
Precordial oppression	H			A	V Elek	V
Heart failure				N	V	
Diuresis	1694, 1733, 1789, H			N		
Dizziness/Giddiness	1845A, H			VN		V
Sneezing (nasal use)	1586A,1657, 1752, H	A	A	AV		
Watery eyes	H (Inflammation)		A			V
Dimness of vision	1845A, (blindness), H	V	A	AV	V	V
Dilated pupils	1845A, H	V		AVN		
Spasms of ocular muscles	1568, H, eyes start out of head			A	V	
Difficult in swallowing, dry mouth.	H		A		V	V

Hellebore Adverse Events	Reports prior to 1852	Dispensatory of the USA 1858	Lewin 1881	King's American Dispensatory 1898	SE of Drugs 1952	ADR 2007
Somnolence	78 AD	V		V		
Headache	H	V			V	
Skin eruption	783A,1789, H Redness of face		A (local use)			N (local use)
Skin pricking (local use)			A			
Cold sweat	1789,1845N, H			AVN	V Elek	V
Tinnitus	H					N
Fever	1752, 1789,		A	V		
Death	370 BC, 1568, 1651, 1662, 1667, 1798.	N	A	AVN		V

Hahnemann (1825) quotes in his 2nd edition for Veratrum Album from 26 different historical sources and there are 716 symptoms written in the vernacular from 5 provers, which makes their interpretation difficult (Hahnemann, 1825). He doesn't mention stupor, fever or death, but does add more than 6 reports of cough and chilliness (?fever). There were 4 reports of dilated pupils and 4 for contracted pupils, other than these and reports concerning the pulse (no measurements of rate) there was nothing to indicate that a physical examination had occurred.

SE of Drugs 1952 = Meyler's Side Effects of Drugs 1st edition 1952 also mentions renal damage, pulmonary oedema and cerebral oedema.

Elek = Separate paper by Elek et al in 1953, placed here for convenience.

Hellebore is no longer mentioned in the British Pharmacopoeia, but it was in the US pharmacopoeia of 1898. In 1889 it was said to be no longer used, as it was obsolete, but still used in domestic animals. The active alkaloids in Veratrum viride or American hellebore were isolated in 1943 and by 1946 and became a product named 'Vertavis' and was used in clinical practice for hypertension. The adverse effects of these alkaloids were: Fall in blood pressure with collapse, bradycardia, nausea and vomiting, tightness in the chest, excess salivation, parathesia about the mouth, joints, hands and feet, and transient blurring of vision (Holley & Koffler, 1950). It was still use in 1962 in hypertension. It is also still available (Micromedex, 2008) in the USA as part of a mixture containing Veratrum viride, hyoscyamus and phenobarbitone or combined with Rauwolfia. It is difficult to date its demise from general use, but it was probably due to the change in medical philosophy in that it was no longer believed that purging patients or making them vomit was helpful. It wasn't until after Hellebore went out of fashion that the means to discover the mechanisms for the ADRs were discovered.

The early reports are often general comments and not specific: Dangerous 370 BC, 1491, 1619; fatal 370 BC, 1491; Poison 49 BC, 47 BC; too violent 1586; perilous 1657; unhappy remedy 23 BC; not to be taken 78 AD by old men, weaklings, etc. and frequently the early reports do not differentiate between the various types of hellebore. Present day evidence emphasises salivation, burning in the mouth and throat as well as bradycardia, but these are not mentioned prior to 1881. Again the different phraseology makes it difficult to know whether the ancients were describing the same thing as the modern writers. Reports by different authors tend to confirm that an event was caused by the drug, but several authors have been known to copy verbatim from previous authors so it is not absolute confirmation.

Chapter 10. Henbane

Indications: Inflammation, gout, pain, eye diseases, to stop bleeding, palpitations, excessive lacrimation, helping eyelids to grow, toothache, earache, insanity, epilepsy, and black bile (Lev & Amar, 2008).

Table 4. Adverse reactions to Henbane

*= Scopolamine   **bold** type indicates a symptom mentioned in aphorism (p259)

Henbane Adverse events	Before 1790	Wood-ville 1790	Dispens. Edin. 1804	Dispens. USA 1858	Harley 1869	Lewin 1881	King's 1898	SED 1952	2007
Dry mouth/ throat	1756						x	x	
Thirst	1729, 1763	x				x			x
Nausea	1780		x			x	x		
Increased pulse	1752 (very slow!)						x	x	x
Fever	1776								x
Arrhythmia	1751, 1776	x							x
BP ⇅									x
Pupils dilated	1763		x	x	x	x	x		x
Vasodilatation	1751, 1776	x			x	x	x		x
Disturbed vision	873A, 1729, 1763, 1776, 1780, 1781	x		x			x	x	x
Loss of speech	1776, 1790	x		x		x	x		
Mad	2500 BC, 354 BC, 1306, 1542, 1546, 1565, 1752, 1789	x							
Troubles in reason	77, 100, 150, 873, 1398, 1610, 1649, 1652, 1676, 1729, 1733, 1752, 1776, 1781								
Loss of memory	1781						x		x

Henbane Adverse events	Before 1790	Wood-ville 1790	Dispens. Edin. 1804	Dispens. USA 1858	Harley 1869	Lewin 1881	King's 1898	SED 1952	2007
Delirium	1751, 1752	x				x	x	x	x
Hallucinations			x				x	x	
Irritability	1776		x			x	x		
Aggressive rage	1619, 1657, 1671, 1776, 1781	x							x
Drunk	1590, 1597, 1619, 1751, 1776		x	x		x			
Dysphagia	1756, 1776, 1781			x		x		x	x
Abdominal cramps	1756, 1763, 1776		x	x			x		x
Diarrhoea	1776			x			x		
Dysarthria							x		x
Urine retention									x
Diuresis			x	x					
Rash		x	x	x		x			x
Allergic symptoms	Tongue swells 1873							x	
Sweating (cold)			x	x			x		
Weakness	1763, 1652,					x		x	x
Headache	1776		x	x			x		x
Body aches/pains	1776								x
Dizziness/giddiness	1751	x				x	x		x
Ataxia/staggering	1763,1751, 1781	x				x			x
Vertigo	873, 1776, 1780		x	x					
Tachypnea						x			x
Confusion	1756						x		x
Convulsions	370BC, 1756, 1776, 1789	x	x	x		x	x		x
Paralysis	1776	x		x		x	x		x
Disturbed sleep	1597, 1619, 1756, 1763, 1776								
Respiratory depression						x	x		x
Coma		x		x			x		x

257

Henbane Adverse events	Before 1790	Woodville 1790	Dispens. Edin. 1804	Dispens. USA 1858	Harley 1869	Lewin 1881	King's 1898	SED 1952	2007
Death	370BC, 777, 1595, 1619, 1733, 1789	x		x			x		x

Allergic symptoms = pulmonary oedema and, oedema of glottis and uvula

Although the first mention of the use of Henbane was in 1550 BC it is not until the 18th century that most adverse events, other than mental problems, are reported. Prior to 1790 there is no mention of dry mouth, *Loss of memory, hallucinations*, increased pulse, *irritability, dysarthria*, urine retention, *diuresis,* rash, sweating, headache, *tachypnea, confusion*, paralysis, *respiratory depression* or coma. Those in italics are those that could be explained by scientific terms not in use then. In the King's American dispensatory 1898 it says *'On account of not producing headache, it is preferred to opium'*, although it goes on to say that henbane can cause it. This may mean that it is rare. The aphorism 'hot as a hare, blind as a bat, dry as a bone, red as a beet, mad as a hen' (Morton, 1939) and originally applied to atropine also applies to hyoscyamus (bold in the table). Yet 'dry mouth' is not mentioned until 1898. The many mentions of disturbed sleep before contrasts with the period afterwards where there is no mention.

There is a steadily increasing awareness of all the ADRs with the passing years and by 1898 we have a full picture. Again it is difficult to pair off the graphic descriptions of symptoms of bygone years with our more precise terminology, e.g. *'maketh man mad and foolish'* could come under the heading of 'mad' or ' troubles' in reason'. Douce, meanwhile, wrote of the ability of the plant to send people mad: *'Henbane, called insana, mad, for the use thereof is perillous, for it if be eate or dronke, it breedeth madness, or slowe lykenss of sleepe'*. (Thiselton-Dyer, 1994) Some of the now known AE could not have been discovered before 1700, as the necessary instruments had not been invented: the mercury thermometer in 1714, an easily used sphygmomanometer in 1896. It is more difficult to understand why 'dry mouth', and 'headache' were not documented prior to 1898 and 1804 respectively. Without knowing the frequency of a specific adverse event it is not possible to appreciate why an AE was not reported earlier.

Alexander quotes cases of oedema of the uvula and glottis due to scopolamine (Alexander, 1955).

Chapter 11. Mercury

The analysis of mercury ADRs is complicated by the large number of variations in chemicals, methods of treatment, combinations of drugs used, doses, duration of treatment, diseases treated, mixtures used, prescribers, formulations and excipients used. In the following table these have been all merged together.

Inorganic compounds:

Quicksilver (Hg) also as Blue Pill (Pilula Hydrargyri), Mercurial plaster (Emplastrum Hydragyri) = Hg + sublimed S + lead plaster, Grey Powder = Hg + prepared Chalk, Mercury Ointment (Ung[165]. `Hydragyri) = Hg, Compound Mercury Ointment (Ung. hydrargyri Compositum) = Ung. Hydrargyri + Yellow bee's wax + Camphor + Olive oil.

Corrosive sublimate (Liquor Hydrargyri Perchloridum–$HgCl_2$) also given as a subcutaneous injection.

Calomel (Hydrargyri Subchloridum–HgCl also as Calomel Ointment and Plummer's Pill).

Red Precipitate (Hydrargyri Oxidum Rubrum–HgO also as ointment.

White Precipitate (Ammoniated Mercury (Ung. Hydrargyri Ammoniati = $HgCl_2$ + solution of ammonia).

Yellow Precipitate (Hydrargyri Oxidum Flavum–HgO also as ointment - Oleated Mercury = Yellow mercuric oxide + Oleic acid).

Green Precipitate. This may be mercurous iodide Hg_2I_2 since it turns from yellow to green over time.

Cinnabar (HgS) Used as fumigation in a hot cabinet.

Cyanide of Mercury $Hg(CN)_2$. Twenty minims of a 1% solution given intravenously three times a week or applied externally.

Mercurated asses' milk.

Sulphide. Hydrargyri Sulphidum Rubrum.

Bromide.

Iodide (Hydrargyri Iodidum Rubrum - HgI_2 also as ointment) or as a mixture with arsenic - Liquor Arsenii et Hydrargryri Iodidi.

---

[165] ung. = unguentum = ointment

Mercurous nitrate $Hg_2(NO_3)_2$ Ungentum Hydrargyri Nitratis Dilutum.

Organic compounds: Phenylhydragyri nitras, merthiolate (Sodium ethyl mercurithiosalicylate), mercuhydrin, mercurophylline.

Benjamin Bell said '...*The preparations of mercury are accordingly very numerous: upwards of five hundred might be enumerated*'. The main chemicals have different ADRs, but have been merged for the table.

Methods of treatment: fumigation, friction, clyster (enema), suppositories (Suppositoria Hydrargyri), plaister (Emplastrum Hydrargi), internally (pills, drops, etc.). Injections: subcutaneous introduced in 1863, intramuscular introduced in 1886, intravenous introduced in 1896. Any one patient might have a combination of these methods.

Combinations with other treatments: antimony from 2500 BC, opium, lignum vitae (Guaiaci lignum) introduced in 1517, China root *Smilax sinensuis* brought by the Portuguese from Goa in 1535, Sarsaparilla from *Smilax Ornata (Decoct Sarsæ Co. Con)* already in use in 1537, Mezereon from *Daphne mezereon*, which is very toxic, Sassafras (*Sassafras officinale)*, potassium iodide (KI) introduced 1835, bismuth (introduced 1884), sulphur, Atoxyl introduced in 1863 alternating with mercury over 13 weeks, arsphenamine introduced in 1910.

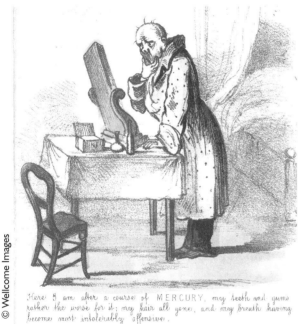

Figure 4. Mercury's effects

Here I am after a course of MERCURY my teeth and gums rather the worse for it, my hair all gone, and my breath having become most intolerably offensive

Doses: titration to salivation. There was a tendency to reduce the dose over the centuries, but during the 19th century the dosage increased (Tiles & Wallach, 1996). Hydragyri Oxidum Rubrum 5 grains (325 mgm) Calomel 5 grains (325 mgm). Seven or eight Blue pills per day. Lewin quotes the use of 500 G daily of Mercurial ointment.

Diseases treated: hysteria, intestinal manifestations, and obstructions, scrofula, infertility, asthma, elephantiasis, scorbutic ulcer, psoriasis, impetigo, leprosy, palsy, cancer, gout, scabies, lichen planus, obstructions of the liver, torpidity of the liver, women's disorders, the green sickness, dripping urine, calculi, and for killing lice and fleas (Lev & Amar, 2008).

Duration (courses): mercurial plasters every 2–3 days, inunction with mercurial liniment for 15–31 days; Zittmann's for ten days; Fournier in 1890 advised treatment spread out over two years. Mercury ointment ½ʒ over 3–5 days; mercury ointment in a hot room for 20–30 days; for at least 100 days; until cured. The duration depended on the severity of the lesions and it would appear that there was a wide variation of individual choices.

Mixtures: Donovan's solution (Liquor Arsenii et Hydrargyri Iodidi); Plummer's Pill (HgCl + sulphurated Antimony + Guiacum resin); Liniment of Mercury = Hg + solution of ammonia + liniment of Camphor, sodium chloride, saltpeter (KNO_3), lead plaster; Unguentum Saracenicum (Euphorbium + Larkspur + yellow oxide of lead + Hg + pig's grease); Zittmann Decoction No 1 (sarsaparilla, calomel, cinnabar, anise, fennel, senna and liquorice). Medicines weren't the only source of mercury: mercurial cakes, mercurial chocolate, mercurials cigarettes, mercurial foot baths and mercurial flannels (Tilles & Wallach, 1996). Added to these were the treatments for the mercurial symptoms.

Users: surgeons, physicians, charlatans, barbers, butchers, farriers, sow-gelders, etc. Physicians tended to concentrate on the internal structure whilst surgeons performed operations and dealt with the outside of the body, e.g. skin.

Formulations: ointment, pills, drops, lotions (Lotio Hydrargyri flava, Lotio Hydrargyri Nigra), cataplasms (poultice), clysters,

Excipients: lard, olive oil, solution of lime, glycerine, liquid paraffin, gum acacia, tragacanth, syrup of glucose, yellow bees wax, and camphor.

Table 5. Adverse reactions to Mercury

Mercury Adverse events	Prior to 1810 B=Bell	Matthias 1810	Francis 1815	Hamil-ton 1819	Colles 1837	Habe-shon 1860	Lewin 1881	SE of Drugs 1952	SE of Drugs 2007	Toxicology Bidstrup Johnstone MBuckell
Poison	77, 1579, 1590									
Hypersalivation	1298, 1363 1500, 1530 1544, 1590 1657, 1676 1711, 1712 1723, 1732 1733, 1736 1737, 1739 1747, 1752 1759, 1782 1788, 1789 1793B, 1797 1804	x	x	x	x		x	x	x	MB, J, B
Metallic taste	1793B, 1797	x		x		x	x		x	J
Gingivitis Stomatitis	1502, 1590 1596, 1711 1739, 1747 1787, 1788, 1793B	x	x			x	x	x	x	J, B
Foetid breath	1533, 1590 1787, 1788 1793B, 1804	x		x	x	x	x	x	2000	
Swollen tongue	1711, 1736 1739, 1747	x			x					J
Ulceration of gums	1533, 1590 1737, 1752 1782, 1787 1793B, 1804	x		x	x		x	x	x	MB
Loose teeth	1363, 1497 1519, 1533 1590, 1737 1739, 1747 1752		x		x	x	x	x	x	
Trismus	1736, 1737 1747,									
Dysarthria	1533, 1711 1737, 1739	x	x	x	x	x			x	J
Thirst	1533, 1711 1718 1756 1804					x				

Mercury Adverse events	Prior to 1810 B=Bell	Matthias 1810	Francis 1815	Hamilton 1819	Colles 1837	Habeshon 1860	Lewin 1881	SE of Drugs 1952	SE of Drugs 2007	Toxicology Bidstrup Johnstone MBuckell
Fever	1590, 1711 1733 1739 1765, 1787, 1788, 1793B, 1804, 1806	x			x	x				J
Emaciation	1733, 1737 1739, 1804			x			x			
Erethism	1711, 1733 1788, 1793B 1804, 1806			x		x	x		x	MB, B
Tremors	1497, 1533 1590, 1657 1711, 1718 1733, 1736 1752, 1756 1788, 1804	x		x			x	x	x	MB, B
Vertigo	1711, 1733 1787, 1788						x	Ataxia	2000	
'Enemy of the nerves'	1657, 1676 1719, 1733 1736, 1752							x		
Parathesia	Part of the above						x		x	
Deafness	1590, 1711 1736		x							
Paralysis / palsy	1497, 1657 1711, 1733 1752, 1756 1797	x		x						
Polyneuropathy	enemy of the nerves							x		
Twitching Vellications	1711, 1718								x	
Epilepsy convulsions	1590, 1596 1711, 1718 1733, 1734 1736, 1747 1756, 1765	x	x	x						J
Intellectual deterioration	1733 grown mad	x	x	x						
Psychosis	1533, 1733 1747	x		x			x	x	x	
Delirium	1765			x		x	x	x		

Mercury Adverse events	Prior to 1810 B=Bell	Matthias 1810	Francis 1815	Hamilton 1819	Colles 1837	Habeshon 1860	Lewin 1881	SE of Drugs 1952	SE of Drugs 2007	Toxicology Bidstrup Johnstone MBuckell
Diarrhoea + blood	1530, 1590 1711, 1718 1733, 1737 1739, 1747, 1752, 1756 1765, 1782, 1786, 1788, 1793B, 1797, 1804	x	x	x	x	x	x	x	x	MB, J
Abdominal cramp	1363, 1590 1676, 1711 1718, 1732, 1733, 1734 1739, 1747 1756, 1786, 1788, 1793B, 1797, 1804		Haema-temesis	x	x	x	x	x	x	MB, J
Constipation	1797, 1804					x			2000	
Nausea + vomiting	1590, 1711 1718, 1739 1756, 1787 1793B, 1797 1804, 1806		x		x	x	x	x	x	MB, J
Anorexia	1533, 1590 1711, 1787		x		x	x			x	B
Insomnia	1711					x	x	x	x	
Headache	1711, 1733 1736, 1752 1788, 1797 1804, 1806	x			x	x	x	x	x	MB
Pulse increase	1737, 1787 1793B, 1797 1804, 1806	x			x	x				
Swollen ankles	1590, 1732, 1787									
Lassitude debility	1711, 1733 1782, 1793B, 1797, 1804	x	x				x			B
Renal damage	1533 couldn't piss		x				x	x	x	MB, J, B
Liver damage	1590							x		J

Mercury Adverse events	Prior to 1810 B=Bell	Matthias 1810	Francis 1815	Hamilton 1819	Colles 1837	Habeshon 1860	Lewin 1881	SE of Drugs 1952	SE of Drugs 2007	Toxicology Bidstrup Johnstone MBuckell
Increased urine	1737, 1793B, 1782	x				x				
Erythema mercuriale	1590, 1793B 1804, 1806			x	x	x		x A	x	MB
Sweating	1662, 1711 1718, 1733 1736, 1737 1739, 1756 1782, 1787 1788, 1793B					x			x	MB
Joint pains	1590, 1787, 1788 1793B	x		x			x	xA		
Rheumatic swelling (face and extremities)	1733, 1736 1739, 1747 1787 (lips)	x			x			x		
Swelling glands (Salivary)	1711, 1733 1739, 1747 1773, 1793B, 1797				x			A		MB
Hair loss	1711,					x		x		
Respiratory problem Suffocation strangulation	1533, 1590 1657, 1711 1733, 1736, 1739 (asthma) 1804, 1806					x		A		J
Cough	1590, 1804 1806					x				
Conjunctivitis	1797							xA	x	B
Mercurialentis										B
Acrodynia								X	x	
Coma / Stupor	1657					x				
Death	1533, 1590 1711, 1733 1737, 1747 1752, 1804					x		A		

Matthias 'The mercurial disease. An enquiry into the history and nature of the disease produced in the human constitution by the use of mercury, with observations on its connection with lues veneria' by Andrew Matthias, 1810

Francis 'The effects of mercury in its natural state and on its abuse in certain diseases'. The Medical and Physical Journal, 1815, 207.

Hamilton 'Observations on the use and abuse of mercurial medicines in various diseases' by James Hamilton. 1819

Alley *'Observations on the Hydargyria or that vesicular disease arising from the exhibition of mercury' by George Alley, 1804.*

Colles *Abraham. 'Practical observations on the venereal disease, and on the use of mercury'. Tracts 339. Dublin 1837.*

Habershon *'On the injurious effects of mercury in the treatment of disease' by S O Habershon, 1860.*

Lewin *'Nebenwirkungen der Arzneimittel: Pharmakologisch–Klinisch Handbuch Lewin Louis', 1881.*

Meyler *Meyler's Side Effects of Drugs 14th edition, 2000.*

Erythema mercuriale was described in great detail in Berenguier's thesis in 1874.

SE of Drugs 1952 Meyler's 1st Edition translated from the Dutch. He also includes: various inflammations–gastritis, colitis, rhinitis, parotitis, bronchitis, laryngitis, urethritis, endometritis, vaginitis and more skin problems–oedema, exfoliative dermatitis, herpes zoster and erythema multiforme. Blood disorders - leucopenia, agranulocytosis, eosinophilia and finally thrombocytopenic purpura. 'Enemy of the nerves'- delerium, hallucinations, psychosis, polyradiculitis and meningo-encephalopathy.

SE of Drugs 2000 In addition: hypertension, hypotension, arteritis of the legs, hypochondria, hyperacusis, polyneuropathy/ parathesia of the extremities (Enemy of the nerves), dysmenorrhoea, hyperthyroidism, hypochromic anaemia, erythrocytosis, lymphocytosis, neutropenia, aplastic anaemia, tylotic[166] eczema, dry skin, skin ulceration, erythroderma, corneal opacities and ulceration.

A *= 'Reactions with Drug Therapy' by Harry L Alexander, who also includes: contact dermatitis, urticaria, scarlatinform maculopapular eruptions, purpura, exfoliative dermatitis, and stomatitis, fever, shock, granulocytopenia, and polyarthritis nodosa.*

B Bell Benjamin. 'A treatise on gonorrhea virulenta and lues venere'. Edinburgh. 1793, volume 2, 288.

J *= Johnstone. Mercury Poisoning. Can Med Ass J. April 1931.*

B *= Bidstrup PL. 'Toxicity of mercury and its compounds'. Levier publishing Company, 1964.*

MB *= Monamy Buckell et al. Chronic mercury poisoning. British Journal of Industrial Medicine.*

Prior to 1800 the modern terms: dysarthria, parathesia, polyneuropathy, acrodynia, conjunctivitis and hydrargia were not known.

Acrodynia (Pink disease) = sweat, pink scaling palms and soles, pruritus, flushed cheeks, photophobia, irritability, insomnia, wasting weakness, hypertension, tachycardia, diminished reflexes; all due to teething powders.

Erethism = great depression of strength, anxiety about the precordium, irregular action of the heart, frequent sighing, trembling, a small, quick and sometimes intermitting pulse, occasional vomiting, pale shrunken countenance, and a sense of coldness (Oke, 1856).

Vellications = twitching

Hydrargia = mercury poisoning

Erythema mercuriale = miliary rash somewhat resembling measles, whilst in others it is considerably raised. Hot and itchy. Local application can produce a pustular rash (Bell, 1793). Parcelsus includes leprosy and lupus vulgaris.

Mercurialentis = Greyish-brown or yellow haze on the anterior surface of the lens (Bidstrup, 1964).

Jarisch-Herxheimer reaction = sudden release of inflammatory cytokines giving headache, myalgia, chills, fever, worsening of pre-existing symptoms,

---

[166] tylotic eczema= hyperkeratotic (thick skinned) eczema usually of the hands

hyperventilation, hypertension later hypotension and tachycardia. Resolves in 6–12 hours (Jarische, 1895; Herxheimer, 1902).

Excluded are: laboratory test abnormalities, effects of inhalation, and effects of organic mercuric compounds. Some of the adverse effects were occupational and therefore chronic.

The loss of hair has only been reported with mercury as a consequence of eczema mercuriale and then only after repeated desquamation . It is much more likely to be due to secondary syphilis. Matthias said *'alopecia, or falling of the hair is not a symptom of mercurial disease, but due to debility'* he went on to say *'I am convinced that in Europe there is no other remedy* (other than calomel) *which has the least effect in subduing the venereal irritation...it* (calomel) *has the power of suppressing, but not of curing the venereal action'* ... *It is, perhaps, capable of curing syphilis in every form'*. (Mathias, 1810).

Discussion

The lack of early references is probably due to the use of mercury being delayed until syphilis arrived in Europe in December 1494 and perhaps partially to fact that it would not have been described in a 'Herbal' being a mineral.

If we examine the ADRs discovered in the centuries after 1500 we can see a pattern:

- 1500s: hypersalivation, gingivitis, fetid breath, ulceration of the gums, loose teeth, dysarthria, thirst, tremors, deafness, epilepsy, madness, anorexia and death.

- 1600s: enemy of the nerves, palsy, abdominal cramp, sweating, strangulation and coma.

- 1700s: metallic taste, fever, emaciation, erethism, vertigo, twitching, intellectual deterioration, hallucinations, diarrhoea, constipation, nausea and vomiting, insomnia, headache, increased pulse, swollen ankles, lassitude, increased urine, erythema mercuriale, joint pains, swollen glands, and rheumatic swellings of the face.

- 1800s: cough, parathesia, renal damage and hair loss (the latter is probably not an ADR, but due to syphilis).

- 1900s: polyneuropathy, liver damage, conjunctivitis and acrodynia.

The commonest ADRs were published before 1600 and during the next century few new ADRs were discovered. There seems to have been a general concern about the early 1700s as to the dangers of mercury and many new ADRs were mentioned. This great surge in the 1700s may be partly due to the advent of medical journals in 1665. It is surprising that nausea and vomiting, and constipation were not mentioned earlier and I can think of no easy explanation. Diarrhoea may not have been considered as adverse, but rather as a treatment for constipation and 'increased urine' similarly as it was used as a diuretic. For some ADRs their absence was possibly due to medical terms not coming into frequent use until later or that with increase in knowledge a more suitable term was devised covering several symptoms. Renal damage and liver damage referring to biochemical evidence and, therefore, not available at that time; but why no mention of conjunctivitis? The word conjunctivitis was used in the 17th century and its presence would have been obvious, but it might only be caused by elemental mercury. Perhaps compared with the other side-effects minor inconveniencies were not deemed important. One of mercury's effects, e.g. diarrhoea has an unexpected beneficial effect in that it clears the bowel of any retained mercury and thereby prevents further absorption and its inherent toxicity. The increased urine first noted in 1737 was re-discovered in 1919 by Alfred Vogl with Novasurol and henceforth was used as a diuretic (Vogl, 1950). In 1924 Mersalyl was discovered and became the main drug used to produce diuresis.

Quicksilver is barely absorbed during its passage through the gut with the result that it collects just above the anal sphincter and if the tone of the sphincter is relaxed for a moment a spray of glistening globules is seen on the floor. 'During a dance at a public assembly a lady was thought to have dropped her pearls, but when her escort went to pick them up he found, much to the lady's confusion, that they were globules of mercury'. (Abraham, 1948).

The monstrous adverse drug reactions of mercury must be balanced by its efficacy. Although the treating physicians and surgeons believed that it cured syphilis they may have been mistaken, since there was a spontaneous resolution of both primary and secondary syphilis. The course of untreated syphilis had been investigated in a study in Oslo (1891–1951) which had 1,978 patients and, more recently, in the unethical Tuskegee study in American male negroes[167] (1932–1972). The primary chancre resolved in 2–6 weeks and the secondary stage developed about 6 weeks after the healing of the primary lesion and consisted of a generalised rash, headaches,

---

[167] Tuskegee Study. 399 poor male negroes, and 201 healthy controls were followed up for 40 years. 28 died from syphilis, 100 died from conditions related to their syphilis, 28 wives were infected and 19 children had congenital syphilis.

fever, malaise, joint and muscle aches and more rarely alopecia, laryngitis, hepatitis, nephrotic syndrome, bone pain and uveitis. All these resolved spontaneously. During the period prior to the tertiary phase the syphilis was latent and in about 60% it remained latent for the remainder of the patient's life. The tertiary lesions included: cutaneous gummas, mucosal gummas, bone syphilis, visceral syphilis (liver, eyes, stomach, lungs, testis, haemolytic anaemia) and neurosyphilis (Wright & Csonka, 1996). The doctors may well have mistaken the spontaneous resolution of the primary and secondary phases as being due to mercury treatment. Since the disease remained latent how can one tell when a cure occurs? This differentiation only became possible when a laboratory test, the Wasserman reaction, was discovered in 1906. The tests have increased in their sophistication since then. It was in 1905 that the discovery of the responsible organism, *Treponema pallidum,* was made by Fritz Schaudinn and Eric Hoffman. Cure involved the conversion of a positive Wasserman to a negative response. In view of the high spontaneous cure rate the efficacy of mercury could only have been found by a controlled clinical trial against placebo and monitored by following the Wassermann conversion rates. Many would have considered this to be unethical as equipoise would not have been present. Arsphenamine had appeared in 1910 and was believed to be the answer to syphilis, but no controlled clinical trials were performed comparing it with mercury.

Hyman in 1941 evaluated the routine conservative treatment of syphilis, which included mercury, bismuth and arsenic. He concluded: Paragraph 5: The 'spontaneous' course of early syphilis tends to "cure" in approximately 43 per cent of all patients, and an additional 22 per cent will remain clinically well with positive serology. Thus, two patients in three, afflicted with early syphilis, may be expected to live their lives and eventually succumb without clinical manifestation of the infection. Paragraph 17: The great triumph of specific chemotherapy in syphilis seems sharply limited to those patients with early syphilis (constituting perhaps 16 per cent of Wassermann-positive individuals) who have persisted through continuous and continued forms of therapy (5% of those who initiate therapy) (Hyman, 1941).

I can find no evidence that there were any clinical trials comparing Mercury with Arsphenamine, again because of lack of equipoise; Arsphenamine was believed to be very superior to mercury treatments. I conclude that mercury may have been better than placebo, if given correctly for a long period, but only if given early in primary syphilis and then only in a few patients.

Fernel comments in 1579 that all the late symptoms of syphilis were really due to mercurial poisoning (Abraham, 1948) were probably an exaggeration and the converse might have been true. Dr Swediaur said *'To distinguish complaints arising from mercury from real venereal ones great judgement is required'.* (Swediaur, 1788).

Mercury was used for other diseases, e.g. skin diseases, and examination of the adverse events reported in these circumstances might clarify the situation as to which ADRs could be attributable to mercury, but unfortunately there are not many studies. A study of mercury ointment in psoriasis in 24 patients over 6 weeks showed no symptoms of toxicity despite 13 patients having toxic mercury levels (Inman et al., 1956).

The ADRs reported in books and articles on toxicology might be thought to be relevant, but on the whole these tend to be those symptoms produced by vapour from mercury used in industry (Buckell et al., 1946) or from suicide attempts where the patients have taken corrosive sublimate ($HgCl_2$) in such large doses that the initial symptoms progress rapidly to renal failure. These reports of suicide cases might not contain the more subtle symptoms (Johnstone, 1931).

Mercury caused tremendous suffering over 450 years without the recompense of curing the disease and was thereby the greatest drug disaster yet known.

Chapter 12. Opium

Indications: Pain, aided digestion, jaundice, acute fever, palpitations, loss of teeth, cough, liver and intestines, malaria, eye disease, syphilis, strengthening the teeth and gums, and mental illness (Lev & Amar, 2008).

Table 6. Adverse reactions to Opium

Opium Adverse events	Before 1800	Dispens. Edin. 1804	Dispens. USA 1858	Lewin 1881	King's 1898	SE of Drugs 1952 Morphine	2007 Morphine
Nausea	1763,1776, 1793		x	x	x	x	70%
Vomiting	1763, 1786, 1788, 1793		x	x	x	x	7%
Anorexia				x			
Constipation	1712, 1764, 1776, 1785, 1789	x	x		x		5-10%
Diarrhoea (Higher dose—10-12 Gr)	1763, 1785, 1788						5-10%
Stertorous breathing	130 BC, 1306 strangleth., 1776, 1793,	x	x		x	x	x
Dyspnoea	47AD, 1763, 1776						5-10%
Respiratory depression					x	x	x
Euphoria	1652, 1763, 1789	x			x		
Dysphoria	47BC, 1586, 1652, 1763, 1786		x	x	x		x
Loss of memory	1586, 1619,1763				x		

Opium Adverse events	Before 1800	Dispens. Edin. 1804	Dispens. USA 1858	Lewin 1881	King's 1898	SE of Drugs 1952 Morphine	2007 Morphine
Imperfect speech	1763						
Miosis	(1763 dilatation of pupil)				x		x
Amblyopia	9th century, 1776			x			<5%
Dizziness/giddiness	9th cent. 1652, 1763, 1785, 1788, 1789			x	x		x
Vertigo	47 BC, 1763, 1786, 1793	x		x			
Tinnitus				x			
Drowsiness/sleep	130 BC, 78AD, 9th century, 1326, 1568, 1580, 1586, 1619, 1652, 1763, 1786, 1789, 1793			x	x		x
Insomnia	1763, 1788 with disagreeable dreams			x			5-10%
Urine retention	1763				x	x	x
Biliary tract spasm	?1788 colicky pains					x	x
Paralytic ileus							x
Exacerbation pancreatitis				Abd. Pain			x
Cramps	1788			x			5-10%
Hiccups	9th century, 1763, 1788						<5%
Flushing of face	1652, 1763, 1789		x	x	x		x
Cold extremities	47AD, 130 BC, 1763	x			x		

Opium Adverse events	Before 1800	Dispens. Edin. 1804	Dispens. USA 1858	Lewin 1881	King's 1898	SE of Drugs 1952 Morphine	2007 Morphine
Itching / Pruritus Opii'	78, 1516, 1551, 1568, 1662, 1752, 1763, 1788		x	x	x	x	< 80%
Contact dermatitis				Spots	Rash	x A	5-10%
Urticaria	Itching rash 1788			x		x A	5-10%
Anaphylaxis							x
Asthma						x A	
Hallucinations					x		x
Delirium	1788 kind of intoxication	x	x		x		x
Decreased libido	1553						x
Bradycardia	1763, 1765, 1785				x		x
Tachycardia	1793, 1788						x
Hypotension				x			<5%
Syncope	1763						
Convulsions	9th century, 1678, 1763, 1786	x		x	x		x
Transient paralysis	1586, 1597, 1619, 1652, 1657			x			
Weakness	1786			x	x		5-10%
Sweating	130 BC, 47AD, 1652, 1662, 1712, 1752, 1763, 1788			x	x		
Salivation	1544, 1763, 1776, 1785	x		x	x		5-10%
Swollen lips	130 BC, 1763, 1789						
Thirst	1662, 1786	x					
Oedema						x	5-10%

Opium Adverse events	Before 1800	Dispens. Edin. 1804	Dispens. USA 1858	Lewin 1881	King's 1898	SE of Drugs 1952 Morphine	2007 Morphine
Antidiuretic effect	1776 urine insensible, 1763 stoppage of urine), 1785 (increased secretion) 1786 (increased urine)					x	x
Fever				x			5-10%
Headache	47 BC, 1763, 1774, 1785, 1786, 1793	x	x	x	x	x	>10%
Backache							5-10%
Relaxation of joints	130 BC, 1652, 1763, 1789				x		
Tremor	1657, 1785, 1793		x	x	x		x
Uncoordinated movements	1652			x	x		x
Abortion	1763						
Cardiac arrest	1788 palpitations			x			
Stupor/coma	147AD, 580	x		x	x	x	x
Death	130 BC, 77AD, 78AD, 1533, 1586, 1619, 1652, 1657, 1678, 1763, 1789	x			x		x

A = 'Reactions with Drug Therapy' by Harry L. Alexander who also gives papular eruption, scarlatiniform eruption, exfoliative dermatitis, erythematous eruption and angio-oedema.

Prior to 130 BC I have found no mention of adverse effects. From then until 1800 the events were described graphically, but did not describe the physiological changes, which are implied by modern terminology.

There are some noticeable absences before 1881: no skin problems, no oedema, no fever or backache, although they are supposed to have an incidence of 5–10%. The delays in recognition of some adverse events until post-1800 are understandable in that the means to diagnose them were not developed or that the terminology of some of the mental symptoms could be included under 'dysphoria' (disquiet, restlessness, malaise, agitation and anguish).

Chapter 13. Aspirin

Most abnormal laboratory values occurring as ADRs have been
omitted. Events specifically associated with poisoning are in
italics. As one of the first modern drugs there are many more
literature references than for the previous examples.

Table 7. Adverse reactions to Aspirin

Aspirin Adverse events	Other Salicylates M=Micromedex	First Pub. Date	Siefert 1915	Meyler's SED Vol. Date	Feinman 1994 Rainsford	Meyler's 2006 (Type A/B)	Micromedex Inchem Martindales 2007
Salicylate intoxication *	1948□	1965[38]		VII 1972		A	
GI Tract Gastric ulcer *	1876[17]	1920[14]		I 1952	F	x A	MID
Peritoneal irritation		1948[20]		I 1952			
GI perforation		1965[69]		VIII 1975		x A	M
Dyspepsia *# abdominal Pain, heartburn	1882[82], 1898[36], 1879[66], 1945[89], 1953*, 1954#,	1899[63, 87] 1906[64]	x	I	F R	x A	MID
Diarrhoea	1880[77], 1898[36], 2007M	1905[97], 1964[94],		I 1952			
Nausea/vomiting# Anorexia	1876[2], 1877[3] 1898[36], 1945[59], 1948□, 1953*, 1954#, 2007M	1905[96], 1949[88]	x	I 1952	F R	x A	MID
Dysphagia	1945[89]	1903[73]	x				
Pancreatitis		1963[32]		V 1966	F		M
Repulsive taste	1879[66], 1881[37], 1898[55], 1954#						

Aspirin Adverse events	Other Salicylates M=Micromedex	First Pub. Date	Siefert 1915	Meyler's SED Vol. Date	Feinman 1994 Rainsford	Meyler's 2006 (Type A/B)	Micromedex Inchem Martindales 2007
Burning/grating in mouth	1898[36], 1881[37]		x				
Saliva increased	1898[36]		x				
Ear Nose Throat Tinnitus*#	1855[35], 1876[12,92],1877[3], 1898[36], 1945 [59], 1948□, 1953*, 1954# 2007M,	1899[48,49]	x	I 1952	FR	x A	MID
Dizziness	1855[35], 1876[2,92], 2007M	1905[96], 1949[88]	x	I 1952	F	x A	MI
Hearing loss/deafness *	1855[35], 1876[2, 12,92], 1898[36], 1945[59], 1948□ 1953*, 1954#	1949[88]	X	I 1952	F R	x A	MID
Vertigo *	1880[77], 1948□, 1954#,	1954#	x	XV 2006	F		
General *Sweating *#*	1855[35], 1876[2,12], 1932[60], 1948□, 1954#,	1899[49], 1936[72]	x	11952	x R	x A	I
Thirst	1945[89], 2007M	1936[72]			x		M
Hypothermia	1945[88], 1876[92]	1949[88],		V 1966			M
*Fever *#* *Hyperthermia*	1876[6], 1880[85], 1887[76],1932[60], 1954#	1946[23]		III 1960	R		MID
Death *	1953*	1933[41]		I 1952	F R	x A	I D
Metabolic *Dehydration **	1945[89],	1949[88]			R		MID
*Metabolic acidosis *#*	1945[89], 1953*, 2007M	1949[27]		I 1952	R	x A	MID
*Respiratory alkalosis **	1948□, (1949[88]) 2007M	1931[103], 1932[60], 1949[27]		I 1952	R		MID
Hypoglycemia		1962[43]		V 1966	R	x A	MID
Hyperglycaemia		1962[43]		VI 1968	R		MI

Aspirin Adverse events	Other Salicylates M=Micromedex	First Pub. Date	Siefert 1915	Meyler's SED Vol. Date	Feinman 1994 Rainsford	Meyler's 2006 (Type A/B)	Micromedex Inchem Martindales 2007
Sod. Bicarbonate Interaction	1944[104], 1945[105]	1949[15]					Stockley
Respiratory Asphyxia / choking	1898[36]	1903[73], 1936[72]			F		
Pulmonary oedema *	1953*, 1948□	1948[14]		I 1952	F R	x A	MI
Hurried respiration *# Hyperpnoea	1876[92] (82), 1898[36], 1945[59], 1948□ 1953*, 1954#, 2007 M	1903[73], 1945[59]		I 1957	F R	x A	M ID
Cardiovascular Angina (variant)#	1898[36]	1933[90] 1983[58], 1979[62]				x	
Cardiac insufficiency / failure /depression	1880[77], 1880[85], 1945[88]	1930[101], 1947[81]		I 1952	F		
Oedema *	1876[6], 1945[89], 1949[88],	1949[88]	x		x F		
Collapse/ shock *#	1876[1], 1876[17,92], 1898[36] #	1949[88]		II 1958	x R		ID
Redness of face/ * Vasodilatation	1898[36], 1953*, 1954#, 1948□	1900[51], 1903[73]		I 1952			I
Dysrhythmias, palpitations	1900[51]	1905[52]	X				MI
Tachycardia#	1879[66], 1945[59],	1899[49], 1903[73]		I 1952			MI
Bradycardia *		1956[56]		II 1958			
BP□ ↑		1947[63,24]				x A	
BP□*↓		1949[88]					MI
Mental Delirium *	1876[92], 1884[84], 1898[36] 1947[25],1953*, 1900[51], 2007M	1932[47]	X	I 1952	F R		I
Depression	1877[3], 1880[85],				F		I
Insomnia	1880[85], 1900[51],	1938[46]					

Aspirin Adverse events	Other Salicylates M=Micromedex	First Pub. Date	Siefert 1915	Meyler's SED Vol. Date	Feinman 1994 Rainsford	Meyler's 2006 (Type A/B)	Micromedex Inchem Martindales 2007
Drowsiness	1909[101], 1945[59], 1948[□], 1954[#], 2007M	1954#,	x	VI 1968		x	
Psychosis		1955[29]			+anxiety		I
Confusion	Psychical disturbance. 1948[□], 2007M			I 1952	F R	x A	MID
Agitation/excitment/ restlessness	1884[84], 1954[#], 1900[51], 1948[□]	1905[53], 1938[46], 1949[88]			R		
Hallucinations# Delusions	1875[4], 1876[2], 1900[51], 1945[59], 1953[*], 1954[#], 2007M	1932[47] 1949[88]		1952	F R		I
Excess debility/ lassitude *	1876[92], 1898[36], 1945[59]	1905[52]			F R	x A	M
Neurological Headache#	1876[2], 1877[3], 1898[36], 1948[□],1953[*], 2007M	1899[49]	x		F	x A	M
Tingling	1898[36]					-	
Dystonia	1877[3]						
Muscle weakness	1877[3]						
Tremors/asterixis *	1877[3], 1880[77], 1884[84], 1898[36], 1965[38],	1965[38] 1981[40]		VII 1972	F R	-	I
Convulsions, Coma*#	1909[101], 1954[#], 2007M	1938[46] 1947[24]	x	I 1952	F R	x A	MI
Cerebral oedema					x		MI
Slurred speech/ dysarthria		1994F			F		
Aphonia		1945[89],					

Aspirin Adverse events	Other Salicylates M=Micromedex	First Pub. Date	Siefert 1915	Meyler's SED Vol. Date	Feinman 1994 Rainsford	Meyler's 2006 (Type A/B)	Micromedex Inchem Martindales 2007
Eyes Dimness of vision	1877[13], 1881[5], 1898[36], 953*,1954#, 2007M				F	Myopia	Myopia
Ptosis	1898[36]	1905[53]					
Strabismus	1898[36]						
Amaurosis/amblyopia	1881[78], 1884[86], 1898[36], 1954#	1946[22]		I 1952			
Raised Intraocular Tension		1962[67], 1974[50]					
Papilloedema	1965[38],	1965[38]					
Myopia		1962[67], 1974[50]					I[50]
Conjunctivitis		2002[99]			-	-	
Renal *Albuminuria#*	1876[1, 6, 92], 1877[3], 1879[9], 1898[36], 1916[45], 1945[59], 1948□ 1953*,	1919[70] 1949[88]		I 1952			M
Dark green urine	1898[25]	1905[52]					
Polyuria	1898[36], 1945[89],	1948[18]		I 1952	F		
Kidney lesions	1898[36], 1953*	1938[46]		I 1952	xF		M*
Rhabdomyolysis		1989[42]					M
*Renal failure /anuria / oliguria**	1877[3],1945[89,] 1953*	1916[45]		I 1952	FR	x	MI
Analgesic nephropathy		1974[31], 1951[21]		I 1952		x	D
Endocrine Cushing's syndrome		1950[26] 1954#		VIII 1975			
Delayed gestation		1976[61]		I 1952			M
Blood Increased bleeding* prothrombin time↑	1880[77], 1948□, 1953*, 1954#, 2007M	1905[96], 1916[80] 1949[15]		I 1952	F R	x A	MID
Bleeding from stomach	1845[89]	1938[98]					

Aspirin Adverse events	Other Salicylates M=Micromedex	First Pub. Date	Siefert 1915	Meyler's SED Vol. Date	Feinman 1994 Rainsford	Meyler's 2006 (Type A/B)	Micromedex Inchem Martindales 2007
DIC	1973[74]	1973[74]		VIII 1975			M
Blood dyscrasia	1954#	1988[91]			x R	x B	
Haemolytic anaemia		1960[57]		III 1960		x B	D
Haematuria	1877[7], 1948□	1930[101], 1949[88]		I 1952			
Thrombocytopenia/ Purpura	1884[83], 1945[89], 1953*	1948[16]		I 1952	F	Bx	MD
Agranulocytosis		1945[89] 1968[68]				x B	D
Neutropenia/ Leukopenia		1935, 1943[100] 1964[94]				x B	
Aplastic anaemia		1985			F	x B	D
Pancytopenia		1966[33]		VI 1968	F		D
Megaloblastic anaemia		1969[30]		VI 1968			
Liver Hepatitis	1953*	1965[74], 1973[64]		VIII 1975	F		M
Reye's syndrome		1962[43]				x B	MID
Hepatic necrosis				XV 2006		x A	I D
Skin Rash petechial	1878[8], 1896[75], 1954#	1944		I 1952	x	x B	
Miscellaneous rashes*	1876[6], 1881[11], 1884[84], 1900[51], 1945[89], 1948□, 2007M	1905[96,108], 1919[70], 1922[44]	x	I 1952	EM R	x B	I
Alopecia		1968[34]		VII 1972			
Itching*	1878[10,8]	1903[73], 1956[95]		II 1958			
Allergy Asthma#	1945[89]	1922[44]		I 1952 H	x	x B	MID
Hypersensitivity	1945[89]	1937[19]		I 1952 H	x	x B	MD

Aspirin Adverse events	Other Salicylates M=Micromedex	First Pub. Date	Siefert 1915	Meyler's SED Vol. Date	Feinman 1994 Rainsford	Meyler's 2006 (Type A/B)	Micromedex Inchem Martindales 2007
Laryngeal oedema	Oedema glottis[89]	1963[79], 1990[65]		I 1952 H			M
Anaphylactoid reaction	1876[6]	1902[28]		IV 1963 H		x A	M
Allergic Rhinitis[#]		1922[44]		I 1952		x B	ID
Urticaria[#]	1876[6], 1879[9], 1955H	1902[28], 1903[73]	x	I 1952 H	x R	x B	MID
Angio-oedema[#]	1878[10], 1945[89], 1955H	1902[28], 1903[73], 1905[53]	X	I 1952 H	x	x B	MID

Abbreviations

A = Type A ADR

B = Type B ADR

BP = Blood Pressure

IOP = Intraocular Pressure

EM = Erythema Multiforme

DIC = Disseminated Intravascular Coagulation

Micromedex: Micromedex Health Care Systems; Thomson. DrugDex, 2007.

Inchem: International Programme on Chemical Safety, 2007.

D = MartinDales, 2007

SED = Meyler's Side Effects of Drugs. Volume and year.

F = Feinman = Beneficial and Toxic Effects of Aspirin. Ed. S E Feinman. CRC Press. 1994

* = Maladies Médicamenteuses d'ordre Thérapeutique et Accidentel [Drug-induced diseases by Claude Albahary 1953. Deals with sodium salicylate and Aspirin.

 # = Le Risque Therapeutique, prevention et traitment des accidents. [The therapeutic risk, prevention and treatment of adverse drug events] By Guy Duchesney. Doin G et Cie. 1954. Deals with Sodium salicylate and Aspirin.

H = Reactions with Drug Therapy by Harry L Alexander. Aspirin precursors: urticaria, angio-oedema, erythema multiforme, erythema nodosum, eczematous dermatitis, fixed eruptions, bullous eruptions, scarlatiniform eruptions, and morbilliform eruptions.

R = Rainsford K.D. Aspirin and Related Drugs. 2004.

□ = The Toxic Manifestations of sodium salicylate Therapy. Quarterly Journal of Medicine. 41, 153. 1948

Salicylate Evidence ADR. www.aapcc.org/DiscGuidelines/Guidelines Tables/ Salicylate Evidence Table.pdf

Stockley IH. Drug Interactions, Pharmaceutical Press. 5th edition, 2000.

Salicylate References with symptoms

1. *Ned Tijdschrift Geneesk* 1920; 64. Gastric hyperaemia and oedema with ulceration.

2. Riegel F. Ueber die innerliche Anwendung der Salicylsäure [concerning the internal administration of salicylic acid]. *Berliner Klinische Wochenscrift* 1876 April 3rd; 14: 182. Salicylic acid was given as either a powder or latterly as an aqueous solution of the sodium salt; the dose varying between 4 and 6 G, but this dose was sometimes repeated on the same day. Headache, vomiting, tinnitus, deafness, sweating, dizziness and transient delusions.

3. Müller G. Beitrag zur Wirkung des salicylsauren Natron beim Diabeten mellitus [Report on the effect of sodium salicylate on diabetes mellitus]. *Berliner Klinische Wochenscrift* 1877; 29. Tinnitus, headache, albuminuria, unsteadiness, dystonia, depression, hesitant speech, tremor, weakness, anorexia, oliguria, after 15 grammes daily for nine days to a diabetic. There was a positive rechallenge with all these symptoms.

4. Schuhmacher. *Deutsche Med Wochenscrift* 1875; No. 18. Visual hallucinations.

5. Knapp *Berliner Klinische Wochenscrift* 1881; 1237. Diminution of vision and contraction of retinal vessels.

6. Lührmann. Nur eine kurze Bemerkung zur salicylsauren Natrons [Only a short comment on the effect of salicylic acid]. *Berliner Klinische Wochenscrift* 1876 August 14th; 33: 477. High fever, tinnitus, tachycardia, increased respiratory rate, oedema of axillae and legs with a positive rechallenge after a dose of 4 grammes.

7. Balz. *Archiv. F. Heilkunde.* 1877; XVIII: 63. Albuminuria and haematuria after the acid and sodium salt.

8. Freudenberg F. Ueber ein neues Arzneiexanthem [On a new drug-induced rash]. *Berliner Klinische Wochenscrift* 1878; 630. Petechial exanthem and ecchymoses with burning and itching after 5 grammes (75gr) sodium salicylate, daily for 5 days, with positive rechallenge.

9. Leube W. Urticaria mit Albuminurie [Urticaria with albuminuria]. Thiring. *Arch of Dermatol Res* 1879; 6 (1): Corr.-B1. VII. 5. p. 95. Single case: urticaria and albuminuria after 4 grammes (61.6 grs) of the sodium salt.

10. Heinlein. *Arztl Intelligenzblatt* 1878 April. Itching, diffuse redness and oedema with a positive rechallenge, after 4 grammes of the sodium salt.

11. Rathery. *Gazette des hôpit* 1881; 149. Pemphigus-like eruption after sodium salt.

12. Stricker. Nachtrag. Ueber die Resultate der Behandlung der Polyarthritis rheumatica mit Salicylsäure [On the results of treating polyarthritis rheumatica with salicylic acid]. *Berliner Klinische Wochenscrift.* 1876; No. 8. Buzzing in the ears, difficulty of hearing, and perspiration.

13. Riess. *Berliner Klinische Wochenscrift.* 1877; 29. Dimness of vision and flickering before the eyes. Also *Lancet* January 8th 1876 Perspiration, tinnitus and vomiting.

14. Graham JDP and Parker WA. The toxic manifestations of sodium salicylate therapy. *Quart J Med* 1948; 41: 153. Survey of 40 cases of toxicity. A single case of pulmonary oedema without details.

15. Hoffman WS, Pomeranc M, Volini IF and Nobe C. Treatment of acute rheumatic fever with aspirin. *Amer J Med* 1949; 6. The prothrombin concentration was only slightly affected by aspirin therapy.

16. Daneo V and Sisto LD. Porpora trombocitopenica da acide acetil-salicilico [Thrombocytopenic purpura from acetylsalicylic acid]. *Minerva Med (Torino)* 1948; 49. Thrombocytopenic purpura.

17. Goltdammer. Zur inneren Anwendung der Salicylsäure [On the internal administration of salicylic acid]. *Berliner Klinische Wochenscrift* 1876; 47. Several cases of collapse after 5 gramme doses.

18. Sollman T. A Manual of Pharmacology and its Application to Therapeutics and Toxicology. 1948; 537. Dehydration, polyuria, oliguria and nephrosis.

19. Prickman LE and Buchstein HF. Hypersensitivity to acetyl-salicylic acid (Aspirin) *JAMA* 1937;108(6): 445. Cases of asthma, angioneurotic oedema, vasomotor rhinitis, purpura, abdominal cramps and salivation.

20. *Wien Klinische Wochenschrift* 1948; 60: 175. Shock, coma and peritoneal irritation.

21. Davison F R, Synopsis of Materia Medica, Toxicology and Pharmacology, St Louis, 1946; p 325. Deafness and blindness.

22. Manchester RC. Rheumatic fever in naval enlisted personnel: III The physiological and toxic effects of intensive salicylate therapy in acute cases *JAMA* 1946; 131: 209, Hyperpyrexia, renal colic.

23. Staff meeting. *Proc Mayo Clin* 1947; 22: 391. Single case of convulsions and coma with a positive rechallenge as part of drug allergy.

24. Krasnoff SO and Bernstein M. Acetylsalicylic acid poisoning. *JAMA* 1947; 135: 712. Single fatal case with confusion, incoherent, restlessness, flushed, petechiae, BP 96/60–170/90 mmHg., Temp 107° F.

25. Cochran J.B, Watson R.D and Reid J. Mild Cushing's syndrome due to Aspirin. *BMJ* 1950; II: 1411. Single case: Cushing's syndrome with glycosuria, acne, water and salt retention.

26. *Amer J Med Sci* 1949; 217: 256. Acidosis and respiratory alkalosis.

27. Hirschberg. Mittheilung über ein Fall von Nebenwirkung des Aspirin [Communication on a case of side effects of aspirin]. *Deutsche Med Wochenschr* 1902; 28: 416. Anaphylactoid reaction to Aspirin.

28. Sarwer-Foner GJ and Morrison GH. Acute toxic psychosis due to acetyl-salicylic acid. *Canadian Services Medical Journal* 1955; 11(9): 599–606. Single case report of visual and auditory hallucinations with paranoia.

29. Williams JO, Mengel CE, Sullivan LW and Haq AS. Megaloblastic anaemia associated with chronic ingestion of an analgesic. *New Engl J Med* 1969; 280(6): 312–3. Concerned aspirin, salicylamide and caffeine in a single case.

30. Macklon AF, Craft AW, Thompson M and Kerr DN. Aspirin and analgesic nephropathy. *BMJ* 1974 1; 597–600. Aspirin rarely if ever causes analgesic nephropathy.

31. Sussman S. Severe salicylism and acute pancreatitis. *Calif. Med.* 1963 99; 29–32.

32. Wijnja L, Snijder JAM and Nieweg HO. Acetylsalicylic Acid as a cause of pancytopenia from bone marrow damage, *Lancet* 1966; 2: 768–770. Five patients with positive dechallenge and in two cases positive rechallenge.

33. Rannsley HM and Shelley WB. Salicylate ingestion and idiopathic hair loss. *Lancet* 1968; 1: 567. Seventy five percent of patients with idiopathic hair loss were consistently taking aspirin or salicylates compared with controls at 14% and 18%.

34. Bertagnini C. Sulle alterationi che alcuni acidi subiscono nell'organismo animale [On the deterioration that some acids produce in animal organisms]. *Il Nuovo Cimento*. Marson, G Pasero, 1855; 1: 363–72. Tried it on himself *'continuous noise in the ears and a kind of dizziness'*.

35. King's American Dispensatory by HW Felter and JU Lloyd. Ohio Valley Co. 1898. '*ptosis, and strabismus are not uncommon results from its use.*'

36. 'Untoward Effects of Drugs' by Lewin L. Pub. George S. Davis. USA, 1883.

37. Greer HD, Ward HP and Corbin KB. Chronic Salicylic intoxication in adults. *JAMA* 1965; 193(7): 555–558. Five patients with chronic intoxication. Three with tremors and one with asterixis and papilloedema.

38. Wigley RD. Aspirin Kidney Study. *Aust N Z Med* 1973; 3: 425.

39. Anderson RJ. Asterixis as a manifestation of salicylate toxicity. *Ann Intern Med* 1981; 95: 185–189. Four patients on chronic therapy had asterixis ('liver flap') three of them with confusion. Positive dechallenges.

40. Dysart BR. Death following ingestion of 5 grammes of Acetylsalicylic Acid. *J Allergy* 1933; 6: 504.

41. Leventhal L.J., Koritsky L. Ginsburg R and Bomalaski JB. Salicylate-induced rhabdomyolysis. *Am J Emerg Med* 1989; 7: 409–410.

42. Mortimer E.A. and Lepow M.L. Varicella with hypoglycaemia possibly due to Aspirin. *Am J Dis Child* 1962;103: 583. Four fatal cases of varicella with hypoglycaemia following large amounts of salicylates in three of them (80, 80 and 160 mgm, 3–4 times a day respectively). Now thought to be Reye's syndrome.

43. Widal F, Abrami P and Lermoyez J. Anaphylaxis et idiosyncrasie. *Presse Médicale* 1922; 30: 189–193. First description of aspirin idiosyncrasy-asthma-nasal polyposis syndrome. Single case of pruritus, urticaria, spasmodic coryza, asthma, headache and fever with positive rechallenge.

44. Scott RW and Hanzlik PJ. The salicylates: salicylate albuminuria. *JAMA* 1916; 67: 1838–1842. Sweating causing oliguria.

45. Biddle E. Aspirin Poisoning, *BMJ* 1938 June 25th. Single fatal case–restlessness, sweating, dehydration, hyperpnoea and terminal convulsions.

46. Balazs J. Acetylsalisäure Vergiftung [Poisoning with acetylsalicylic acid]. *Samml Vergiftungsf* 1932; 3: 201. Hallucinations and delirium.

47. Dreser H. Pharmacologisches über Aspirin (Acetylsalicylsäure) [Pharmacological details on aspirin]. *Pflugers Archiv. Für die Geschichte der Physiologie* 1899; 76:305–318, Bonn, Emil Srauss.

48. Floeckinger F C. *BMJ* Dec. 9th 96, 1899 also in *Med. News* November 18th 1899. Violent headache, tinnitus, sweats, tachycardia and flashes of light after 135 grs of Aspirin.

49. Sandford-Smith JH. Transient myopia after Aspirin. *Br J Opthalmol* 1974; 58(7): 698–700. Single case also with raised intraocular pressure, coloured vision and retinal oedema following 2.7 G Aspirin.

50. Heffernan HH. A case of sodium salicylate poisoning. *BMJ* 1900 Jan 6th: 16. After 130 gr Sodium salicylate had palpitations, delirium, tinnitus, visual and auditory hallucinations, restlessness, sweating, dilated pupils, insomnia, tachycardia and tachypnoea.

51. Barnett HN. Aspirin in rheumatism: a warning. *BMJ* 1905 July 1st. Palpitations, difficult respirations, weakness and dark green urine after 15 gr Aspirin. Positive rechallenge.

52. Dockray JS. Some toxic effects of Aspirin. *BMJ* 1905 Dec. 30th. Single case with some bizarre symptoms: tinnitus, drowsiness, numbness of gums, tongue and pharynx; dysphagia, choking sensation, numbness over whole body, right ptosis, yellow vision and ear problems. Dose of aspirin = 10gr 3 hourly.

53. Mackey E. Aspirin. *BMJ* 1906 Jan 13th. Repudiating previous paper but adding '*I have also heard in private practice of dyspepsia caused by ordinary doses*'.

54. Hopkins FG. In Materia Medica, Pharmacy, Pharmacology, and Therapeutics by William Hale-White, 1898 Pub P Blakiston's Son. '*Salicylate of soda has, as is well known, an unpleasant sickly sweet quality.*'

55. Dowdle E. The reaction of patients with typhoid fever to the administration of aspirin. *S Afr Med J* 1956; 30: 474. '*Five cases of shock phenomena, with sweating, slow pulse and low temperature.*'

56. Szeinberg A, Kellermann J, Adam A, Sheba C, Ramot B. Haemolytic jaundice following aspirin. administration to a patient with a deficiency of glucose-6-phosphate dehydrogenase in erythrocytes. *Acta Haematologica* 1960; 23:58–64. Single case, 19 year old male, with glucose-6-phosphate dehydrogenase deficiency after 1.5 G Aspirin.

57. Al-Abbasi AH. Salicylate-induced variant angina. *Am Heart J* 1983; 106(6): 1450.

58. Wégria R and Smull K. *JAMA* 1945; 129(7): 485–490. Toxic over 50 mgm per 100cc. Tinnitus, deafness, nausea and vomiting, hyperpnoea, sinus tachycardia, apathy, drowsiness, auditory and visual hallucinations, stuporous and unconscious.

59. Odin M. *Acta Med Scand* 1932; Suppl. 50:177. Respiratory alkalosis.

60. Shapiro S, Siskind V, Monson RR, Heinonen OP, Kaufman DW, Slone D. Perinatal mortality and birth-weight in relation to aspirin taken during pregnancy. *Lancet* 1976; 1: 1375–1376.

61. Miwa K, Kambaka H and Kawai C. Variant angina aggravated by aspirin. *Lancet* 1979; Dec. 22/29:1382. Single case against control.

62. Wohlgemuth. Aspirin. BMJ 1899 July 1st and Therap Monat 1899 May. One of 10 cases: *'Aspirin 3 grammes daily in dilute alcoholic solution. Pains at once relieved. After a few days the patient complained of pain in the stomach; this immediately subsided when the medicine was stopped. There was no loss of appetite or tinnitus. The pain in the stomach was no doubt due to the alcohol; the patient at the time disliked the strong smell of alcohol in the medicine'.* The promotional booklet 'L'Aspirine' published by Bayer c1900 referred to these cases as *'un succès complet et n'observa jamais d'effets secondaires fâcheux'* [A complete success and he has never observed any annoying side effects].

63. Rich RR and Johnson JS. Calculate hepatotoxicity in patients with juvenile rheumatoid arthritis. *Arthritis Rheum* 1973;16: 1-9. Six patients.

64. Velo GP and Milanino R. Non-gastrointestinal adverse reactions to NSAID. *Journal of Rheumatology* 1990; Suppl 2017: 42–45.

65. Maclagan TJ. The treatment of acute rheumatism by salicin and salicylic acid. *Lancet* 1879 June 21st. Salicylic acid caused irritation of the throat and stomach, and also alarming depression. Its taste was disagreeably sweet and nauseous. It also gave copious perspiration…. and increasing the pulse rate and singing in the ears.

66. Korol E A. *Zdravookhr Beloruss* 1962; 8: 66. Single case of myopia with raised intraocular tension.

67. Pretty HM. Gosselin G. Colpron G. Long LA. Agranulocytosis: a report of 30 cases. *Can Med Assoc J* 1965 Nov 13; 93(20): 1058–1064.

68. Duggan JM. The relationship between perforated peptic ulcer and aspirin ingestion. *Med J of Aust*. 1965 Oct 16; 2(16): 659–662.

69. Karunaratne WAE. A case of Aspirin idiosyncrasy. *BMJ* 1919 July 12th; 42. Oedema of the face, forehead and neck, erythematous rash, albuminuria, a sensation of choking, and skin irritation. Positive rechallenge.

70. Myers ABR. Salicin in acute rheumatism. *Lancet* 1876 November 11th; 676. Several cases of haemorrhagic erosions in mucous membrane of the stomach and intestines seen at post-mortem.

71. Neale AV. Aspirin poisoning. *BMJ* 1936; 1, 109-110. Five cases: sweating, disorientated, perspiring, thirst, convulsions, delirious, albuminuria, vision streaked and a choking sensation.

72. Franke. Vergiftungserscheinungen nach Aspirin [Symptoms of poisoning after aspirin]. *Muencher Medizinische Wochenschrift* 1903 July 28th. Single case (the author): 1 gramme (15.4 grs) Aspirin: swallowing difficulties, strangulation, face red, tachycardia of 160 beats per minute, urticaria and sweating.

73. Pinedo HM, Van de Putte LB and Loeliger EH. Salicylate-induced consumption coagulopathy. *Ann Rheum Dis* 1973; 32: 66-68. Single case with liver damage and coagulopathy with positive rechallenge.

74. Okumura H, Takayama K, Obayashi K, Ichikawa T. and Aramaki T. Chronic toxic hepatitis caused by aspirin. *Japanese Journal of Clinical Medicine* 1965; 23(8): 1633–1636.

75. Sheperd FJ. Remarkable case of purpuric eruption ending in gangrene apparently caused by sodium salicylate. The New Sydenham Society; selected essays and Monographs. 1896 , 367–375. After Sodium salicylate 20 grs t.d.s for three days developed eruption on body and extremities very much like urticaria which became petechial, and which left a raised and indurated ulcer.

76. Broadbent. *BMJ* 1887 5th February. '*Cases… temperature suddenly rises, ushering in furious delirium and hyperpyrexia.*'

77. Greenhow EH. The treatment of Rheumatic fever with salicin and salicylate of soda. *Transactions of the Clinical Society of London* 1880, Spottiswoode & Co. London. '*Some symptoms of cardiac failure, calling for withdrawal of the drug.*'

78. *Wiener Allgem Med. Zeitung*. 20th December 1881. Took 8 grammes (about 120gr) sodium salicylate: headache, blind, mydriasis, deafness and somnolence. Lasted 10 hours (see 86).

79. Rushton DG. Salicylates. An International Symposium. 1963. J & A Churchill Ltd. Post-mortem oedema of larynx.

80. Gregersen JP. Occult blood in faeces of patients on oral salicylate. *Ugeskr Laeg* 1916; 78, 697: 1197–1266.

81. York CL and Fischer WJH, Jnr. *New Engl J Med* 1947; 237: 477. Cardiac failure, sodium intake increased, plasma volume increased, sodium retention, potassium loss, hypokalemia and increased cardiac output.

82. Coupland. The treatment of acute rheumatism by salicin and the salicylates. *Proceedings of the Medical Society of London* 1884; VI: 100–105. Twenty-four cases: vertigo 2, headache 8, tinnitus 10, deafness 11, delirium 2, vomiting 3, abdominal pain 2, retention of urine 3. albuminuria 1.

83. Millican. *Proceedings of the Medical Society of London* 1884; VI: 126. Two out of six cases: purpura and haematuria; albuminuria.

84. Fagge CH. *Proceedings of the Medical Society of London* 1884; VI: 50–61. Nausea and vomiting, deafness, mental excitement, giddiness, papular rash, pustular rash, delirium tremens, tremors and headache.

85. Sinclair R. The alkaline, salicin and salicylate of Soda treatment of acute rheumatism. *Lancet* 7th February 1880; 201–3: 244–246, 281–282. Headache, giddiness, tinnitus, sleeplessness, delirium, disagreeable taste, cardiac depression, perspiration, depression, dimness of vision, vomiting, deafness and unconsciousness.

86. Owen I. *Proceedings of the Medical Society of London* 1884; VI: 61-73. Single case: headache, transient blindness, somnolence, mydriasis and deafness after 120 gr sodium salicylate.

87. *Witthauer Die Heilkunde* 1899 April. '*It can be given without deranging the stomach…. Ringing in the ears is hardly ever observed with aspirin.*'

88. Leveson I. Aspirin Poisoning. *BMJ* 1949 September 17th: 628–630.

89. Sable HZ. Toxic reactions following salicylate therapy. *Can Med Assoc J* 1945 Feb; 52:153–159. Dimness of vision, thirst, dehydration, bradycardia, hypotension, oliguria, heart failure, granulocytopenia, dyspnoea, gastric retention, maculopapular rash, pustular acne, convulsions, psychosis, irritability, aphonia, dysphagia, asthma, glottic oedema, angioneurotic oedema, purpura, diarrhoea, perspiration,

depression of bone marrow function, albuminuria, headache, dizziness, tinnitus, impaired hearing, weakness, collapse, delirium, subnormal temperature, nausea and vomiting.

90. Shokhoff C and Lieberman D L. Hypersensitiveness to acetyl salicylic acid expressed by angina pectoris syndrome, with and without urticaria. *J. Allergy*, S. Louis 1933; 4: 506–512.

91. Dukes MNG. Antipyretic-analgesics. In: Meyler's Side Effects of Drugs. 11th edition. 1988, 156–169. Severe blood dyscrasias.

92. Quincke H. Zur Kenntniss der Salcylsäure Wirkung [Identification of the effect of salicylic acid], *Berl klin Wchnschr* 1882; 19: 709–711. Deep breathing.

93. *J La Med Soc* 1961; 113: 292. Single case: anaphylactic shock, urticaria and itching.

94. *Med Letter* 1964; 6(14): (MRL L5.325) Leucopenia mentioned.

95. *J Indian Med Assoc* 1956; 27: 19. Single case: itching, bullous exanthema, urticaria and angioneurotic oedema.

96. Notes, short comments and answers to correspondents. *Lancet* 1905 November; 1518.

97. Tirard Nestor Some clinical observations with new remedies. *Lancet* 1905; 73: 83-4. Dyspeptic symptoms, diarrhoea and perspiration.

98. Douthwaite AH and Lintott GAM. Gastroscopic observation of the effect of aspirin and certain other substances on the stomach. *Lancet;* ii: 1222-5. Gastric submucosal haemorrhage.

99. Fernandez-Rivas and Miranda I. Unusual NSAID hypersensitivity. *Allergy* 2002; 57: 183–184, *Reactions* 2002; 899: 13. Conjunctivitis with positive rechallenge also with diclofenac.

100. Hawkinson O and Kerr EK. A case of granulocytopenia with severe anaemia and staphylococcemia. *Illinois Med J* 1943; 81: 168–170. Single complicated case after long-term use of 40–60 grain Aspirin daily.

101. Balazs J. Uber Acetylsalicylsäure (Aspirin) [On acetylsalicylic acid (Aspirin)]. *Vergiftungen Med Klin* 1930; 26: 1664–1666. Cardiac depression.

102. Lees DB. The effective treatment of acute and subacute rheumatism. *Proc R Soc Med* 1909; 2: 34–48. Coma, air-hunger, vomiting, deafness, vertigo and delirium.

103. Gebert Karl. Die Atmung nach Therapeutische Salicylgaben [Respiration after therapeutic administration of salicyl]. Thesis, Friedrich-Wilhelm Univ. Berlin. 1931. Respiratory alkalosis.

104. *Merck G. Reports* 1904.Tympanic congestion, erythematous patches, oedema and sore throat.

105. Smull K, Wegria R and Leland J. Effect of sodium bicarbonate on serum salicylate level during salicylate therapy of patients with rheumatic fever. *JAMA* 1944; 125: 1173–1175 (August 26th). Addition of sodium bicarbonate lowered salicylate blood level.

106. Coombs FS. Toxicity of salicylates. *News Letter. AAF Rheumatic Fever Control Program* 1945; 2: 11–12 (April). Effect of sodium bicarbonate lowers salicylate blood level by increasing urinary excretion.

107. Freund R. Arzneiexanthem nach Aspirin [drug-induced rash after aspirin]. *Münch Med Wschr* 1905; 52: 707. Fixed drug eruption with positive rechallenge.

Unsubstantiated Adverse events

Strabismus, ptosis, megaloblastic anaemia, increased saliva, tingling, teratogenicity and analgesic nephropathy.

Side Effects of Drugs, Meyler's 1st Edition, 1952. This covers all salicylates: aspirin, salicylic acid, sodium salicylate, methyl salicylate and phenyl salicylate (Salol). The miscellaneous rashes are: maculo-papular exanthema, urticaria, fixed drug eruption, erythema nodosum, erythema multiforme (EM), pigmentation and haemorrhagic exanthemata.

Side Effects of Drugs 2006 15th Edition. This refers only to Aspirin.

a) Dermatological events (Type B events): the miscellaneous rashes include: purpura, Henoch-Scönlein purpura, haemorrhagic vasculitis, erythema multiforme, Stevens-Johnson syndrome, Lyell's Syndrome (TEN), eczematous dermatitis, exanthematic eruption, erythematous, scarlatiniform and morbilliform eruptions, bullous eruptions, pomphylox, dishydrosis-like lesions, and fixed drug eruptions. There is supporting evidence for these skin reactions in Litt's Drug Eruptions Reference Manual 9th edition: angio-oedema 1–5%, erythema multiforme < 1%, erythema Nodosum < 1%, fixed drug eruption < 1%, Stevens-Johnson Syndrome, Lyells syndrome < 1%, urticaria 1–10%, rash 1–10%, bullous eruption < 1 % and purpura.

b) Opthalmological events (Type B events): ptosis, strabismus and amaurosis may only be relevant to salicylic acid as I have found no confirmation of a causal association with aspirin. There have been two reports of myopia and raised intraocular pressure, but these are only likely to have been tested if there were other ocular symptoms, which had been referred to an ophthalmologist. Similarly papilloedema. They might be more frequent than this figure suggests.

c) Aspirin idiosyncrasy (Type B events): these are substantiated by many papers, but the mechanism is not certain. It is likely that hypotension is secondary to anaphylactoid shock (or poisoning) and that hypersensitivity is part of the same syndrome, which is not an allergy since no antigen–antibody reactions have been identified. This situation is usually referred to as a 'pseudo-allergic reaction' (Freie, 2000).

d) Haematological events (Type B events): there is some evidence supporting thrombocytopenia, agranulocytosis and aplastic anaemia. The relative risks were 1.9 and 2.9 respectively and, according to Dr Shapiro, the results were equivocal (IAAAS, 1986): slightly elevated, but the relative risks were of borderline statistical significance (Scrip, 1986).

e) Renal events: oliguria, renal failure, acute and/or chronic interstitial nephritis, acute tubular necrosis, papillary necrosis, analgesic nephropathy: haematuria, nocturia, symptoms of urinary tract infection, renal colic, renal calculi, renal failure, dehydration, acidosis, anaemia, hypertension, dyspepsia, peptic ulcers with haemorrhage are common. *'Reported in a considerable number of patients who have consumed a large amount of aspirin.'* (Wigley, 1973).

f) Salicylism - mild chronic intoxication (Type A events): tinnitus, dizziness, diminished vision, hearing loss, headache, feeling of intoxication, nausea and vomiting. The onset of these symptoms indicates that the plasma concentration was approaching 35 mg per 100cc. (Graham & Parker, 1948). To keep below the threshold for salicylism a dose of 12 to 20 gr every 4 hours to start with and then every six hours maintained a plasma salicylate value of 20–25 mgm per 100cc. The threshold for salicylism was 30 mgm per 100cc. (Hoffman et al., 1949).

g) Reproductive events (Type A events): prolonged labour, teratogenicity (animals only), increased bleeding.

h) Reye's syndrome is a rare paediatric disorder characterized by an initial febrile illness, commonly influenza or varicella (chickenpox), followed after several days by vomiting, disorientation, seizures and loss of consciousness. Signs–liver histology, hyperammonemia, lactic acidemia, elevated free fatty acids and amino acids (Reye et al, 1963). Most of the children died within a few days and at autopsy there was diffuse fatty infiltrate of the liver and severe cerebral oedema. The clinical and pathological features of the syndrome were first clearly defined by Dr. Reye and his associates in 1963 in Australia. Numerous cases were subsequently reported throughout the world. In the USA three epidemiologic studies were done in the late 1970's and early 1980's, which showed a statistical association between Reye's syndrome and the use of aspirin for treatment of febrile illnesses in children. In the early 1980's warnings were issued to the public and physicians about the possible association between the use of aspirin and Reye's syndrome. Heated controversies developed concerning the validity of the studies between physicians, public advocates, US Public Health Service, pharmaceutical manufacturers and others. Aspirin use was voluntarily severely curtailed and the incidence of Reye's syndrome fell dramatically. In the peak year of 1980 there were 555 cases reported in the USA, by 1987 only 36 and in the late 1990's only two to three per year. However there is still debate as to its causal factors; firstly, many cases were the result of misdiagnosis and secondly, there were flaws in the methodology and antiemetics have also been suggested as a factor. It has been written that aspirin is definitely not the cause of Reye's syndrome (Orlowski et al, 2002). The fact that the syndrome almost disappeared after the warnings were given although suggestive might also be accounted for by another factor, such as an epidemic of a viral disease. The same reasoning applies to acrodynia (see under Mercury) and deaths associated with isoprenaline inhalers. That there is an association between Aspirin and Reye's syndrome is indisputable, but whether it a causal relationship has been disputed (Glasgow, 2006); (Orlowski et al., 2002). Waller and Suvarna, both of whom either worked or had worked for the MHRA, responded to Orlowski et al. acknowledgeing that causality could not be proved, but stating that the probability of a causal relationship was strong enough to warrant the action taken, bearing in mind the availability of alternative drugs (Waller and Suvarna, 2004). Orlowski et al. replied to this with a reiteration of their arguments (Orlowski et al., 2004). The Aspirin Foundation (supported by Aspirin manufacturers) concludes; there is a lack of convincing evidence that aspirin causes Reye's syndrome: it may be one of many possible factors but many cases currently reported are probably due to inborn errors of metabolism. These arguments highlight the importance of considering the pros and cons for all the alternative treatments for a particular patient. The doubts about the safety of aspirin for children warrants its restriction to those over the age of sixteen years.

i) Acute salicylate poisoning (Type A events): headache, dizziness, nausea & vomiting, deafness, tinnitus, vertigo, visual disturbance, sweating, thirst, hyperventilation, dehydration, abnormal acid base balance, hyperpyrexia, depressed consciousness, convulsions, hyper & hypoglycaemia, pulmonary oedema, acute tubular necrosis, tremor, weakness, ataxia, dysarthria, parathesia, diplopia, hallucinations, papilloedema, confusion and agitation (Greer et al, 1965). Albuminuria, haematuria and heart failure (Balazs, 1930) It is rare below 40mgm per 100cc (Grollman, 1951).

Bayer Pamphlet (28 pages) dated probably early 1901

Includes (translated from the French):

Dosage: 3 grammes per day taken as 50 centigrammes every four hours. The innocuity of Aspirin is absolute: no action on the stomach or the digestive tract… the gastric tolerance is absolute… It is almost always useless to give more than 3 gr. Not because there is any fear of a side effect whatever, but simply because at that dose Aspirin produces generally its maximum effect… it has been possible to state the complete innocuity of the medication; of 43 patients, two only have not tolerated it because it provoked a loss of appetite and a heaviness of the stomach; but they were two badly affected cardiac patients who could not tolerate any medicine and even had difficulty with milk…We can confirm that there was a slight increase in blood pressure in the hour and during 4 hours following its ingestion… We have nothing to reproach this medicine, concerning side effects, no gastric pain, no tinnitus. Only sweating has been established, sometimes considerable. (see comments in 1899).

Patient Information leaflet (UK 2004)

Possible side effects: irritation to or bleeding of the stomach, difficulty breathing or asthma attacks in patients with a history of these, and allergic skin reactions. There is no mention of the most likely symptoms of salicylism with high doses. This is minimal information but does cover the most important ADRs at normal doses.

Summary of Product Characteristics (SPC) Electric Medicines Compendium: Boots Aspirin

Dyspepsia, nausea, vomiting. Less commonly irritation of the gastrointestinal mucosa may lead to erosion, ulceration, gastrointestinal bleeding. Hepatotoxicity occurs rarely.

Hypersensitivity reactions including urticaria, rhinitis, angioneurotic oedema and severe bronchospasm.

Aspirin may cause salt and water retention as well as deterioration in renal function.

Overdose

Salicylate poisoning is usually associated with plasma concentrations >350 mg/L (2.5 mmol/L). Most adult deaths occur in patients whose concentrations exceed 700 mg/L (5.1 mmol/L). Single doses less than 100 mg/kg are unlikely to cause serious poisoning.

Common features of salicylate poisoning include vomiting, dehydration, tinnitus, vertigo, deafness, sweating, warm extremities with bounding pulses, increased respiratory rate and hyperventilation. Some degree of acid-base disturbance is present in most cases.

A mixed respiratory alkalosis and metabolic acidosis with normal or high arterial pH (normal or reduced hydrogen ion concentration) is usual in adults and children over the age of 4 years. In children aged 4 years or less, a dominant metabolic acidosis with low arterial pH (raised hydrogen ion concentration) is common. Acidosis may increase salicylate transfer across the blood brain barrier.

Uncommon features of salicylate poisoning include haematemesis, hyperpyrexia, hypoglycaemia, hypokalaemia, thrombocytopaenia, increased INR/PTR[168], intravascular coagulation, renal failure and non-cardiac pulmonary oedema.

Central nervous system features including confusion, disorientation, coma and convulsions are less common in adults than in children.

British National Formulary (BNF)

Gastro-intestinal irritation with slight asymptomatic blood loss, increased bleeding time, bronchospasm and skin reactions in hypersensitive patients. The chief features of salicylate poisoning are hyperventilation, tinnitus, deafness, vasodilatation, and sweating. Coma is uncommon but indicates very severe poisoning. The associated acid-base disturbances are complex.

---

[168] INR/PTR = international normalised ratio/prothrombin time ratio = measures of blood coagulation

Bearing in mind the BNF and SPC are both intended to supply the prescriber with sufficient information, the difference between them is large. One of the possible reasons for this is size; the SPC is a very large volume which is rather too big to fit comfortably on a desk, whilst the BNF is pocket size.

Comments

The long list of AEs is partly due to listing symptoms that are part of syndromes or diseases, and are to that extent duplicated.

The number of ADRs caused when used for short periods at the correct dose are few and many of the ADRs mentioned are due to chronic use in diseases such as rheumatoid arthritis when it is used at maximum (in)tolerable dosage or are occasioned by accidental and deliberate overdosage.

A few AEs are either specific to salicylic acid/sodium salicylate, e.g. repulsive taste or are probably not ADRs, e.g. strabismus.

Many of the AEs are part of common physio-pathological processes and therefore unlikely to occur singly.

Many of the AEs mentioned under Aspirin precursors are also ADRs of Aspirin.

Common ADRs tend to be discovered in the first few years whilst the rare serious events were discovered late in the history of aspirin. Even ADRs, which are very familiar, are surprisingly rare, e.g. gross haemorrhage– absolute risk increase 0.6% (0.2%–1.0%); proven ulcer 0.06% (0%–1.2%) (Gøtzsche, 2000). For rare ADRs such as agranulocytosis and aplastic anemia the rate ratio estimates were for salicylates 1.6 (1.0–2.7) and 1.0 (0.6–1.6) respectively. The authors said of the agranulocytosis result that the statistical significance was borderline and it must be interpreted with caution and of aplastic anemia results that the rate ratio was somewhat elevated but that the result could have been due to chance (IAAAS, 1986).

As Owen Wade pointed out it is strange that the recognition of the relationship between the consumption of aspirin or other salicylates and massive gastrointestinal bleeding didn't come until the late 1930s and 1940s (Wade, 1970). Douthwaite and Lintott first showed bleeding from the stomach via a gastroscope in 1938. The semi-flexible gastroscope only having been invented in 1932 (Douthwaite and Lintott, 1938).

The terminology in the 1900s was not as specific as that used in the present century, e.g. agranulocytosis was first described in 1922 as angina agranulocytotics (Hess et al, 1983), although aplastic anemia was described as early as 1888 by Erlich (Erlich, 1888). Many of the early reports were couched in terms of symptoms such as dimness of vision, albuminuria and rashes, which were later, specified as individual specific disorders.

In the various listings it is difficult to separate the ADRs occurring at normal therapeutic doses from those where an overdose has taken place due to large variations in individual responses.

The sources for 2006 and 2007 (Meyler's, Micromedex, Inchem and Martindale's) do not mention peritoneal irritation, diarrhoea, vertigo, cardiac insufficiency, bradycardia, insomnia, agitation, dysarthria, polyuria, Cushing's syndrome, haematuria, megaloblastic anemia, alopecia or conjunctivitis. Although 11 of these were mentioned in earlier Meyler's. In all I have traced 65 adverse events: Meyler's; prior to 2006; mentioned 56; Meyler's 2006–40; Martindale 2007–28; Inchem 2007–40. There are probably several reasons why they have not included all of them: too rare, doubtful ADR or dealt with under a broader term.

In planning any pharmacovigilance with a new drug one needs to examine the prior probabilities, which will be partly based on drugs of the same class, i.e. other salicylates. How soon were the predictable ADRs recognised with aspirin?

I contacted Bayer Archives with a view to obtaining more information about aspirin ADRs, but I was unsuccessful.

Relating serum salicylate concentration to symptoms

For treatment of acute rheumatic fever the maintenance level should be 30–35 mg. per 100cc. (Hoffman et al., 1949). The Mayo clinic considers the optimum level for rheumatoid arthritis to be 18–20 mg per 100cc., but may need from 60–125 grains (3.9 to 8.1 gm) a day (Greer et al., 1965). A single dose of Aspirin of 2 gm. gave levels of 10 mg. per 100cc. A dose of 12 to 20 gr. (0.8 to 1.3 gm) every four hours until the desired level had been reached and then the same dose every six hours maintained levels of between 20 and 25 mg. per 100cc. (Hoffman et al., 1949). The toxic dose of sodium salicylate is between 12 and 30 gr (0.78 gm to 1.95 gm) in a single dose (Duchesney, 1954).

Table 8. Aspirin serum concentrations and symptoms

Mg/dl	Grading	Symptoms
20-30	Salicylism	Aspirin: no symptoms (Hoffman et al., 1949) Sodium Salicylate: erythema, tinnitus, deafness, nausea, vomiting (Graham & Parker, 1948)
30-40	Salicylism	Aspirin: tinnitus, partial deafness, nausea/vomiting, general feeling of intoxication (Hoffman et al., 1949) Sodium salicylate: albuminuria, hyperventilation, sweating and headache (Graham & Parker, 1948)
40-50	Intoxication	Sodium Salicylate: vertigo, drowsiness, haematuria, confusion, excitement, severe dyspnoea (Graham & Parker, 1948)
50-80	Mild	Aspirin: hyperpnoea, marked lethargy and/ or excitability; hypocapnia without acidosis (Rainsford, 2004)
80-100	Moderate	Aspirin: severe hypopnoea, marked lethargy and/ or excitability, vomiting in children, compensated metabolic acidosis (Rainsford, 2004)
110	Severe	Aspirin: coma, possible convulsions, uncompensated metabolic acidosis in children after 12 hours (Rainsford, 2004)
160	Usually lethal	Aspirin (Rainsford, 2004)

Relating dosage to symptoms

The following 4 categories are helpful for assessing the potential severity and morbidity of an acute, single event, non enteric-coated, salicylate ingestion:

1. Less than 150 mg/kg – Spectrum ranges from no toxicity to mild toxicity
2. From 150-300 mg/kg – Mild-to-moderate toxicity
3. From 301-500 mg/kg – Serious toxicity
4. Greater than 500 mg/kg – Potentially lethal toxicity (http://www.emedicine.com/emerg/byname/toxicity-salicylate.htm)

It was said that the raison d'etre for Aspirin was that it had less gastric problems that its predecessors, but it was in fact more toxic to the stomach, as Rainsford points out, the Gastric lesion index in rats was 63.0 for Aspirin whilst for salicylic acid it was 16.0 and for sodium salicylate it was 10.6. As was seen with mercury one of the adverse effects of Aspirin has a unexpected benefit in that with some suicidal attempts the resultant gastric irritation is so severe that the patient promptly vomits up the stomach including a lot of the Aspirin so saving the patient's life.

Chapter 14. Streptomycin

Streptomycin was originally discovered in January, 1944, by Schatz, Bugie and Waksman. It was extracted from colonies of *Actnomyces griseus*, but its purity varied. It is scarcely absorbed at all by mouth and was given either subcutaneously, intramuscularly, intravenously or intrathecally. The main problem has been the development of resistance. In the beginning supplies were very scarce and only a few US hospitals had supplies. Reports of its activity for the treatment of tuberculosis in humans date from 1945.

Animal toxicity

Guinea pigs and mice – well tolerated (Molitor, 1947).

Monkeys and dogs–transient anaemia, proteinuria with casts and blood in the urine. Dogs showed signs of vestibular dysfunction (Hinshaw and Feldman, 1948) Fatty metamorphoses in parenchymal cells of the liver and tubular epithelium of the kidneys.

1944 January Schatz, Bugie and Waksman discovered Streptomycin (Schatz et al., 1944).

1944 September

Streptomycin first used clinically.

1945 September

First report of its use. Thirty four patients had a dose between 800,000–1,200,000 Streptomycin units per kilogram per day (1,000,000 streptomycin units = 1 Gram streptomycin).

1. Histamine reactions: throbbing headache and flushing.
2. Mild malaise, myalgia, and rarely arthralgia.
3. Four patients with fever.
4. One case of transient deafness and three cases of disturbed vestibular function (Hinshaw and Feldman, 1945).

1945 Ten patients

1. Toxic effects: headache, flushes, palpitations, urticaria and fever (Zintel et al., 1945).

Irritation at the injection site, chills and fever, flushing, toxic erythema, urticaria, joint pains, nausea, albuminuria and microscopic haematuria (Heilman et al., 1945).

1945 October Three patients.

1. Peculiar taste in the mouth, headache, flushing, and two had nausea.
2. Soreness and induration of the injection site (Anderson & Jewell, 1945).

1945 December

Four typhoid carriers were treated:
1. Fever and inflammation at injection site.
2. Depression of blood pressure (Rutstein et al., 1945).

1946 January Forty-five patients treated. Two had a bad taste in the mouth, dizziness and respiratory difficulty and lost consciousness for 3-5 minutes. Thirteen of the remaining patients had toxic symptoms: fever - 3, rash -2, generalised aching, weakness and pain the joints - 9, and one had swelling of her wrists. Others had flushing of the skin, headache and a sense of fullness in the head shortly after injection (Buggs et al., 1946).

1946 March Nine patients. Differing doses.

1. Histamine reactions: flushing, headache, fall in blood pressure (2).
2. Fever (4), myalgias and arthralgias (3).
3. Skin eruption (2).
4. Local reactions: pain and tenderness.
5. Urine: two patients had formed elements and one haematuria (Hettig & Adcock, 1946).

1946 June US Veterans Administration started clinical trials using 1.8 gm daily and in December 1946 the dose was increased to 2.0 Gm daily.

1946 September

4th Eighth Nerve Toxicity. Twenty three patients. The dose used is uncertain.

1. Equilibrium problems: dizziness, lightheadedness and giddiness produced by turning over in bed or sitting up for meals; several complained of nausea and one vomited and one had spontaneous nystagmus. Caloric stimulation indicated a decrease in labyrinthine function usually bilateral. After stopping treatment because of dizziness labyrinthine function doesn't return to normal but compensation takes place.
2. Hearing problems: Five had some degree of hearing loss and five cases had tinnitus. If the treatment was stopped the hearing usually improved. There was no cochlea dysfunction at 1-2 grams daily (Brown & Hinshaw, 1946).

1946 September 14th

One thousand patients. Incidence of ADRs was 20.5 %
1. Sensitization reactions: skin eruptions (erythematous, urticarial, maculopapular or haemorrhagic)[49], fever (49), eosinophilia (Nine of eleven patients).
2. Histamine reactions: headache (55), flushing (43), nausea and vomiting (1), fall in blood pressure (1)
3. Neurological Disturbances: vertigo (33), tinnitus (13), deafness (6).
4. Local irritation: pain, soreness and induration (15) tingling (2) and parathesias (3).
5. Miscellaneous problems: diarrhoea (1), albuminuria and casts (2), purpura haemorrhagica (1) and arthralgia (1).
6. Urine: Nine out of ten had hyaline and granular casts. Information given on time to onset and duration of ADRs. Overall 20.5% of patients had adverse reactions and at 3G daily 46% had reactions, whilst at ≥ 4 G 60% had reactions. When the average daily dose exceeded 1 Gm there was an increase in the number of ADRs. (Keefer et al., 1946).

1946 September 28th

One hundred and four patients. No individual ADR mentioned. Dose between 1 and 3G daily.

General mention: nausea, malaise, fever, renal irritation, arthralgia, local reactions at site of injection (possibly due to impurities), tinnitus and dizziness, skin reactions (urticaria, maculopapular or generalized dermatitis) (Nichols & Herrell, 1946).

1946 November 30th

One hundred patients. Dose 1–3 gm daily. No individual ADRs.

1. Vestibular damage with frequent persistence of diminished response to caloric stimulation for at least several weeks after dechallenge.
2. Irritation at site of injection and is inversely proportional to the purity of the product.
3. Histamine-like reactions caused by impurities (Hinshaw et al, 1946).

1947 January 11th

Otic Complications. One hundred and sixty one patients. Dose 3 gm daily. There was definite toxicity in 3% of patients.

1. Hearing problems: 65% had high tone loss and 13.6 % of these also had low tone loss whilst 32.1% had normal hearing.
2. Vestibular function: Caloric stimulation showed a normal response in 80.2% of patients (Fowler & Seligman, 1947).

1947 June 21st

Thirty one patients received 3 gm of highly purified streptomycin daily for 120 days.

1. Two patients had 'anaphylactic[169]' reactions: fever, maculopapular rash, nausea and vomiting, hypotension and eosinophilia (14 out of 16).
2. One patient had acute synovitis of the interphalangeal joints.
3. Casts (cylindruria) occurred in the urine of 14 out of 17 patients.
4. Disturbed vestibular function appeared in all patients.
5. Leucopenia in two patients.
6. Two patients had tinnitus and hearing impairment (Farrington et al., 1947).

There were no histamine reactions or injection site reactions.

1947 June Deafness occurred in 7 patients out of one hundred; five of these had intrathecal streptomycin for meningitis and the other two had doses greater than 3 gm daily. The other factor may be renal insufficiency (McDermott, 1947).

---

[169] anaphylactic = Usually refers to immediate hypersensitivity reaction in which the exposure of a *sensitized* individual to a specific antigen or hapten results in urticaria, pruritus and angioedema followed by vascular collapse, however here it probably refers to the development of hypersensitivity induced by exposure to a specific antigen which results, after a latent period of 1–3 weeks, in an allergic manifestation

1947 Five patients with miliary tuberculosis. Possible renal tubular damage in one patient (Haggenstoss et al., 1947).

1947 Pharmacology Review

1. Circulatory effects: Histamine like - vaso-dilatation, fall in blood pressure, increased secretion of gastric juice, temporary inhibition of water diuresis, contraction of the isolated intestine and uterus, due to impurities. In man these are manifest as headache, nausea, reddening of the skin, and occasionally fainting spells.
2. Hepatic changes: none in man.
3. Renal effects: albuminuria, haematuria, appearance of casts due to tubular degeneration and necrosis.
4. Neurotoxic properties: vestibular and auditory disturbance.
5. Others: rashes, temporary elevation of body temperature, pain in the joints and injection site discomfort which may be due to impurities (Moliter, 1947).

1947 July Review:

1. Histamine reactions: flushing, headache and fall in blood pressure.
2. 'Anaphylactic' reactions.
3. Disturbance of vestibular function and occasional deafness.
4. Irritation of the kidney (Leader BMJ, 1947).

1947 Forty patients. Dose 3.0 gm daily

1. Histamine reactions: flushing, headache and fall in blood pressure. Probably due to impurities.
2. Irritation at injection site: pain, soreness and induration, which was probably due to impurities.
3. 'Anaphylactic' manifestations: fever, dermatitis (about 5%) and eosinophilia (14 of 16 patients).
4. Renal irritation: cylindruria, albuminuria, reduction of renal function (1–3%).
5. Neurological Disturbances: vestibular dysfunction varies with dose and duration of treatment, headache, heavy headiness, vertigo, nausea, and vomiting.
   Deafness (7%) was dose related and more common in those who have had intrathecal streptomycin.
6. Miscellaneous reactions: leucopenia with relative

granulocytopenia; and one case of thrombocytopenia (McDermott, 1947).

1947 Miliary Tuberculosis. 5 patients
One patient became deaf and others developed confusion and delerium and these were probably disease related.

1947 November 8th

Five hundred and forty three patients (Veteran's Administration). Dose used varied between 1.8 and 2.0 G daily.
Preliminary statement.
Toxic manifestations required 6% to stop treatment. Medical staff developed contact dermatitis.
1. Local irritation due to intrathecal injections caused temporary partial paraplegia in 3.3% of patients.
2. Minor toxic reactions: fever was rare, circumoral parathesia was commonly observed and nausea and vomiting occurred occasionally.
3. Jaundice, psychosis and blood dyscrasias: jaundice (2), psychosis (1), mild leucopenia with neutropenia (5), agranulocytosis (3) quite definitely due to streptomycin.
4. Sensitivity Reactions: eosinophilia (10-20%) skin eruptions (0.80%).
5. Renal damage: casts and albumin almost routinely found. Increasing renal dysfunction (2.1%).
6. Damage to the eighth nerve: vertigo (96%) deafness (1.1%) (Veterans Administration, 1947).

1947 December 6th

One hundred and eighteen patient with tuberculous meningitis.
1. General toxic disturbances: somnolence and clouding of the mind may be caused by the drug. Deafness in 15 of patients.
2. Cutaneous reactions: transient erythema with fever.
3. Meningeal reactions: stiff neck, pain on each injection, severe convulsions with opisthotonos (Debré, 1947).
Reaction most frequently encountered is disturbance of equilibrium which is uncomfortable, but not usually dangerous; deafness–usually in patients with meningitis, mild irritation of the kidneys (Riggins and Hinshaw, 1947)

1948 January 17th

Review

The vestibular disturbance is dose dependent–at a dose of 1 Gm daily fewer than 30% will have symptoms but at 2 Gm daily this increases to at least 90%. Including erythematous rash, fever, eosinophilia and abnormal urinary elements (Feldman & Hinshaw, 1948).

1948 April George Orwell, author of '*Animal Farm*' and '*Nineteen Eighty Four*'

His Doctor: 'He was given 1g of Streptomycin daily and appeared to be making some clinical response, but after a few weeks he developed a severe allergic reaction with dermatitis and stomatitis. He wrote an excellent description of this in his notebook, he could not receive any more of this drug'.

George Orwell: 'I forget them; it is worth writing down the secondary symptoms produced by streptomycin when I was treated with it last year. Streptomycin was then almost a new drug & had never been used at that hospital before. The symptoms in my case were quite different from those described in the American medical journal in which we read the subject up beforehand.

At first, though the streptomycin seemed to produce an almost immediate improvement in my health, there were no secondary symptoms, except that a sort of discoloration appeared at the base of my fingers & toe nails. Then my face became noticeably redder & the skin had a tendency to flake off, & a sort of rash appeared all over my body, especially down my back. There was no itching associated with this. After about 3 weeks I got a severe sore throat, which did not go away & was not affected by sucking penicillin lozenges. It was very painful to swallow & I had to have a special diet for some weeks. There was now ulceration with blisters in my throat & in the insides of my cheeks, & the blood kept coming up into little blisters on my lips. At night these burst & bled considerably, so that in the morning my lips were always stuck together with blood & I had to bathe them before I could open my mouth. Meanwhile my nails had disintegrated at the roots & the disintegration grew, as it were, up the nail, new nails forming beneath meanwhile. My hair began to come out,

& one or two patches of quite white hair appeared at the back
(previously it was only speckled with grey).

   After 50 days the streptomycin, which had been injected at the
rate of 1 gramme a day, was discontinued. The lips etc. healed
almost immediately & the rash went away, though not quite so
promptly. My hair stopped coming out & went back to its normal
colour, though I think with more grey in it than before. The old
nails ended by dropping out altogether, & some months after
leaving hospital I had only ragged tips, which kept splitting, to
the new nails. Some of the toenails did not drop out. Even now
my nails are not normal. They are much more corrugated than
before, & a great deal thinner, with a constant tendency to split
if I do not keep them very short. At that time the Board of Trade
would not give import permits for streptomycin, except to a few
hospitals for experimental purposes. One had to get hold of it
by some kind of wire-pulling. It cost £1 a gramme, plus 60%
Purchase Tax'. He could not tolerate the side effects and he died
from lack of chemotherapy (Crofton, 2009).

1948 July Review
   1. Histamine reaction: flushing, headache and fall in blood
      pressure? due to impurities.
   2. Soreness and induration after intramuscular injection. ? due
      to impurities.
   3. Hypersensitivity with fever and dermatitis, including one
      case of exfoliative dermatitis. Eosinophilia in large number of
      patients.
   4. Renal toxicity with albuminuria, decrease in renal function
      (urea clearance ↓, Blood urea nitrogen ↑).
   5. Neurotoxicity. Almost all patients on prolonged courses will
      develop vestibular damage. 96% at 2 gm daily for 120 days.
      Daily dose of 1 gm daily reduces incidence by 20%.
   6. Deafness is not common, but is dose related and partly
      reversible.
   7. Blood dyscrasias: Eight cases reported: five mild leukopenia
      with neutropenia, three cases of agranulocytosis.
      Thrombocytopenia was rare (Farber and Eagle, 1948).

1948 August Canada. The drug became available on May 2nd 1947 but in
such limited supplies that only the most serious cases could

be treated. The dosage started at 3 gm daily but by November had been reduced to 1 gm daily. Case series of 100 patients: there were 6 deaths and 32 patients suffered ADRs: minor skin lesions, slight dizziness, nausea and occasional vomiting. One patient had severe dizziness, which reversed on dechallenge, and three others had severe nausea, vomiting and dizziness; two of whom died and the other recovered from the toxic effect. One patient after local application developed an itchy erythematous rash with positive rechallenge. Original dose 3 gm daily then reduced to 2 gm daily and finally 1 gm daily.

Comment: No precise numbers of patients suffering individual events. No mention of any dose-relationship (Kincade et al, 1948). No controlled trials had been undertaken in the US.

1948 October MRC Streptomycin in Tuberculosis Trials Committee. Streptomycin treatment of pulmonary tuberculosis. Randomised control trial. Total number of patients 107; 52 on bed rest only and 55 on bed rest plus streptomycin at a dose of 2 gm daily. The duration of the study was 6 months.

'Toxic effects' were observed in many patients and 'the effects will only be described briefly because they have already been described by other investigators'.

1. Giddiness was noticed by 36 out of 55 patients with nystagmus coming on after 6 weeks in some patients.
2. Two cases of high-tone deafness.
3. Many patients suffered from nausea and vomiting.
4. Albuminuria and casts in urine and raised blood urea.
5. Pruritus, urticarial rash and eosinophilia.
6. Yellow vision after injection.
7. Circumoral numbness (Streptomycin in Tuberculosis Trials Committee, 1948).

'By far the most important toxic effect was the damage to the vestibular apparatus. Giddiness was a frequent first symptom; it was noticed by 36 of the 55 patients, and first appeared on sitting up in bed or turning the head suddenly. It appeared usually in the fourth or fifth week of therapy, and persisted for periods varying from one week to several months. Spontaneous nystagmus on lateral vision was another frequent sign of vestibular disturbance; blurring of vision was less common. Tests

for vestibular dysfunction were not carried out in all centres with sufficient regularity and uniformity to permit analysis of grouped results, but it is possible to say that absence or reduction of caloric response was not found with the frequency reported in many American investigations, and that in some patients loss of response was temporary only. No standard functional tests at the ends of treatment were performed; many patients are reported as having unsteadiness of gait, which improved gradually with visual compensation but remained a handicap in the dark, crossing a congested street, or walking in a moving train. It is highly desirable that standard tests be adopted for assessment of vestibular dysfunction. No loss of hearing was reported, except for two cases of high-tone deafness' (MRC Council, 1948).

Comment: there was no comparison with the control group as far as adverse effects were concerned; no information on grouping of symptoms; many adverse events have no numbers attached; no comparison with previous studies in the discussion section; no grading of severity (MRC, 1948). The clinical trial form (A) requested symptoms on admission and these included vertigo, giddiness and deafness (These had already been established as ADRs in the USA). This form also asked for *'Previous treatment for present illness (dates, place, nature and duration of treatment)'*, but no request for details of treatments for other illnesses. The final summary form (A3) had space for 'Evidence of toxicity' and remarks, so that it presumed that the investigator's opinion as to attribution was correct. Form (C) Clinical Record said *'Record here symptoms and clinical findings not recorded on sheets A or B. Symptoms attributable to streptomycin toxicity should be underlined'.* Form (D) was a record of treatment. Although vestibular disturbance and deafness were predictable insufficient testing was performed to allow a true assessment of the damage done. No analysis of the reversibility of these ADRs was published. In 1951 a paper on the return of the vestibular function following streptomycin toxaemia was published. Of 62 patients who had taken 2 gm daily for 110 days: 42 had complete loss of caloric stimulation and in the majority of cases response returned in varying degrees over a period of two years and 89% had mild decrease in

vestibular function at the end of six weeks. These were followed
up and at one year 25 patients had negative responses, at 2
years 5 patients and at three years 3 patients had no response
to caloric tests, but in the older group (over 45 years) in a small
percentage there was never a return to normal. Those over 45
years of age suffered more than younger patients. These figures
give a percentage of 68% for diagnosis by caloric stimulation of
vestibular dysfunction compared with 65% for clinical diagnosis
in the MRC study. In 215 patients taking the lower dose of
1gm per day for 110 days the figures at the end of treatment
was 18 negative responses (complete loss of response to caloric
stimulation), two had negative responses after one year and
none had negative responses after three years (Chase, 1951). In
the MRC study neither the streptomycin group nor the control
group knew that they were in a clinical trial (Crofton, 2006)
and therefore it would have been unacceptable to have carried
out tests which did not have a direct connection with their
treatment. However this would not have prevented them from
monitoring the streptomycin group for their vestibular function
and hearing. Neither the MRC nor the National Archives could
find copies of the protocol and the safety results (MRC, 2009).

1949 Nausea and vomiting occurred in 17(35%) of 49 patients, but
this could be prevented by 'Benadryl', an antihistamine with
anticholinergic properties (Bignall & Crofton, 1949).

1951 During trials at the Brompton hospital in the above study 76
patients were treated with streptomycin and of these 14% on 2G
daily had giddiness with an average time to onset of 45 days,
whilst of those on 1G daily 7% complained of giddiness and the
time to onset was halved at 22 days (Bignall et al., 1951).

1953 Patients developing hypersensitivity could be desentised and so
continue with treatment, but this did not come in time to save
George Orwell (Crofton, 1953).

1961 A review of 3,148 patients found 7 cases of hearing impairment;
all were older than 40 years and had normal renal function.
The dosage used was 1G either daily or twice weekly, plus para-
aminosalicylic acid (PAS) 3 G twice or four times a day. Isoniazid
(INAH) at a dosage of 100 or 150 mgm twice daily. They quoted

other papers giving incidences of vestibular damage: 12%, 20%, 24%, 21%, 14%. In their study 1.6% of patients discontinued streptomycin because of vestibular dysfunction (n = 2,660) with an overall figure of 6%. Factors: age (> 45 years), size of the dose, duration of treatment and purity of drug (Kalinowski et al., 1961).

2006 Side effect of Drugs

Peripheral neuritis rarely, neuromuscular blockade with respiratory depression, disturbance of vision, anosmia, circumoral anaesthesia, temporary loss of concentration, drug fever, hypotension, Stevens-Johnson syndrome, haemolytic anaemia (which is very rare), vestibular damage in 30% of patients on 1 gm daily and high-frequency deafness in 5–15% of patients. Exanthematous skin reactions in about 5% of patients. Intrathecal injection has been followed by radiculitis, myelitis and other neurological complications.

2008 Micromedex

Haematological: blood coagulation, eosinophilia (common), leucopenia, thrombocytopenia and pancytopenia.

Dermatological: urticaria, purpura, pruritus, exfoliative dermatitis, anaphylactic reaction, Stevens-Johnson syndrome, and mouth ulcers.

Neurological: encephalopathy, arachnoiditis, peripheral neuritis, optic nerve dysfunction, neuromuscular blockade with respiratory paralysis and facial parathesia (common).

Ototoxicity: tinnitus, vertigo, hearing loss, dizziness, giddiness and ataxia.

Renal: nephrotoxicity.

Other: fever (common).

Dose effect

3 gm - Severe perceptive deafness and vertigo.

2 gm–68% had vestibular damage.

1 gm–8.4 % had vestibular damage.

Symptoms are unlikely to occur if the dose does not exceed 0.5 Gm a day (Cawthorne & Ranger, 1957).

SED refers to the editions of Meyler's 'Side effects of Drugs'.

Table 9. Adverse reactions to Streptomycin

ADRs of Streptomycin	1945	1946	1947	1948	SED Ia 1952	SED Ib 1957	SED 2 1958	SED 3 1960	SED 4 1964	SED 5 1966	SED 6 1968	SED 7 1972	SED 14 2000	2008
Histamine release	x	x	x	x	x									
Anaphylaxis					x		x	x	x	x	x	x	.	x
Asthma				x					x	x		x		
Vestibular effects	x	x	x	x	x	x		x	x	x	x		x	
Deafness	x	x	x	x	x	x	x	x	x		x		x	
Injection reaction	x	x	x	x	x									
Fever	x	x	x	x	x						x			x
Malaise	x	x				x			x					
Nausea/ vomiting	x	x	x	x	x	x			x	x				
Myalgia	x	x	x		x				x					
Taste in mouth	x	x			x			x						
Arthralgia	x	x	x		x									
Myocarditis								x	x	x				
Eosinophilia		x	x		x					x				x
Leucopenia		x	x	x	x									x
Agranulo-cytosis			x	x	x									
Thrombo-cytopenia			x	x	x									x
Pancytopenia									x					x
Aplastic anaemia					1951			x	x					
Haemolytic anaemia													x	x
Purpura		x			x									x
Coagulation problem		x			x									
Renal–Casts		x	x	x	x									
Albuminuria	x	x	x	x	x									
Renal dysfunction		x	x	x	x	x	x							x
Vision–Yellow				x			x							

ADRs of Streptomycin	1945	1946	1947	1948	SED Ia 1952	SED Ib 1957	SED 2 1958	SED 3 1960	SED 4 1964	SED 5 1966	SED 6 1968	SED 7 1972	SED 14 2000	2008
Disturbed vision		x			x	x	x	x		x			x	x
Hypotension	x	x	x		x				x					
Skin eruption	Urti-caria	x	x	x	x	x		x		x				
SJ syndrome/ TEN	Toxic ery-thema												x	x
Urticaria	x	x		x	x									x
Pruritus		x	x	x	x						x			x
Oral lesions				x										
Anosmia													x	
Jaundice		x			x									
Psychosis		x			x		x	x	x					
CNS Facial parathesia		x	x		x	x	x	x		x			x	x
Peripheral neuritis													x	x
Encepha-lopathy					1952				x					x
Neuro-muscular block							x	x	x	x	x	x	x	x

Histamine release = Headache, flushing and fall in blood pressure.

Injection site reaction = pain, soreness, induration and lipodystrophy.

Intrathecal injection reactions = headache, nausea and vomiting, nystagmus, slow respiration, retention of urine, delerium, loss of weight and meningeal irritation.

Deafness = deafness and tinnitus.

Vestibular effects = Vertigo, dizziness, giddiness, ataxia and cochlear toxicity.

Neuromuscular blockade = impaired vision, respiratory paralysis (1961) and muscular weakness (1965).

Skin eruptions = urticaria, angioneurotic oedema, purpura, erythroderma; roseola, follicular, maculo-papular, scarlatiniform, morbilliform and bullous exanthemas.

Facial parathesia = usually circumoral.

Oral lesions = stomatitis, erosions, ulcers and leucokeratosis.

Disturbed vision = included ambylopia, diminished accommodation, diplopia and optic neuritis (Walker, 1961).

Renal dysfunction = raised blood urea nitrogen.

Myocarditis = Fiedler's myocarditis (Chatterjee & Thakre, 1958).

2 gm - Vertigo in 75% but no deafness.

1 gm - Vertigo in about 15% (Ormerod, 1954).

Comment

Was the dosage of streptomycin used unduly high for too long? The Canadians reduced their dosage from 2 G daily to 1G daily on November 1st 1947, but McDermott in 1947 said that it was probable that 3G represented the upper limit of the safe daily dose. Other papers published at this time did not suggest reducing the dosage. The MRC study started recruiting patients in January 1947 and the dosage of 2 G daily had been decided after speaking with Dr HC Henshaw, who had a wide experience and in his paper of 17th January 1948 he suggested that in TB the average daily dose be approximately 1G for a patient of average weight, but in November 1946 he had recommended for adults 1 to 3G per twenty-four hours. The difficulty in choosing a safe dose may have been due to:

1. The numerous forms of TB which demanded different doses, e.g. miliary TB, TB meningitis, different sites of the TB infection and a wide range of severity.
2. Causal factors for vestibular dysfunction: patient aged over 45 years, size of dose, duration of treatment, patient's weight, a difference between complaints of giddiness on a single daily dose compared with divided doses during the day,
3. Varying purity and three different salts: Glaxo–S calcium chloride complex, Merck–S hydrochloride and Pfizer - S sulphate.

Although the MRC study made little effort in exploring the adverse effects of streptomycin most of the relevant facts had been established by the previous case series.

Histamine release due to impurities suggests an anaphylactoid reaction due to instant release of histamine without developing hypersensitivity whereas the anaphylactic reactions only occurred after prior hypersensitzation. The injection site reactions also seem to have been due to impurities and also do not occur after 1948, The fact that fever is not mentioned after 1948 suggests that too maybe due to impurities but not connected with injection site reaction as its time to onset and duration are rather too long and there is no mention of a relationship. Renal casts and albuminuria are not mentioned after 1948 when purified streptomycin became available so they too may have been due to impurities. Nausea and vomiting developed abouts six weeks after the start of the trial and they were also thought to be due to impurities as they ceased when the pure streptomycin became available (Crofton, 2009) Asthma, pancytopenia, aplastic anaemia, haemolytic anaemia, Stevens-Johnson syndrome, peripheral neuritis, encephalopathy, neuromuscular block, anosmia and loss of concentration were all discovered after 1957 suggesting that they might be very rare. Fiedler's myocarditis was probably a single case (Chatterjee & Thakre, 1958). The case series prior to 1948 seem to have been effective in discovering the commoner ADRs.

Of those ADR not discovered before 2000:

Stevens-Johnson Syndrome. There was a single case published in 1982 (Sarker et al., 1982) A case of toxic erythema with generalising follicular pustules with a positive rechallenge appeared in 1981 (Shimoto & Aoki, 1981).

Anosmia. A survey of 300 patients found 8 cases of anosmia and 13 cases of hyposmia, but all but two had had anosmia before streptomycin (Kerekovic & Curkevic, 1971) an allusion to 5 case of olfactory disturbance was made in 2003 (Welge-Luessen & Wolfensberaed, 2003).

Haemolytic anaemia. A single case of immune haemolytic anaemia and renal failure was reported in 1977 (Martinez-L et al., 1977) and a similar case in 1962 (Nachman et al., 1962).

Peripheral neuritis. First reported in 1971 (Herishany & Tauste, 1971).

The small number of patients involved in these late reported cases suggests that they are rare and that their discovery probably resulted from the large number of patients treated over the years. Most of the ADRs were discovered via individual reports or small case series and the MRC Trial added little to our knowledge of the ADRs. In the USA where they had started with individual cases and case series the dramatic improvements meant that controlled studies would be unethical, but the dramatic improvement only became clear after a controlled study had started and since there was sufficient drug available to treat patients the placebo control study was unethical and was stopped. The situation was different in the UK as there was insufficient drug to treat all the patients so a placebo group was ethical (Green, 1954). The advent of streptomycin made little difference to the already declining death rate of tuberculosis (McKeown, 1976).

Ideal knowledge of an ADR

How much do we know about the most common reactions for the first five marker drugs compared with a modern drug–Streptomycin (Type A reaction characteristics in italics that will alter with dose)

The manifestation (clinical or laboratory) both subjective and objective

Graded both for severity and seriousness

Frequency or incidence, both absolute and relative to similar drugs with confidence intervals

Mechanism of action
Causality
Predisposing factors
Treatment and its effect
Reversibility or sequelae

Table 10. Knowledge of adverse reactions to the marker drugs

Attributes	Hellebore	Henbane	Mercury	Opium	Aspirin	Streptomycin
Manifestation	Vomiting	Madness	Salivation or ptyalism	Nausea	Tinnitus	VIII cranial nerve. Giddiness usually appearing in the 4/5th week. Deafness (rare)
Severity	+++	Variable	Variable	Vomiting	+	+++
Seriousness	Potentially	+++	No	+	No	+++
Incidence	Dose related	Dose related	Dose related	Dose related	Dose related	65% - 68%
Absolute	Dose related	Dose related	Dose related	Dose related	9 of 58	36 of 55
Relative to competitors	More than most other emetics	?	Not with other syphilis treatments	Affects 2/3 of patients	Occurs with all salicylates	More than dihydro-streptomycin
Cls	?	?	?	?	?	?
Mechanism	Type 'A'	Type 'A'	Type 'A'	Type 'A'	Type 'A'	Type 'A'
Causality	Certain	Certain	Certain	Certain	Certain	Certain
Factors	Dose (see 78,1619, 1652 & 1694)	Dose	Dose, age	Dose	Dose	Renal function, age, weight (see above)
Treatment	Stop	Stop	Reduce dose	Anti-emetic or reduce dose	Reduce dose	Reduce dose
Effective	Yes	Yes	Yes	Yes	Yes	Usually
Reversible	Yes	Yes	Yes	Yes	Yes	Not always
Sequelae	Dehydration	?	Nil	Dehydration	Nil	Possible

By choosing the most common ADRs one automatically rules out most type B reactions and some of the categories are not relevant. In type 'A' reactions confidence limits for incidences would only be relevant at a standard dosage. Although under 'factors' only dose is mentioned there may also be idiosyncratic predisposition, e.g. salivation with mercury.

Regulatory responses to adverse drug reactions

Usually herbs and drugs disappear from the scene quietly as the cost/benefit ratio is superseded by that of a new drug and the pharmaceutical company realises that it is no longer commercially viable. Many of the herbs that dominated the therapeutic market until the 19th century have persisted, aided by outworn philosophies, whilst some have had active principles that have been extracted and have joined the standard pharmaceutical armamentarium. It was not until a central authority took an interest in pharmaceuticals that action was taken on a nationwide basis to deal with unsafe drugs. Between the initiation of voluntary withdrawal by the company and the official withdrawal by the regulatory authority there remains the grey area where the interaction between the two parties results in the company withdrawing the drug under pressure from the regulatory authority.

The ultimate sanction is the withdrawal of a drug from the market for all indications, but before this occurs there are several alternative actions that can be taken:

Warning of adverse effects

Restrictions on dose and dosage forms

Restrictions on indications

Restrictions on prescription

Restrictions on use of 'inactive' drug constituents (Bakke et al., 1984)

Despite these actions the prescribers may not heed them and the regulatory authority will be forced to withdraw the drug, e.g. amidopyrine, bromfenac, cisapride, ebronidine and troglitazone (Smalley, 2001; NAO[170], 2003). The whole area of regulatory response to adverse events was secret *'The CSM's policy on non-disclosure of adverse drug reaction data, agreed at a meeting in June 1989, is itself an official secret'* (Medawar, 1990); *'data handled by regulatory authorities are highly confidential'.* (Hancher, 1989). The confidentiality laws are included within the 1968 Medicines Act.

Regulatory authorities

The dates when different countries have undertaken some kind of control of drugs on the market have been given earlier in the book, but for many countries it is unknown. Many of the drugs mentioned in Part 3 were removed after 1960 and their removal from a specific market depended on whether there was an active regulatory authority in that country at the time of the drug problem. As a marker for the date when a country's regulatory system was viable, I have taken the year of entry to the WHO programme.

---

[170] NAO = Nation Audit Office (UK)

For those countries where there was an active system prior to joining the WHO programme the earliest date known for that country is in brackets

1968: Canada (1965), Denmark, Germany (1958), Ireland, Netherlands (1963), Sweden (1934), UK, USA (1938)

1971: Norway (1928)

1972: Poland, Japan

1973: Israel

1974: Finland (1966), Yugoslavia

1975: Italy, Bulgaria

1976: Roumania

1977: Belgium

1984: Spain, Thailand

1986: France (1975)

1987: Turkey

1990: Greece, Hungary, Iceland, Malaysia, Indonesia

1991: Switzerland, Australia, Austria, Costa Rica

1992: South Africa, Republic of Korea, Morocco, Croatia, Czech Republic

1993: Tunisia, Portugal, Singapore, Slovakia, Tanzania

1994: Cuba, Argentina

1995: Oman, Philippines, Venezuela

1996: Chile

1997: Bangladesh set up an ADR advisory committee.

1998: Zimbabwe, Russia, Iran, Estonia, China, India

1999: Mexico, Fiji, Vietnam (1994)

2000: Cyprus, Macedonia, Serbia and Montenegro, Sri Lanka.

2001: Brazil, Egypt, Ghana, Uruguay, Armenia

2002: Ukraine, Peru, Latvia (1996), Jordan, Guatemala.

2003: Kyrrgystan (1998), Moldova (1996)

2004: Columbia (1996), Malta, Nigeria.

2005: Mozambique (1999)

2006: Sierra Leone, Uzbekistan (1970), Belarus, Nepal (1979)

2007: Surinam (2006)

2008: Kazakistan, Barbadoa, Adorra, Lithuania (1995) (WHO Uppsala reports, 2004)

However, countries were able to withdraw drugs from the market before the dates given above. It is difficult to pinpoint the moment when any particular country was in the position to be able to assess all the data and take regulatory action.

Part 3. Regulatory responses to adverse reactions

Drugs that were introduced prior to 1960 and later withdrawn or restricted

In order to assess the pharmacovigilance aspects of drug withdrawals and restrictions it is necessary to establish the dates when the relevant ADRs were first mentioned, subsequent cases as described in Meyler's Side Effects of Drugs (SED) 1952, 1957, 1958 and 1960, and then the dates when the drug was withdrawn. Unfortunately, it is difficult to find out whether a drug was on the market in any other countries, other than those where it is stated that it has been withdrawn. It is likely that those countries that have a strong pharmaceutical research background will also be those countries that pick up any ADR problems and withdraw the drug. These countries are: USA, UK, Japan, France, Germany, Switzerland, Netherlands, Belgium, Sweden and Italy (Ballance, 1992). The other countries may then follow suit later. The main sources of information used are the 'Multi country survey on banned and restricted pharmaceuticals' Health Action International August 2008 and the 'Consolidated list of products whose consumption and/or sale have been banned, severely restricted or not approved by governments; WHO/EDH/QSM/99.2. Two drugs, acetanilide and antipyrine, have been omitted despite their having been withdrawn from one and three countries respectively. (see page 208) This is because the evidence of their causing blood dyscrasias is unreliable.

370 BC Datura (Stramonium containing atropine and scopolamine)

Also known as Jimson weed or Thorn apple was introduced as a cigarette for asthma in 1802 in India (Salter,1859; Sims, 1812). Datura itself was used since the time of Hippocrates. Lewin referred to its intoxicating powers in 1928 (Lewin, 1928). In the 1970s a favourite asthma treatment was 'Potter's Asthma Remedy, the active ingredient was Datura strammonium and it was abused both in the USA and in the UK (Barnett et al., 1977).

Use: asthma as cigarettes and pipe mixture. Smoking a cigarette made from about 1 gram of crushed datura relaxes bronchial muscles, calming the symptoms of asthma. This treatment is still preferred by many elderly French asthmatics. It was used in Bengal by thieves by combining it with sweetmeats aiming to stupify the victim (Leader, 1842).

ADR: It was said to produce aggravation of the dyspnoea, paralytic tremblings, epilepsy, headache, and apoplexy (Salter, 1859). The poisonous effects were: headache, agitation, choreic trembling of the arms, dilatation of the pupils, weakness of sight, dry red tongue, a strong tumultuous pulse, and finally collapse (Kuborn, 1866). Abuse (Morano, 1972; Bethel, 1978) anticholinergic syndrome (Shervette et al., 1979). Three teenagers died in France in 1992 (Leader New Scientist, 1992). Datura has been linked to a number of murders in southwestern France where a number of young men were ritually killed in the early 1990s.

SED 1952: no mention

Withdrawn: in France in 1992 because of abuse and causing the anticholinergic syndrome (New Scientist (22 August 1992), but ten cases reported the following year (Roblot et al., 1993).

Availability: Australia (in combination with potassium iodide), France, Brazil, Germany, Netherlands, Spain and Switzerland (Martindale).

Lifespan: 72 years (as cigarette), c2, 300 year (as a drug)

Delay in recognition: its abuse has always been recognised.

Delay in regulatory action: none following the deaths in France.

Comment: the recognition by the media as a 'good' story has frequently been a spur to action by the regulatory authorities.

429–347 BC Mercury

Mercurous Chloride, Hg_2cl_2, (Calomel, Stedman's teething powders) first mention found in 1676.

Use: eye salve, purgative, eczema, psoriasis and syphilis.

ADR: acrodynia (symptoms: pink-coloured rash, irritability, photophobia, painful and swollen extremities, hyperkeratosis, and hypersecretion of sweat glands [Aw & Vale, 1996]). It was first recognised by Zahorski in 1922 (Tzanck, 1953) and confirmed in 1949 (Launay et al., 1949), but it was probably a series of 28 case published in 1951(Warkany et al., 1951) that initiated the regulatory action. Warkany also said in 1949 that almost all the individual manifestations in the form of acrodynia had been known long ago as manifestations of mercurialism (Warkany, 1951) SED 1952: There are signs which may serve as evidence that Feer's disease, acrodynia, is caused by chronic mercury poisoning. The children concerned had had calomel previously in the form of a dental powder or as an ointment, or by mouth. The condition had been recognized in Australia in 1890 (Akabane, 1983) and in 1903 Selter reported eight cases of the syndrome among children between one and three years of age (Selter, 1903). Selter used the term 'trophodermatoneurose', and his cases exhibited the characteristic picture of the syndrome. The neurologic aspects of acrodynia were emphasized by Swift in Australia in 1914 (Swift, 1914) and by Feer in Switzerland in 1923 (Feer, 1923). The condition was established as a clinical entity in the British and American literature by Byfield and Bilderback in 1920 (Bilderback, 1920).

Withdrawn: during the time of Plato the physicians of Greece were prohibited under penalty of death, from prescribing mercury and other drugs of a poisonous nature (Abramowitz, 1934). In 1495 Mercury was introduced for syphilis.

Withdrawn world wide in 1953 because of Pink disease (acrodynia).

Availability: still available in the USA. Calomel is still available in Hungary in the form of a wound powder (Martindale).

Drug lifespan: more than 458 years.

Delay in recognition: 2, 269 years, but if taken from appearance of syphilis then 427 years.

Delay in regulatory action: (time between first mention of the ADR and the first withdrawal): 31 years.

Comment: the severe side effects of mercury were tolerated when there was no other apparent effective treatments for syphilis, but the advent of Salvarsan in 1907 made it obsolete. Its continued use as an antiseptic was not warranted since it was absorbed through the skin and there were better alternatives. Its contemporary use in vaccines is dealt with under Thiomersal. It has been suggested that there are other factors which interact with mercury to produce acrodynia, e.g. avitaminosis. *'If one does not admit, in effect, a favourable background, nothing would allow the explanation that so many children taking in one form or another mercurial medication and at doses extremely varied following the indication, without ever presenting the picture of acrodynia.'* (Launay et al., 1949).

The delay seems to be in the identification of a syndrome rather than in the individual signs and symptoms, which had been known for a long time.

78 AD Antimony

It is said to have been known to the Chaldeans in 4000 BC, and that its sulphide had been found in an Egyptian cosmetic case of 2,500 BC as a rouge to be brushed on the lips (Thorwald, 1962)

Use: It had been used as an emetic in the form of antimony potassium tartrate (Tartar Emetic) by Dioscorides, so use in this form dates back to at least 78 AD and it was later recommended by the Prophet Muhammad, for ophthalmia. Roger Bacon used it for gout, leprosy, stroke, dropsy, epilepsy, consumption, fever and pestilence. It was also advocated by Paracelsus in 1564. Mentioned in 1664 as a cure for syphilis, melancholy, chest pains, fever and the plague (Sneader, 2005; Valentine, 1604). In the 19th century it was used in fevers and for pneumonia.

ADR: a large dose (15 grains) of tartar emetic given to a 19 year old female produced: a cold sweat, convulsive twitchings of facial muscles, a quick weak pulse, violent sickness and diarrhoea, very difficult breathing, tremors and occasional fainting. Two grains given to a two year old child killed her after causing cold sweats, insensibility, tremor and convulsions, whilst four grains given to a 50-60 year old female for 'flu killed her after cold sweats, violent vomiting and purging, faintings and a scarcely palpable pulse (Blackburne, 1788). *'The internal administration of...antimony is sometimes followed, especially in children, by a condition resembling collapse, owing to the very pronounced property of antimony in*

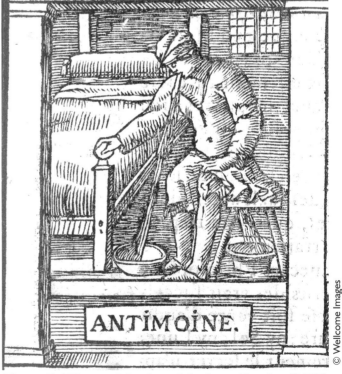

© Wellcome Images

Figure 5. Effects of Antimonials, from Bartlet (1657)

causing a lowering of the frequency and force of the heart beat' (Lewin, 1883). It also caused nausea and vomiting (N & V), diarrhoea, hepatitis, renal failure, red cell toxicity, cardiovascular collapse and death (Duffin & René, 1991). *'Antimony given in large doses: enormous evacuations both up and down with atrocious pain, convulsions, dyspnoea, haemorrhage, swelling of the lower abdomen, inflammation, erosion and gangrene of the stomach and the intestines and which finishes by death' …'Devouring heat and wrenching in the region of the epigastrium, switching from syncope to convulsive agitation followed closely by violent vomiting of frothy yellow matter and sometimes mixed with streaks of blood… frequent fainting fits and painful cramps in the legs.'* (Magendie, 1813).

SED 1952 N & V, diarrhoea, cyanosis, anaphylactic shock, asthma, cough, dizziness, urticaria, oedema of the glottis, muscle & joint pains, headache, bradycardia, pyrexia, hepatitis, albuminuria, herpes zoster, rash, glandular swellings, necrosis of gingival mucosa and pulmonary infiltrations.

SED 1957 Stilbophen caused haemolytic anaemia leading to shock.

Withdrawn: on 3rd August 1566 the Paris Faculty of Medicine forbade its use on the grounds that it was a dangerous poison and had caused several deaths and that it should not be taken internally. This was a result of a quarrel between the more modern medical faculty of Montpellier, which favoured iatrochemistry and that of Paris, which was very conservative and favoured the old fashioned Galenical outlook. It was also banned at Heidelberg University from 1558 until 1655, In Augsberg in 1567, Vienna from 1569 to 1667 and in parts of Italy. In 1611 the Royal College of Physicians (London) issued a certificate condemning as dangerous to life a medicine that contained antimony or one of its ingredients.

The French ban was rescinded in 1666 when the Paris faculty voted 92 to 102 in favour of its restoration, which was probably related to the fact that Louis XIV was cured of typhoid fever by antimony (tartar emetic) in 1657. In a series of decrees and court cases this powerful body tried to forbid any use of chemistry in medicine (MacCallum, 1999; Pilpoul, 1928)). Pentavalent sodium stibogluconate (pentostam) is still used in leishmaniasis and trivalent antimony potassium tartrate (tartar emetic) in schistosomiasis.

Availability: the trivalent and/or pentavalent forms are available in

Brazil, France, Spain, Venezuela, Austria, Germany, Thailand and Italy (Martindale).

Comment: the side effects were severe in comparison with those of other emetics of the time and later in the 19th century it was used for fevers especially bronchitis and pneumonia and the fact that it has some *in vitro* antimicrobial activity supports this usage (Duffin & René, 1991) and its more specific use in parasitic disorders was demonstrated in 1910 (Camac, 1911) which warranted its continuation until better drugs became available.

Drug lifespan: 1,488 years

Delay in recognition: not known

Delay in regulatory action: not known

Time span of withdrawals: 23 years

1831 Chloroform (Phedros)

In 1847 was used as an anaesthetic by Simpson of Edinburgh for use in childbirth.

Use: originally it was introduced as a general anaesthetic, but it was later widely used in pharmaceutical preparations as a solvent and preservative.

ADR: in 1842 it was reported to have caused instantaneous death in four patients by 'paralysing the heart' during anaesthesia (Sibson, 1848). In 1848 Professor Simpson said that a death was due to congestion of the lungs from the effects of chloroform (Simpson, 1848). In 1858 John Snow having used chloroform on 50 patients considered the various possible causes of death:

    Falling back of the tongue

    Sitting position

    Alleged exhaustion from struggling

    Alleged closure of the glottis

    Alleged exclusion of the air

    Alleged impurities in the chloroform

    Idiosyncrasy

    Supposed effect of the surgeon's knife

    Sudden death from other causes

He did not come to any conclusion. However, we can now see that numbers 3 and 8 would have caused increased secretion of adrenaline, which is now known to be a factor in producing the ventricular fibrillation (Snow, 1989).

The BMA in 1877 appointed a committee to investigate the actions of anaesthetics and they concluded that chloroform could cause sudden stoppage of the heart and of respiration, and that ether was less dangerous than chloroform (McKendrick, 1880). Others disagreed and a Surgeon Major E Laurie who was the Residency surgeon at Hyderabad established the Hyderabad Commission on Chloroform which reported that deaths from chloroform are due to asphyxia and that as long as respiration was attended to there was no problem of sudden death; this itself was disputed and a second Hyderabad Chloroform Committee was appointed and they reported that chloroform did not affect the heart to any critical extent (Brunton, 1890). The results were hampered by the absence of the use of electrocardiograms that had only been discovered in 1887 and by the difficulties of extrapolating from animals to man, since all the committee's investigations were in animals. In 1911 the ECG evidence for ventricular fibrillation was established (Levy, 1911). Some members of the medical profession (physicians, nurses and pharmacists) became addicted to chloroform (Lewin, 1893).

SED 1952: No mention of sudden death during anaesthesia or of carcinogenicity. In the 1976 the National Cancer Institute of the USA, found malignant kidney tumours in rats and hepatocellular carcinoma in mice as a part of the programme of carcinogenicity in pharmaceuticals and concluded that the overall evaluation was that it was carcinogenic and possibly carcinogenic in humans.

Withdrawn: in the USA, Greece, Turkey, Japan, Panama in 1976; Brazil and Saudi Arabia in 1977; Italy, Canada, Norway, Philippines in 1978; UK in 1979; New Zealand in 1980; Denmark, Ethiopia and Zimbabwe in 1981; Germany and Bangladesh in 1982; Belgium and Dominica in 1983; Nigeria in 1985; Ireland in 1989; Oman as an excipient.

Drug lifespan: 145 years

Delay in recognition: 45 years

Delay in regulatory action: nil

Time span of withdrawals: 16 years

Comment: anaesthetists gradually adopted safer anaesthetics and only its use as a solvent, preservative or flavouring continued until its carcinogenicity was shown.

1869 Chloral Hydrate (CCl_3CHO)

Synthesised in 1832 by Justus von Liebig, but only marketed in 1869 (Welldorm, Noctec, Somnos). It was also known as 'Mickey Finn' or 'Knock Out Drops'.

Use: hypnotic and sedative

ADR: 1881 *'Its habitual use as particularly noted in England and America, even in 'chloral drinkers' causes no habituation to the effects of the drug, and gives rise to no deleterious consequences so long as the standard doses are not exceeded.'* (Lewin, 1881). A 1896 Dictionary of Domestic Medicine states: *'Unfortunately the properties of chloral render it liable to great abuse and many persons have seriously injured their health by frequent and large doses; in some instances death has resulted from one overdose, inadvertently or intentionally taken.'* (Thomson et al., 1896). *'The tendency to habituation to chloral exists as for all the other narcotics. In many of the subjects, the habituation and the progression in dosage hasn't taken place as quickly as with morphine.'* (Lewin, 1928).

SED 1952: habituation causes symptoms of insomnia and delerium tremens (Fühner, 1948). Neoplastic lesions found in mice in 1986 (Rijhsinghani et al., 1986). The IARC[171] (1995) evaluated the carcinogenicity data for chloral hydrate and it was concluded that there was inadequate evidence in humans and limited evidence in experimental animals for the carcinogenicity of chloral hydrate. A two-year study in which male mice were treated with chloral hydrate in drinking water showed increases in hepatocellular adenomas among all treated groups (George *et al.*, 2000). In 2003 the Reproductive and Cancer Hazard Assessment Section Office of Environmental Health Hazard Assessment of the California Environmental Protection Agency said that *'there is evidence indicating the carcinogenic potential of this chemical, including the carcinogenicity findings in the animal bioassays, extensive observations of genetic toxicity, and chemical structural analogies with known carcinogens'.* The first report of its abuse was in 1880 (Anon, 1880). A cohort study in the USA did not find persuasive evidence to support a causal relationship between chloral hydrate exposure in humans and the development of cancer (Haselkorn et al., 2006).

Withdrawn/Restricted: it was withdrawn in France and the USA in 2001 because it was mutagenic carcinogenic in animals, but a single dose was permitted in the USA for children under 5 years of age. Chloral hydrate is restricted because of the IARC ruling 'not classifiable as to its carcinogenicity to humans (Group 3)'. In France it is restricted to hospital usage and only by prescription.

---

[171] IARC = International Agency for Research on Cancer International Agency for Research on Cancer (World Health Organization). Monographs on the Evaluation of Carcinogenic Risks to Humans. Overall Evaluations of Carcinogenicity: htpp-monographs.iarc.fr-ENG-Monographs-suppl7-suppl7.pdf.url. Accessed 1st November 2008

Availability: Martindale: Available in Canada, USA, Belgium, France, Germany, Italy, Netherlands, Switzerland, Austria, Spain, Australia, Rumania, Hungary and the UK (BNF, 1999).

Drug lifespan: 132 years

Delay in recognition: probably less than 12 years

Delay in regulatory action: 15 years

Time span of withdrawals: zero

Comment: the delay may have been due to the doubts expressed as to its carcinogenicity and its application to humans. Bearing in mind that it was widely known as a drug of abuse in 1896 and that it continued to be on the market for a further 105 years indicates that its removal was for the threat of carcinogenicity and not because of abuse.

1875 Bismuth (insoluble salts, less than 1% absorbed in the gastrointestinal tract)

Bismuth itself was in use in Roman times and spoken of by Paracelsus. Bismuth subnitrate was created in 1748-1817 and bismuth subcarbonate in 1857. The other insoluble salts are the subsalicylate, subcitrate and subgallate.

Use: used since 1733 as a medicinal salve and later in the 1920s for syphilis and amoebiasis. Also used as an antacid and as a treatment for diarrhoea.

ADR: 1881 Bismuth subnitrate can cause vomiting, colicky pains, diarrhoea, a sensation of heat, headache, dizziness and general debility (Lewin, 1881). In 1972 a colostomy association warned the Australian Adverse Drug Reactions Advisory Committee (ADRAC) that there was a possibility that bismuth subgallate powder was causing a neurological condition which is now known as reversible myoclonic encephalopathy (symptoms: malaise, dysaesthesiae, loss of memory, tremor, acute confusion, myoclonus, severe ataxia and dysarthria) and the first report was by Burns et al. in 1974, when he reported on treatment with bismuth subgallate in five Australian cases, where it was used for colostomy patients to reduce the odour and flatulence and to improve the consistency of their motions. 'Reversible encephalopathy' was once a problem in some countries, notably France and Australia; bone and joint toxicity had also occurred, sometimes associated with the encephalopathy. This led to restrictions on the use of bismuth salts and a virtual disappearance of these toxic effects (Burns et al., 1974). There were another 24 similar cases in Australia that year (ADEC,

1974). At the same time in France there were 942 cases with 72 deaths (Martin-Bouyer, 1999). First described in 1973 in French journals (Besle, 1975). In France there was an uneven geographical distribution within France spreading from the Loire Atlantique region and Paris eastwards and south across the country (Le Quesne, 1981) A single bismuth injection for stomatitis caused death (J Belge, 1956). No cases had been reported in the UK or the USA, where the subsalicylate and the subcitrate were used. There were five cases in Switzerland with various salts, 6 cases in Belgium, at least six cases in Spain and some cases in Germany following the use of a cosmetic containing bismuth (Lagier, 1980). It was suggested that an intestinal microorganism was able to convert the insoluble bismuth salt to an absorbable form. It would seem to be dose-related with those with encephalopathy having blood levels above 100μg/l whilst those taking similar doses but not having encephalopathy having levels below 50μg/l (Le Quesne, 1981). Probable factors are: constipation, colostomies/ileostomies, prolonged use and high doses.

SED 1952: CNS symptoms–insomnia, nervousness, parathesiae, incoordination, tetanic convulsions, paralysis, polyneuritis and coma.

SED 1960: no mention

SED 1972: no mention

SED 1975: discolouration of teeth, parathesia, impairment of concentration acuity, dementia, inability to walk, psychoses, hallucinations and convulsions were all reported in France with bismuth sub-nitrate.

Withdrawn: bismuth subgallate was withdrawn in Egypt and became prescription only in Japan in 1975. It was used only in suppository form in Saudi Arabia. It was withdrawn in Greece in 1976. All insoluble salts were suspended in France in 1978 and withdrawn in Austria in 1980. They were banned in Bangladesh and withdrawn in Turkey (except colloidal bismuth K citrate complex) and in Mauritius in 1982. In Cuba bismuth sub-nitrate was prohibited for children. In Sweden they became prescription only products and in Oman antidiarrhoeal preparations containing bismuth were prohibited in 1989. India prohibited their manufacture and sale. Italy warned of prolonged use and high dosage, because of reversible myoclonic encephalopathy. There is restricted usage in the USA–subsalicylate and subcitrate. Health Action International (HAI): banned in 7 and restricted in seven.

Availability: Spain, Mexico, Brazil, Argentina, Germany, USA, Netherlands and South Africa (Martindale). The salts available are: subgallate, subsalicylate, aluminate, subcitrate, oxide, subnitrate, salicylate and subcarbonate. The subgallate is registered in Sri Lanka, Malaysia and Thailand where other bismuth products are also available. Bismuth products are also available in Korea and Thailand (HAI, 2008). The subgallate is available in the UK in suppositories and as an anal ointment–Anusol. Bismuth is still used as antacid (BNF, 1999). Bismuth subsalicylate (Pepto-Bismol 525 mgm q.d.s[172]) is a recommended treatment for traveller's diarrhoea (Hill & Ryan, 2008). It remains an over-the-counter (OTC) product in many parts of the world.

Lifespan: 100 years.

Delay in recognition: 99 years probably because an unknown factor was not present until the early 1970s.

Delay in regulatory action: 1 year.

Time span of withdrawals: 14 years

Comment: there has been a wide variation in the reports from different countries. There were no cases in the UK, but the cases were seen predominantly in France and Australia. The subgallate was the main bismuth product available in Australia and the subnitrate in France. Quite how the previously insoluble salts became soluble enough to be absorbed and reach the brain is not certain. The known factors are: adult, elderly, colonopathy with chronic constipation, colostomy or ileostomy and female (Manigand, 1982). The first action taken after the recognition of a serious ADR may be to withdraw it; but once the causative factors are known and warnings can be given it may be allowed back on the market. There seems to be no reason why this should not apply to insoluble bismuth salts. Further reading: KK Jain's Drug-induced Neurolgical Disorders. Hogrefe & Huber Publishers 2001, 27–28.

1885 Urethane (ethyl carbamate). Trade Names: Pressyl, Surparine, Profenil.

Use: originally used as a hypnotic, but later, when combined with quinine, for sclerosing varicose veins and for malaria: Urethane, an efficient soporific remedy (Kühn, 1894). 'Urethane (dose 15 to 30 grains) is a mild and safe hypnotic, suitable for children (Willcox, 1934). First introduced by Schmiedeberg in 1885 (Schmiedeberg, 1885) Urethane was found by Warburg in 1910 to inhibit cell division in sea urchins. In 1943, clinical trials were started in the Royal Cancer

---

[172] Q.D.S. = quarter die sumendus = four times a day

Hospital. Later in 1946, it was used for the treatment of chronic myeloid leukaemia and then for acute neoplasia.

After 1943, many trials were carried out with it, but by 1950 it had virtually fallen out of use, superseded by the development of so many other chemotherapeutic agents, whose discovery it had helped to stimulate (MacGregor, 1966).

SED 1960: no mention.

ADR: carcinogenicity [pulmonary adenomas in mice](Nettleship et al., 1943). There is inadequate evidence that urethane is carcinogenic in humans, but in animals the evidence is considered to be sufficient (IARC vol 96, 2008) Aplastic anaemia (6%), thrombocytopenia (14.5%), leucopenia (16%) and cytolytic hepatic necrosis (Ohler et al., 1950). Agranulocytosis (Albahary, 1953).

SED 1952: leucopenia, thrombocytopenia and aplastic anaemia (Webster, 1947). *'It has been virtually abandoned for therapeutic use as more efficient tumour chemotherapeutic agents have been found.'* (Bonser, 1967).

Withdrawn: in Brazil and Canada in 1963, Cuba in 1964, Denmark in 1967, Egypt, Japan and Thailand in 1973, the USA in 1977 (injection), Italy in 1979, Greece in 1980, Germany in 1982 and France in 1985,

Availability: still available as an animal anaesthetic. Still used for multiple myeloma in 1966 (Holland et al., 1966).

Lifespan: 100 years

Delay in recognition: 59 years

Delay in regulatory action: 20 years

Time span of withdrawals: 22 years

Comment: it seems to have had four lives, the first as an hypnotic in humans, second as an intravenous injection for varicose veins and malaria, thirdly as an anti-cancer drug and the fourthly as an animal anaesthetic. One might have expected that it would have been replaced by other anti-cancer drugs starting in the main research countries. Its demise was drawn out over a long period without any apparent reason.

1887 Phenacetin (APC)

Use: analgesic. It was usually combined with other drugs, e.g. aspirin and caffeine, hence Aspirin, Phenacetin and Caffeine tablets (APC) and was also in Tabs Codeine. Co. Phenacetin was removed from these two products in 1968.

ADR: the Therapeutic Committee of the British Medical Association conducted *'an inquiry regarding the importance of ill-effects following the use of antipyrin, antifebrin, & Phenacetin'* in 1894 (Leech & Hunter, 1894) and the US Department of Agriculture a similar study in 1909 (Kebler et al., 1909). No indication of Phenacetin nephropathy was found, the latter study quoted the literature and mentioned two cases of haematuria and nephritis and one of uraemic syndrome.

Methaemoglobinaemia was first described in 1909 as *'occurring in an elderly patient as the result of taking phenacetin to excess'* (Jacob, 1909). 1915 Seifert mentions haemoglobinuria and haemorraghic nephritis (Seifert, 1915).

SED 1952: methaemoglobinaemia, No mention of renal problems.

The hypothesis that analgesic drugs containing Phenacetin can cause chronic renal disease was first mooted in 1953. They had noticed that women working in Swiss watch factories took large amounts of analgesic drugs because of occupational aches and pains (Spühler & Zollinger, 1953).

SED 1957: interstitial nephritis reported in 18 patients.

SED 1958: renal insufficiency due to chronic interstitial nephritis (Schweiz Med Wschr, 1956).

In 1959 a cross sectional study of 698 inpatients showed a significant correlation between impaired renal function and the dosage and duration of phenacetin use (Larsen & Moller, 1959; Venning, 1983)

SED 1967: Prescott said ' *nephrotoxicity has not been convincingly demonstrated in respect of phenacetin and since other potentially nephrotoxic drugs are always taken together with it. 'Analgesic nephrotoxicity' is a more accurate term'.*

In 1969 it was reported that it could also cause carcinoma of the renal pelvis (Angervall et al., 1969)

In 1970 Koutsaimanis and Wardener said that it was only phenacetin that caused renal papillary necrosis (Koutsaimanis & Wardener, 1970), but this was disputed by Prescott (Prescott, 1970). The number of UK fatal reports between 1964 and 1980 was 105 and the rate per million of general-practitioner prescriptions was 1.6 (approximately) (Venning I, 1983)

A multicentre case-control study concluded that Phenacetin may increase the risk of chronic renal disease and that its metabolite paracetamol (acetaminophen) was also associated with an increased risk (Sandler et al., 1989).

In 1991 it was shown in an epidemiological study in Switzerland that

Phenacetin caused an increased risk of hypertension, cardiovascular disease, and mortality due to cancer, urological and renal disease; and that the relative risk of death was 2.2 times that of the control group (Dubach et al., 1991). Stolley referred to the lack of histopathological observations in analgesic nephropathy which he thought was due to the late onset of renal failure and therefore by the time a biopsy was done the scarring had so distorted the histology as to make it unclassifiable (Stolley, 1991). Kracke first mentioned Phenacetin as a possible cause of agranulocytosis in 1931 (Kracke, 1931). In Meyler's 14th edition it says *despite withdrawal of phenacetin from the market, analgesic nephropathy has since continued to appear* (Frie, 2000). The incidence of analgesic nephropathy (AN) shows remarkable geographic variation: In Australia addiction to analgesics is more common in Queensland and New South Wales which has been attributed to the poor economic status of these areas. In Scotland the incidence is 25% in Glasgow but only 4.8% in the rest of Scotland and here it was thought to be due to a factory producing the analgesic combination in the locality. In Belgium there is a much higher incidence in the north around Antwerp, where again there are local factories producing the analgesics. There is a similar predisposition in Germany in Northern Germany and around West Berlin and a factor might be different drinking habits of the population. The incidence of analgesic nephropathy around the world is also rather bizarre. It was suggested that this might because of regional peculiarities in the epidemiology of nephropathies.

Table 11. National figures for analgesic nephropathy

AN incidence	% age
Australia	20.0%
Belgium	18.4%
Switzerland	17.5%
USA	7–10.0%
Germany	5.0%
Scandinavia	3.4%
Canada	2.5%
France	1.6%
UK	1.2%
Italy	1.0%

(After Vanherweghem and Even-Adin, 1982)

The American Medical Association had a propaganda department, which in 1909 produced a leaflet for public information stating *'Beware of…. and acetphenetidine (Phenacetin) in ' Headache Cures'. These drugs Depress the heart–Injure the blood–Produce a habit. DANGER.'*
There is limited evidence that phenacetin is carcinogenic in animals (IARC vol 24, 1980).

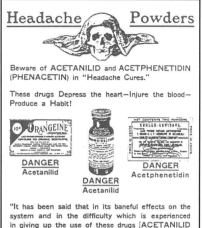

Withdrawn: in Finland in 1965, it was removed from one Australian product in 1967 and the other product in 1975, withdrawn in Italy and Kuwait in 1973, 1974 first UK regulatory warning, but withdrawn in New Zealand and Canada in 1977, Nigeria in 1978, Cyprus and Yemen in 1979, France, Philippines and UK in 1980, Norway, Brazil, Argentina and Israel in 1981, Romania, Turkey, Bangladesh, Mauritius, Sweden, Hongkong, Japan, India, Nepal, Thailand, Rwanda and USA in 1983, Chile, Ethiopia, Greece and Denmark in 1984, Panama, Germany and Malaysia in 1986, Oman in 1987, Austria and Belgium in 1988, and also in Bahrain, Egypt, Switzerland, Ireland, Israel, Netherlands, Saudi Arabia, and Surinam because of analgesic nephropathy (Stolley, 1991). The various reasons for withdrawal included: carcinogenicity, hepatotoxicity, renal toxicity and methemoglobinemia (WHO). HAI: banned in 41 countries and restricted in one.

Availability: Hungary, Spain, Czechoslovakia, and France (Martindale).

Lifespan: 65 years

Delay in recognition: 65 years

Delay in regulatory action: 12 years (since the Spühler & Zollinger paper) or, 56 years after the AMA warning. Venning said that the avoidable delay was 21 years; that is since the Larsen and Moller study in 1959 (Venning II, 1983).

Time span of withdrawals: 23 years

Comment: doubt lingered on as to whether Phenacetin was solely to blame for the nephropathy or whether the other drugs, with which it was combined, might have played a part (Prescott, 1970). This doubt

Source: American Medical Association, copyright 1909

333

seems to have vanished as aspirin and paracetamol have been cleared of responsibility.

1888 Piperazine $C_4H_{10}N_2$ (Antepar, Pripsen)

Was introduced. It was discovered by Schreiber in 1878.

Use: originally for gout and rheumatism because it had been shown in vitro to dissolve urate in stones (Mapother, 1894). Its use as an antihelminthic drug was discovered in 1951.

ADR: marked toxic effects after a drachm or more were reported in 1894 (Stewart, 1894). A booklet published by Pipérazine Midy in 1910 said: *'the innocuity of piperazine is absolute, so tolerance always perfect'* .(Midy, 1910). 1915 Seifert mentioned headache (Seifert,1915). The first gastrointestinal, allergic and neurological side effects were reported in 1952. The neurological symptoms were: lack of coordination resulting in dropping things, sickness, inability to focus and a sense of detachment ? due to overdose (Standen & White, 1952).

SED 1952: no mention. A warning was given in 1956 of neurotoxicity [Worm wobble] (Combes et al., 1956). Severe neurotoxicity (Yohai and Barnett, 1989) consisting of absences and atonic seizures. It also caused hypersensitivity and possible carcinogenicity. It is still considered sufficiently safe for use; although in most industrialised countries it has been abandoned, primarily because of concern about possible carcinogenicity and electroencephalographic changes (Kaddu, 2000). (Parsons, 1971; Belloni, 1967; Miller, 1967; Savage, 1967).

SED 1960 : mention of incoordination, muscle weakness, tremors and headache.

SED 1963 : they had added: Abnormal limb movements, myoclonus, dyskinesia and purpura.

Withdrawn: in Italy in 1977, in Sweden in 1983, Denmark in 1984 (prescription control), Netherlands in 1985, Malaysia and Thailand (use severely restricted) in 1996, Armenia in 2000. It is not manufactured in the USA.

Availability: in some countries where ascariasis is not endemic and where piperazine was used predominantly for the treatment of pinworm it has been withdrawn from use on the grounds that other more effective and less toxic drugs are now available. In other such countries, however, piperazine remains available in over-the-counter preparations: Canada, France, Ireland, Spain, Portugal, Belgium, Thailand, Turkey, Venezuela, Brazil, Mexico, Indonesia and South Africa, (WHO, 2003). It was used in the UK for threadworms and roundworms (BNF, 1999). It is still available in India but with restrictions.

Lifespan: c92 years.

Delay in recognition: 64 years

Delay in regulatory action: 25 years

Time span of withdrawals: 23 years

Comment: the side effects, which are dose-related only appeared after the drug was used as an antihelminthic some 64 years after its appearance on the market for the treatment of gout and this needs some explanation. Piperazine in 1894 cost 12 shillings an ounce–*'scarcely affordable for public practice'* . The dose used then was 5-10 grains three times daily, which in 2008 terms would mean £17. 37 per day (Gordon, 1894), whilst the dose now for round worms is two doses of 4 G or 61. 2 grains, two weeks apart and for thread worms at a dose of 2.5 G daily for seven days. It is probable that piperazine was little used in the treatment of gout because its inefficacy, the price and the availability of colchicum. Some confirmation this is found in the lack of articles in the BMJ of this period and that there is no mention of piperazine in a book of household remedies of 1896. (Thompson et al., 1896). The potential carcinogenicity is based on the possibility that some nitrososamine may be generated in the stomach but it is widely considered that the trace amounts are not relevant (WHO, 2003).

1896 Amidopyrine [US National Formulary]/aminopyrine, [BPC]/ aminophenazone/pyramidone (Cibalgin, Veramon, Pyramidon, Allonal, phenyldim ethylamidopyrazolone)

A thesis dated 22nd February 1897 said that experiments on dogs and guinea-pigs was not able to establish the precise degree of toxicity in man and supposed that doses of 8–10 grammes could be followed by most severe results.

Use: analgesic and antipyretic.

ADR: bone marrow suppression, agranulocytosis, renal damage, toxic epidermal necrosis (Lyell's syndrome) and Stevens-Johnson syndrome. Agranulocytosis was reported with amidopyrine in 1933 (Madison and Squier, 1934), although the first hint was given in 1931 (Kracke, 1931). A leader in the BMJ at the time of the Discombe article said *'Amidopyrine became notorious as a cause of agranulocytosis as long ago as 1922'* (Leader, 1952), but I have been unable to verify this statement. The relationship was finally established in 1935 (Kracke and Parker, 1935). Agranulocytosis–amidopyrine should be restricted to patients having leukocyte counts several times a week (Hoffman et al., 1934; Bohn, 1934; Silver, 1934).

SED 1952: agranulocytosis often occurs after use of compounds containing aminopyrine. It is estimated that 50 patients annually die from agranulocytosis after use of aminopyrine (Lancet 260, 1951, 389). Urticaria, purpura, skin gangrene, albuminuria and optic nerve atrophy.

SED 1957 although agranulocytosis is observed (Gazz Int, 1954) it can cause pancytopenia (Klin Wschr, 1954). The Committee on Safety of Drugs in its annual report in 1966 said that the danger arises when it is given in excessive doses over a long period and that special action was not necessary. It has been suggested that aminopyrine and dipyrone are so similar that there is no reason to suspect that they are not equally likely to produce agranulocytosis. Therefore, an incidence of 0.79% or 1 in 126 for both drugs has been estimated (Huguley, 1964). Others have estimated the figure as 1 in 10,000 (Dameshek & Colmes, 1936) whereas Discombe suggests that where amidopyrine can be obtained freely an incidence of agranulocytosis between 2 and 5 per million may occur (Discombe, 1952). The IAAA study in 1986 did not give figures for amidopyrine specifically, but gave a figure for other pyrazolones which included aminopyrine multivariate rate ratio of 1.2 (CI 0.6-2.5) compared with dipyrone 23.7 (CI 8.7–64.4) The estimates for aminopyrine 'lack validity' (Levy, 1980). A meta-analysis of the IAAAS, a US study and a Thailand study showed a relative risk of 1.4 (CI 0.6–3.2) (Kaufman et al., 1996).

Withdrawn: over-the-counter sales were prohibited in the UK in 1936 and in the USA in 1938. It was banned in 1963 in Canada, 1965 in Australia, 1975 in the UK and France, 1976 in Finland, 1977 in the USA, Germany and Japan, 1978 in Italy (but still in use in 1979), Korea, Thailand and Austria; 1979 in Ireland, Denmark, Kuwait; 1980 in Yemen and Greece, 1981 in Argentina, 1982 in Romania, Sudan, Turkey and Mauritius; 1983 in India, Nepal, Philippines, and Rwanda, 1984 in Ethiopia, Hongkong; 1986 in Malaysia, 1987 in Oman; 1988 in Belgium and Ghana in 1989. Dates of withdrawal were not given for Bahrain, Switzerland, South Korea, Singapore, Sweden, and Venezuela; it had been made a Schedule IV drug (prescription only)(Discombe, 1952). HAI: banned 36 countries and restricted in two.

Availability: Martindale: it was available in France, Germany, Belgium and Switzerland in 1952 and in Hungary, Italy, Venezuela, and Mexico (still in 2001). In 1983 it was still being sold in Africa and the Middle East (Healthy Skepticism, (2008). Still available in Indonesia as injections with Anatalgin and lidocaine (Novamidon, Mutivaldon) (Informasi Spesialite Obat Indonesia, 2005).

Lifespan: 66 years

Delay in recognition: 37 years

Delay in regulatory action: 3 years.

Time span of withdrawals: 53 years

Comment: the problem is that with agranulocytosis the cases are so rare that a very large number of patients need to have taken the drug to provide enough cases for a case-control study and to calculate the excess risk. The other problems are the variation of incidence across different populations and the variation in what is considered as an acceptable risk.

1898 Clioquinol–Iodochlorhydroxyquinoline (Entero-Vioform, Quinoform, Chinoform)

Was introduced in Japan in 1929. It was a derivative of chionline.

Use: amoebic dysentery since 1933 (David et al., 1933) and later Travellers' diarrhoea, despite no evidence of efficacy (It had been available as a topical antiseptic [Vioform] from 1900).

ADR: subacute myelo-optic neuropathy (SMON) and peripheral neuropathy. Up to 15% of people with this ADR ended up in wheelchairs and as many as 30% had their vision affected (Cobert & Biron, 2002). The first case was reported in 1935 in Argentina (Grawitz, 1935; Barros, 1935) and the first probable case in Japan in 1938 (Katahira, 1976). In 1952 Dr Kiyono in Yomagata described the full syndrome (Cobert & Biron, 2002). Convulsions and neurological disorders were seen in cats in 1939. In 1965 animal toxicity showed convulsions and behavioural changes in dogs and cats and in 1966 there was an English report of optic atrophy leading to blindness. By October 1967, 1,452 cases had been reported and this had increased to 1,653 in 1968, to 2,892 by 1969 and to 7,856 by October 1970. The Japanese undertook an investigation in 1968 and concluded that the drug was the cause in August 1970 (Tsubaki et al., 1971) and promptly removed the drug from the market with 186 other halogenated hydroxy-quinolones (Cobert & Biron, 2002). Between 1956 and 1970, there were 10,000 cases of SMON in Japan (Oakley, 1980).

SED 1952: Vioform: agranulocytosis.

SED 1960; SED 1963; SED 1966; and SED 1968: no mention ADRs.

Withdrawn: FDA stopped OTC products in 1961. withdrawn in Japan on 8th September 1970, warning given in Australia in 1971, Withdrawn in the USA in 1973, Norway in 1974, Sweden in 1975, Belgium in 1976, Germany in 1977, Denmark in 1978, France, Argentina and UK in 1981, Nigeria, Philippines and Bangladesh in 1982, Canada, Italy, Nepal, Dominica, Zambia and Spain in 1983, Hongkong and Ethiopia in 1984, Honduras in 1985, Oman in 1987, Pakistan in 1988, Ghana in 1989, Libya in 1990, also in Bahrain, Cuba, Switzerland, Netherlands, Saudi Arabia, Congo, Thailand, Malaysia, Taiwan, and Venezuela, because of subacute myelo-optic neuropathy (SMON). There are many paradoxes: greater use in Indonesia but no epidemic there, retained in India where the disease is rare (Mann, 1986). The role of clioquinol in SMON was not recognised before 1965 when they considered the possibility of infection and allergy, but they noted that it occurred one week or so after the abdominal symptoms, which included diarrhoea (Tsubaki et al., 1965). Australia and Venezuela restricted its use to amoebic dysentery and acrodermatitis enteropathica (Scrip, 1983). HAI: banned it in 23 countries and restricted in three.

Availability: in 1993 in 39 countries including India, Indonesia, Thailand, the Middle East, Egypt, Mexico, Central America, Columbia, Venezuela, Brazil and New Zealand (prescription only) (Drug labelling in developing countries, 1993). Available in the UK as eardrops and as an ingredient in skin preparations – Vioform hydrocortisone (BNF, 1999).

Lifespan: 36 years

Delay in recognition: 36 years

Delay in regulatory action: one month after the SMON Research committee reported.

Time span of withdrawals: 20 years

Comment: the two possible causes were a virus infection and clioquinol. An infectious aetiology is consistent with evidence of seasonal variation in incidence and the clustering of cases in families, institutions, doctors and hospitals. Animal studies suggested that it was a new neuropathic slow virus causing pathological changes including spongy degeneration of the brain (ADEC, 1971). It is unlikely that clioquinol was the only causative factor in the production of SMON as has been pointed out by Meade:

The possibility of protopathic bias since the early symptoms of SMON can be diarrhoea and abdominal pain.

The absence of SMON prior to about 1955 despite being on the market since 1934.

The decline in incidence before the drug was suspended.

A large proportion of patients with SMON had not taken clioquinol.

The virtual absence outside Japan.

Some cases of SMON had not taken clioquinol (Meade, 1975).

On the other hand, there are observations inexplicable by the infection hypothesis:

SMON is a new disease seldom reported in other counties.

Rare in children and high morbidity in middle or old aged women.

The disease was sporadic: it was hard to trace contact between cases.

No fever, rash and other symptoms suggesting infection; blood or spinal fluid showed no abnormality.

Pathohistology No inflammatory change. Changes reminiscent of outcomes of metabolic disorder, vitamin deficiency or intoxication (Kono, 1971). Further reading: KK Jain's Drug-induced Neurological Disoders, Hogrefe & Huber 2001, 435-441.Venning said that there was no satisfactory evidence concerning the incidence of the adverse reaction, but this was almost certainly too low for a cohort approach to post-marketing surveillance to be effective for either alerting or verification (Venning, 1983).

1899 Aspirin

Use: anti-inflammatory agent and analgesic

ADR: Reye's syndrome (acute encephalopathy associated with selective hepatic abnormality and metabolic decompensation).

SED 1952: acetylsalicylic acid should not be given in the first years of life, because young children are particularly sensitive.

Reye's syndrome was named after Dr R Douglas Reye, who along with Dr Graeme Morgan and Dr Jim Baral, reported on a series of children admitted to the Royal Alexandra Hospital for Children in Sydney. The original report by Reye et al (1963) did not mention aspirin use and the author did not believe that it was due to aspirin. However, in a letter to the editor of Pediatrics in 1988, Dr Baral claimed that 11 of the 21 patients in the original study were given aspirin before the onset of their syndrome and that exposure to other sources of salicylates (such as topical creams, gels or shampoos) was possible (Baral 1988). This is in contrast to a statement by Dr Morgan in 1985 that *'We enquired into the use of medications, including aspirin, but the information we obtained did not lend itself to any likely interpretation'*. (Morgan 1985). Arguments against aspirin being a cause were given by an American team (Orlowski et al., 2002), but these were rejected by Waller and Suvarna (Waller & Suvarna, 2004). Initially Orlowski's paper was meant to be one of two, one 'pro' and the other 'anti', but the second paper didn't arrive and so the Orlowski paper was published without its balancing paper. Balancing papers, such as this, inevitably polarise the authors and reduce the possibility of producing a balanced assessment. A later paper favours the causal association (Glasgow, 2006).

SED 1960: there were 49 cases of salicylate intoxication in children (<6 years old) of whom 5 died with hyperpyrexia. There was mention of: ketosis, hyperglycaemia, dehydration and respiratory alkalosis going on to metabolic acidosis.

Restrictions: warnings were given concerning paediatric preparations in Australia in 1972 (Waldman et al., 1972) and in the USA, Mauritius and Bangladesh in 1982, in Switzerland, Iraq, Israel, Italy, France, Ireland, Australia, Spain, Hongkong, Germany, and the UK (This restriction was extended in 2002 to children under 16 years) and Oman in 1986, in Egypt, Nigeria, Chile, Denmark and Singapore in 1987, in Belgium, Sweden and the USA in 1988, Sri Lanka in 1996, France in 1997 (100 mgm tablet for fear of aspiration), in Brazil in 2001, in Spain all paediatric preparations were withdrawn in 2003; warnings were also given in the Netherlands, because of Reyes syndrome.

Availability: Martindale: available in Italy and as suppositories in the USA. Available in Chile, Uruguay and Argentina.

Lifespan: 63 years

Delay in recognition: 81 years

Delay in regulatory action: 2 years.

Time span of restrictions: 31 years

Comment: after 20 years there is little evidence of doubt as to the causal relationship.

1902 Phenolpthalein (Exlax, later reformulated)

Use: originally used for masking the colour of adulterated wine made from the husks of grapes. Now used as a laxative.

ADR: skin reactions, potassium loss, atonia and carcinogenicity in animals. In 1918 it was pointed out that it could cause peculiar eruptions in susceptible persons (Abramowitz, 1918). By 1933 nineteen different cutaneous manifestations were reported (Newman, 1933). A review of animal carcinogenicity studies showed that rats and mice fed high doses – approximately 50 to 100 times the recommended dose for humans – developed a variety of tumours. When fed 30 times the recommended human dose for six months, mice also developed genetic damage (November 1996 as NTP's Technical Report Series, No. 465 (TR-465): Toxicology and Carcinogenesis Studies of Phenolphthalein (CAS No. 77-09-8); HO Drug Information vol.11, 4, 1997). Phenolphthalein is possibly carcinogenic in humans (IARC vol 76, 2000).

Because it undergoes enterohepatic circulation, it is eliminated slowly and it has been associated with adverse effects, notably skin reactions, potassium loss and atonia (WHO, 2003).

SED 1952: erythema exudativum multiforme, pemphigus, erythrodermia, contact dermatitis, fixed eruption, acute nephrosis with anuria, polyneuritis and haemorrhagic diathesis.

Withdrawn: in Norway and Yemen in 1979, UK in 1980, Bangladesh in 1982 and Greece in 1985 probably because of skin reactions, potassium loss and atonia. USA, Canada, France, Morocco and the European Community in 1997, in Oman and Japan in 1998, Saudi Arabia in 1999, Brazil in 2002, also in Poland, South Africa, New Zealand Singapore, and Bahrain, because of potential genotoxicity and carcinogenicity (rats and mice). In the USA, the FDA reclassified the drug from category 1 (safe and effective) to category III (more safety information needed) in response to the animal data and then later withdrew it (Cobert & Biron, 2002). HAI: banned in the EC + 12 countries and restricted in one.

Availability: remains in wide usage often in over-the-counter preparations, e.g. Thailand (HAI, 2008).

Lifespan: 77 years

Delay in recognition: skin reactions > 50 years; carcinogenicity 95 years

Delay in regulatory action: skin reactions > 27 years; carcinogenicity None.

Time span of withdrawals: 23 years

Comment: prior to the discovery of animal carcinogenicity in 1997 there was one spate of withdrawals and then a second spate afterwards.

1908 Cincophen–Cinchophene (Atophan, Cinchphan, Navarrard)

A uricosuric drug, was introduced, but it had been discovered in 1887.

Use: gout and as an analgesic.

ADR: Seifert says that the urine can be dark yellow, reddish or brown with a peculiar smell and also cystitis with dysuria and haematuria (Seifert,1915). Severe hepatitis with subacute hepatic necrosis was first reported in 1923, (Worster-Drought, 1923) and by 1931 thirty four deaths had been reported (Parsons and Kimball, 1931). In 1941 the Council on Pharmacy and Chemistry of the American Medical Association concluded that the case against Cincophen was not proved and that an urgent need existed for controlled clinical studies. Twenty-five years later, such studies had still not been undertaken (Dykes, 1998), but a Lyon University thesis was published in 1954 entitled 'Les Ictères au Cincophen' [The jaundice caused by Cincophen] (Cerf R, 1954). Cirrhosis was reported in 1957; toxic hepatitis was reported in 1957 (Ann Int Med, 1957) and in 1991 (Prieto, 1991). A case of agranulocytosis was first reported in 1936 (Shapiro & Lehman, 1936). Haemolytic anaemia was described in 1937 (Esbach & Bérard, 1937). SED 1952: agranulocytosis, hepatitis and jaundice and yellow atrophy (Lenyer et al., 1947; Cabot & Cabot, 1925).

SED 1957 acute yellow atrophy.

SED 1960 agranulocytosis.

Withdrawn: in Germany in 1991 and in Spain in 1992 for cytolytic hepatotoxicity and cirrhosis, which had a 50% fatality rate (Alvarez-Del-Castillo et al., 1991). Also withdrawn in Italy and South Africa.

Availability: still available in Spain (Prieto et al., 1991), Italy, US and the Netherlands.

Lifespan: 83 years

Delay in recognition: 15 years

Delay in regulatory action: 68 years.

Time span of withdrawals: 1 year

Comment: perhaps the Prieto paper stimulated Germany and Spain to withdraw cincophen, but there was amply evidence of the problem in the 1930s. It would appear that there were two types of hepatitis: the first a benign cholestatic hepatitis, which could come on after dechallenge and was mild, and secondly an allergic hepatitis which sometimes occurred on rechallenge and this might be accompanied by an allergic rash. This could cause a rapid death. Only enormous doses could produce hepatic damage in rabbits (Albahary, 1953).

1912 Phenobarbitone (Luminal)

Synthesised in 1911 by Hörein and introduced the following year, but not in England until 1923 and in France in 1927.

Use: sedative, hypnotic and antiepileptic.

ADR: by 1928 forty-one papers had been published on cutaneous reactions with phenobarbitone; the earliest dating back to 1912 (Menninger, 1928) Severe cutaneous reactions (Lyell's disease and Stevens-Johnson syndrome), fatal poisoning (20 per year in the UK) and abuse. Known to cause habituation in 1928 (Lewin, 1928). *'I have seen a large number of cases where a definite craving for the drug has arisen after repeated daily administration, and the daily use of the drug has been continued inspite of strong medical advice to the contrary. Addiction to the barbituric acid group is different from morphine and heroin in that sudden discontinuation is not followed by severe withdrawal symptoms.'* (Willcox, 1934).

SED 1952: prolonged use may give rise to habituation and addiction. When the drug is stopped abstinence symptoms may occur, even epileptiform attacks have been seen (there was no differentiation between the various barbiturates).

SED 1957: the state induced by the chronic use of barbituric acid derivatives may resemble chronic alcoholism and withdrawal resembles delirium tremens. By 1976 there was a campaign to stop the use of barbiturates as hypnotics (Leader, 1976). Phenobarbital is possibly carcinogenic in humans (IARC vol 79, 2001).

Withdrawn: in Sweden, where it was associated with fatal poisoning and abuse in 1985 and in Argentina in 1996. It was also withdrawn in South Africa and Switzerland. Restricted to epilepsy and anaesthesia in Germany in 1994, USA in 1997 and in France and Mauritius in 2001 (except for epilepsy).

Availability: in the UK it is restricted to epileptic patients (BNF, 1999). Worldwide.

Lifespan: 73 years.

Delay in recognition: 62 years before the campaign to stop its use.

Delay in regulatory action: 9 years

Time span of restrictions: 16 years

Comment: dependence of the 'barbiturate type' has been described as being different from morphine, cocaine and amphetamine types with its own characteristics (Current Practice, 1964).

1921 Dipyrone noramidopyrine/noraminosulfone/metamizole sodium (Novalgin, Baralgin, Analgin, Conmel)

It was also known as 'Mexican Aspirin'.

Use: analgesic

ADR: dipyrone is the sodium sulfonate derivative of aminopyrine and has the same pharmacological properties, so there is no reason to suspect that they are not equally likely to produce agranulocytosis (Huguley, 1964). The first case of agranulocytosis associated with dipyrone was reported in 1935 (Blake, 1935).

SED 1952: rarely causes blood changes. Erythema multiforme, purpura, haemorrhagic exanthemata and other rashes.

SED 1960: *'agranulocytosis is so generally known....'*

Reported as causing agranulocytosis with an incidence of 0.86% in 1952 (Discombe, 1952) and of 0.79% in 1964 (Huguley, 1964), but these papers had major flaws. The International Agranulocytosis and Aplastic Anaemia Study (IAAAS) gave a figure of 1.1 case per million. In Sweden three warnings (February, September and December 1967) were sent by the ADR committee, but it was only after the third warning that there was any drop in sales (Böttiger & Westerholm, 1973).

Withdrawn: there is a large variation in the reasons for withdrawal/restrictions. Canada in 1963, Australia in 1965, Sweden in 1973, Norway in 1976, France, Philippines (but can be used as a last resort), UK, Yemen, USA, Zimbabwe, Colombia, Armenia and Syria in 1977, Kuwait in 1978, Italy and Demark in 1979, Saudi Arabia in 1980 (anaphylactic shock), Argentina in 1981, Sudan and Bangladesh in 1982, Egypt in 1983 (anaphylactic shock), Israel in 1985, Belgium, Malaysia and Germany (prescription only) in 1987, Spain and Ghana in 1989, Netherlands in 1990, Switzerland and Sri Lanka in 1992, Thailand in 1994, Nepal in 1997, Syria, Yemen and Zimbabwe in 1998, Sweden in 1999, Morocco, Armenia, Lithuania, and Colombia in 2000, Pakistan in 1988, Brazil in 2005, Bahrain, Greece, Ireland, Mexico, Peru, Singapore, India, Venezuela and Japan (injection only) in 2006, because of agranulocytosis and anaphylaxis. Banned in Vietnam and Nigeria. It was withdrawn in Sweden in 1974 due to an estimated incidence of agranulocytosis of 1 in 3000 patients (Böttiger & Westholm, 1973) and then the IAAA study put the excess risk at 1.1 cases per million for the combination of Ulm, Berlin and Barcelona, but in the combination Israel, Budapest and Hungary there was no excess risk (IAAAS, 1986) and therefore it was reintroduced in Sweden in 1995 and finally withdrawn in 1999 because of the data presented by Hedenmalm and Spigset showing a figure of 1: 1439 (CI 1:850–1: 4684) (Hedenmalm & Spigset, 2002).The Ministry of Health in Brazil convened a conference in 2001 that decided that the risks of dipyrone are similar, or even lower, than of other analgesic/antipyretic drugs available on the market (Wong, 2002). Restricted in Germany in 1981 to treatment of severe pain and colic, and high fever not controlled by other drugs. HAI: banned it in 27 countries and restricted it in twelve.

Availability: Metamizole is still manufactured in many countries (at least 25), e.g. Germany, France, Spain (1995), the Far East, Africa and Latin and South America (Martindale): available in France, Germany, Thailand, Brazil, Turkey, Czechoslovakia, Argentina, Finland, Hungary, Mexico, Russia, Italy, Sweden, Belgium, South Africa, Austria, Venezuela, Spain, Poland, Israel, and Hongkong. From other sources, which may not be so reliable: Romania, Brazil, Bulgaria, India, and Costa Rica (1993). Still available in Indonesia both as single drug (Pyronal) or combination with vitamins (Neurogesic) vitamins or with vitamins caffeine, chlordiazepoxide and diazepam and caffeine (Metaneuron).

Lifespan: 42 years

Delay in recognition: 23 years

Delay in regulatory action: 14 years.

Time span of withdrawals: 37 years

Comment: a Lancet editorial entitled '*Dipyrone hearing by the German Drug Authority'* illustrates the problem of converting medical evidence into law: *'Political pressure, coupled with the manufacturer's argument that the case-control study would document the safety of the drug, prevented the BGA from taking stronger measures–such as removing the drug from the market or even having it put on prescription...*" The case of dipyrone is the most important example of serious discrepancies in the standards of safety adopted by different national drug regulatory authorities. These discrepancies seem to be due to administrative and political differences rather than to differing standards or competence' (Leader, 1986). Another editorial said that drugs such as metamizole were perhaps unjustly deleted from our pharmacopoeia because of imprecise studies of adverse side effect; some of the older therapeutic agents such as metamizole may be identified as having clinical utility in children (Berlin, 2001). The wide variation in the figures from the different centres (Ulm, Berlin and Barcelona) with the multivariate rate ratio 23.7% whilst for Israel and Budapest it was 0.8%) in this IAAA study suggests that there are other factors at play which may be genetic (IAAAS[173], 1986).

1928 Dioxide (Thorotrast) introduced

Use: radioactive contrast medium containing Thorium

ADR: aplastic anaemia was induced in a rabbit by a large dose of thorium in 1931 (Lambin & Gerard, 1931) and leucopenia in rabbits in 1933 (Gottlieb, 1933) and in 1933 granulomas had been produced in animals (Jörg & Aguirre, 1933). A comment in the BMJ stated that as thorium dioxide is radioactive and that it was known that prolonged radio-activity was known to result in cancer that there was a possibility that Thorotrast might give rise to malignant disease (BMJ leader, 1935) Its carcinogenetic properties were shown in animals in 1938 *'Because of the ultimate danger of malignancy, radio-active substances such as thorotrast should never be introduced into the human body, all the more so since there are other non-toxic radio-opaque substances'.* (Selbie, 1938). A case of aplastic anaemia due to Thorotrast was reported in 1946 (Spier et al., 1947). Acute leukaemia (Artzl Forsch, 1955), pancytopenia, myelofibrosis and also caused liver cirrhosis, hepatocellular carcinomas, intrahepatic cholangiocarcinomas and haemangioendotheliomas of the liver and other tumours. The induction period was from 6 years to 35 years (Bonser, 1967). Its radioactivity consisted almost entirely of very short-range alpha particles with negligible gamma radiation (Jellinek, 2004). It had a half-life of 400 years. It was shown to produce subcutaneous sarcomas in rats and mice in 1938 (Anon, 1938). There were 60 cases of tumours in man in the literature by 1961 (Dahlgren 1961). The increase estimated cumulative incidence for those exposed in the 1950s is 35–86% (Wetzels, 2007).

SED 1952 renal carcinoma, pulmonary carcinoma, liver carcinoma, and aplastic anaemia.

SED 1957 endothelial sarcoma in liver and spleen reported in 1956.

SED 1967 said that its use was condemned in 1932 by the AMA Council on Pharmacy and Chemistry because of the possibility of necrosis or

---

[173] IAAAS = International Agranulocytosis and Aplastic Anaemia Study

malignant change. The latent periods between administration and development of these ADRs was 5 years for granulomas, 15 years for liver fibrosis and 20 years for liver tumours.

Withdrawn: in France in 1936 and in the USA in 1964 (the FDA said that it was unsafe). Withdrawn in the UK in 1955 because of carcinogenicity.

Availability: nil. Still available in 1967 (Granger, 1967).

Lifespan: 27 years

Delay in recognition: 10 years

Delay in regulatory action: the delay of 28 years after being withdrawn in France before withdrawal in the USA is difficult to understand.

Time span of withdrawals: 28 years

Comment: there was ample evidence of its toxicity by 1932 and the regulatory authorities must have been relying on the radiologists to be aware of the toxicity and reserve its use for those whose life expectancy ruled out a problem with latent carcinogenicity. Selbie's warning was ignored.

1930 Mercurothiolate Sodium (Thiomersal, Thiobactal)

Use: antiseptic

ADR: *'the risks from thiomersal-containing vaccines are speculative and inadequately quantified.'* (Bigham & Copes, 2005).

Withdrawn: in Malaysia in 1995 and in Brazil in 2001, USA, and European Union in 1999 because of urothelial cancer, nephrotoxicity and peripheral neuropathy.

Availability: in the USA, Israel, France, Brazil, Spain, Australia, Chile, Italy, Argentina, South Africa, Thailand, Venezuela and Mexico (Martindale). It is still present in vaccines in 2008.

Lifespan: 65 years

Delay in recognition: potential problems were recognised and investigated and no convincing evidence found to ban its use.

Delay in regulatory action: none

Time span of withdrawals: 6 years

Comment: the general rule is Thiomersal free vaccines for rich countries and thiomersal containing vaccines for the developing world (Bigham & Copes, 2005).

1933 Dinitrophenol (2,4-dinitrophenol) (Nox-ben-ol, Nitroment, Nitrophen, Redusols, Formula 17, Slim, Dinitrenalm, Dinitole)

Use: weight reduction (Cutting et al., 1933, Tainter et al., 1934). During the First World War it was used in explosive manufacture and since then it has been used as a pesticide. The ability of dinitrophenol to raise the body temperature together with its toxicity had already been recognised in 1885 when the compound was being used as a food colouring (Parasandola, 1977).

ADR: the first report In July 1935 was on three cases of cataract (Horner et al., 1935) and the author later said *'The ratio of lens changes to the total number of patients taking dinitrophenol is small, probably less than one per cent and perhaps nearer 0.1%.* '(Rodin, 1936). The reaction was confirmed in August 1935 when another seventeen cases were reported (Boardman, 1935). Cataracts in 29 female patients had an average time to onset of 11 months (Rodin, 1936). *'Thousands of women developed aggressive sclerosing cataracts, sometimes requiring enucleation.'* (Temple 1996). Granulocytopenia with thrombocytopenia and anaemia (Imerman & Imerman, 1936), severe skin rashes, jaundice, disturbance of smell and taste. The FDA gave a warning in 1934, but before 1938 it was legal to sell it as a diet potion. The premarketing studies lasted for less than 3 months (FDA, 1987). SED 1952: serious warnings must be issued against the use of this drug. ADRs include bilateral cataracts and agranulocytosis.

Withdrawn: 1938 FDA 2,4-dinitrophenol (DNP) ban as a weight loss drug. On July 6, 1935, the AMA's Council on Pharmacy and Chemistry reported dinitrophenol would not be included in its quasi-official list of acceptable remedies (Report, 1935).

Availability: advertised on the Internet to body builders.

Lifespan: 5 years

Delay in recognition: 1½ years, but the time to onset was about 2 to 12 months after stopping the drug. The recognition was helped by the rapid progression over about a month and the occurrence in a relatively young age group (45–55 years).

Delay in regulatory action: 4 years

Comment: it is difficult to believe that it was only on sale in the USA. The FDA was not able to ban DNP because it was rated as a diet potion and therefore outside their jurisdiction until there was a change in the law.

1937 H$_1$-antihistamines (Oxomemazine–Promethazine–Alimemazine–Mequitaxine)

Use: H$_1$ antihistamine (Phenothiazine derivatives) for coughs, allergic reactions, motion sickness and sedation.

ADR: in 1979, the possibility was raised that the use of phenothiazine antihistamines, particularly promethazine, could be associated with sleep apnoea in young children and with sudden infant death syndrome (SIDS) (Kahn & Blum, 1979, 1982). Studies were carried out subsequently, although they have not established a causal relationship (WHO, 2003).
SED 1952, 1960, 1963, SED 1980, SED 1984, SED 1988, SED 1992 and SED 1996: not mentioned.

Restrictions: should not be used in children below the age of one year, having regard to their possible association with sudden infant death syndrome (WHO, 2003). Warning in the USA in 2005 against use in children under two years of age, the EEC advised in 1991 that they should not be used for children under the age on one year. Switzerland made it prescription only in 1990. In Germany (1987), they were not to be used during pregnancy because of the possibility of pyloric stenosis. Oman said in 2005 that promethazine was contraindicated in children under two years of age.

Availability: as a cough medicine in Belgium, Netherlands, Brazil, Israel, France and Switzerland (Martindale).

Lifespan: 54 years

Delay in recognition: 42 years

Delay in regulatory action: 8 years

Time span of restrictions: one year

Comment: in France BIAM advises that it should not be given to children under one year of age if there is a family history of SIDS.

1938 Diethylstilboestrol (DES) (Distilbene)

Use: prevention of miscarriage since 1941. Approved by the FDA on September 19th 1941 for four indications; Gonorrheal vaginitis, atrophic vaginitis, menopausal symptoms and postpartum lactation suppression. On July 1st 1947, the FDA approved the first supplemental New Drug Application (by Squibb)) adding prevention of miscarriage.

ADR: identified as a carcinogen in animals (adenocarcinoma of the breast in male mice) in 1938. NB before approval (Lacassagne, 1938). Known to have no therapeutic value in pregnant women (Dieckmann et al.,

1953). Adenocarcinoma of the vagina in offspring discovered in 1970 by a case-control study (Herbst et al., 1970; Herbst et al., 1971). A study in a special registry found maternal exposure in 49 cases out of 66 cases of clear-cell cancers of the genital tract (Herbst et al., 1972). Labelled by the FDA 5 months later, by the Netherlands in 1972 and in France in 1977; the UK advised against its use in pregnancy in 1973 (Plamlund, 1993). The estimated tumour risk is 0.14–1.4 per 1000 DES-exposed subjects, but since up to 6 million persons were exposed in utero to DES between 1940 and 1970 the total number may be very high indeed (Dukes, 2000). There was also an increased risk of breast cancer in DES mothers (relative risk >2)(Giusti et al., 1995).

SED 1952: the same side effects as other synthetic substances with an oestrogenic effect.

'However, one is still uncertain concerning the harmlessness of such quantities of drugs on the product of conception, and more especially on its gonadic functions.' (Albahary, 1953).

SED 1960: no mention

SED 1968 (VI) it also causes hepatocellular carcinoma in males.

Withdrawn: FDA banned its use in pregnant women in 1971. It was withdrawn in Panama in 1973, the USA, Netherlands and Australia in 1975, Germany and Austria in 1977, Greece and Kuwait in 1980, Tunisia in 1983, France and Japan in 1997, Spain and Belgium in 1983, also in Italy and Saudi Arabia. In Australia, Greece and Germany, its use is permitted only for the treatment of prostate cancer.

Availability: diethylstilbestrol remains available in many countries; however, only for the treatment of certain hormone-dependent neoplasms including carcinoma of the prostate and postmenopausal breast cancer (WHO, 2003).

Last documented prescription was in Spain in 1983. (Direcks et al.,1991). In the UK it is still used, but rarely, for breast cancer and prostate cancer (BNF, 1999).

Lifespan: 35 years

Delay in recognition: 33 years

Delay in regulatory action: 3 years

Time span of withdrawals: 12 years

Comment: it was the first drug submitted to the FDA after the 1938 Food, Drugs and Cosmetic Act although it had already been identified as a carcinogen. This, plus its lack of efficacy for its intended purpose, which was only discovered in the 1950s, should have prevented its marketing. A pharmacovigilance disaster.

1940 **Pyrithyldione**/diphenhydramine (Dorma; Persedon, Benedorm, diprilone, dihydropyridine)

Use: a sedative/hypnotic

ADR: a case of agranulocytosis was reported in 1949 in the USA (Tyson, 1949) and there were anecdotal cases from the 1960s and 1970s in Germany and from the 1980s in Japan (Ibáñez et al., 2000). Leucopenia had been reported in rabbits in 1940.

SED 1952: agranulocytosis

In Spain between 1980 and 1995, the Pharmacovigilance Centre of the Catalan Institute of Pharmacology received some 280 reports of agranulocytosis. Of these, nine were associated with use of a combination hypnotic-sedative product, pyrithyldione and diphenhydramine. Although evidence was weak, the Centre suspected that agranulocytosis might have been caused by pyrithyldione, and warned that the benefit-risk profile of this product might have been unfavourable as a consequence (Butlletí grog, 1996). The adjusted odds ratio found in a case control study was 200 (CI 95% 22–infinity). There were eight cases of which none were fatal and the National Commission of Pharmacovigilance recommended withdrawal, but the Ministry of Health took more than 2 years to withdraw the drug and six more cases occurred in this time (Ibáñez et al., 2000).

Withdrawn: in Spain in 1997 because of the eight cases of agranulocytosis.

Availability: by the end of the 1980s it was still marketed in Belgium, Denmark, Germany, Sweden and Switzerland (Martindale).

Lifespan: 57 years

Delay in recognition: 9 years

Delay in regulatory action: 48 years

Comment: no trace of further cases.

1941 **Sulfathiazole** (Cibazol, Thiazomide, Tresamide)

Use: an antibacterial drug used for pnemococcus pneumonia, gonorrhoea, staplococcus septicaemia, and urinary tract infections.

ADR: the toxic effects of sulfathiazole on the kidneys (nitrogen retention, haematuria, oliguria and crystals in the urine) were known soon after its discovery in 1939 (Simon & Kaufman, 1943). Agranulocytosis was recognised in 1941 (Hoyne & Larrimore, 1941). Hepatotoxicity in 1942. All sulphonamides can cause hepatitis. (Lederer & Rosenblatt, 1942). Liver lesions include: granulomas and necrosis (Rios Sanchez, 1971). Other ADRs were aplastic anaemia and haemolytic anaemia, exfoliative dermatitis, erythema multiforme and fever.

SED 1952: generalised dermatitis, erythema nodosum, crystalluria, fatal anuria due to damage to the renal parenchyma, hepatitis, thrombocytopenia, haemoglobinuria and necrotising arteritis. The older sulphonamides, e.g. sulfathiazole, are more harmful than the modern preparations. There are no sulphonamides known which cannot cause renal damage.

SED 1960: obstructive anuria with Sulfathiazole and 23 children had haematuria.

Withdrawn: in the USA in 1970, Philippines in 1971 (because of the risk of crystalluria), France and the United Arab Emirates in 1977, and Dominica in 1982.

Availability: in USA, Italy, Spain, Chile, Austria, Germany, Venezuela, Brazil, Argentina and Vietnam (Martindale).

Lifespan: 29 years

Delay in recognition: None

Delay in regulatory action: 29 years

Time span of withdrawals: 12 years

Comment: the problem was finding whether there were sulphonamides that were better than sulfathiazole and it is probable that that caused the delay in withdrawal. Aplastic anaemia, agranulocytosis and thrombocytopenias are sulphonamide class effects (Albahary, 1953).

1944 Di-hydro-streptomycin sulphate

Use: an antibiotic.

ADR: neuropsychiatric problems and ototoxicity. *'Di-hydro-streptomycin is more toxic than streptomycin.'* (Minkenhet, 1950). Clinically the toxicity of di-hydro-streptomycin is much more significant, since it may easily cause partial or complete loss of hearing, whereas streptomycin tends to affect only the vestibular apparatus (Ruef & Blaser, 2000).

SED 1952: some investigators are of the opinion that the toxicity for the vestibular and cochlear nerves is greater after prolonged use of dihydrostreptomycin than is the case with streptomycin (no reference was given).

Withdrawn: in the USA in 1970, Philippines in 1972, Spain in 1983 and also in Dominica and Italy. HAI: banned in 6 countries.

Availability: in Belgium, Poland, Mexico, Portugal, Philippines, Australia, Greece and Ireland (Martindale).

Lifespan: 26 years

Delay in recognition: ≤ 8 years

Delay in regulatory action: ≥ 18 years

Time span of withdrawals: 13 years

Comment: I haven't found a paper which reports on a comparison between the two streptomycins. It was his deafness caused by di-hydro-streptomycin that prompted Leopold Meyler to write his famous textbook 'The Side effects of Drugs'.

1947 Methapyrilene (Rinofol, Thenylene, Histadyl, Nytol)

Use: a type 1 antihistamine.

ADR: produced hepatocellular carcinomas and cholangiocarcinomas in rats (Lijinsky et al., 1980). This was confirmed in 2000 (Cunningham, 2000). Fatalities occurred on over dosage (Winek et al., 1977). It was banned because it could cause liver tumours in rats if given 25 to 30 times the normal human dose throughout the animal's normal life span (Lewis, 1979).

SED 1952: one fatal case in a 16 month child: anuria, cerebral oedema, nephrosis and toxic psychosis (Rives et al., 1949).

SED 1960 and SED 1963: no mention of ADRs.

Withdrawn: in Germany, Italy, Singapore, Hongkong, Domenica, France, UK, USA and Canada in 1979; Australia, Egypt, Brazil, Panama and Philippines in 1980; Argentina in 1981; India in 1983; Oman in 1992; and also withdrawn in Chile, New Zealand and Venezuela. HAI: banned in 19 countries.

Availability: on the internet.

Lifespan: 22 years

Delay in recognition: 27 years

Delay in regulatory action: Nil

Time span of withdrawals: 13 years

Comment: if a drug is left on the market for specific indications it is impossible to police the generalised use in poorer countries.

1948 Chloramphenicol (Chloromycetin)

Was approved in the US on 12th January 1949 and introduced in the UK in August 1949.

Use: an antibiotic, which was originally tested for scrub typhus and now used for typhoid, salmonella, meningitis and rickettsial infections (Sneader, 2005).

ADR: the presence of the nitrobenzene radical in the structure of chloramphenicol led to the suspicion that the drug might be toxic to the haemopoietic system (Smadel, 1949). Three patients showed marrow hypoplasia after chloramphenicol with a positive dechallenge (Volini et al., 1949). The first confirmation of this hypothesis was a single fatal case of aplastic anaemia reported in 1950 (Rich et al., 1950) followed in 1952 by a paper, authored by FDA staff, saying, '*it appears beyond a reasonable doubt that chloramphenicol, in certain susceptible individuals, causes blood dyscrasias, including aplastic anaemia, thrombocytopenic purpura, granulocytopenia and pancytopenia*'. This paper gave details of 19 articles on the subject between 1949 and August 1952. The authors recommended a change in labelling and that the drug should not used for minor infections (Lewis et al., 1952). '*In 1952 when it was realised that chloramphenicol had caused scores of cases of aplastic anaemia and that it had taken three years to appreciate the potential toxicity of the drug*'. (Doll, 1969). In June 1952 the number of cases of blood disorders associated with chloramphicol in the US was 410, but in only 61 cases was the drug the only drug being taken. It was suggested that a case control study should be undertaken but nothing was done. The main problem, which is true with many drugs, was that doctors misuse and over use antibiotics (Marks, http://www.hopkinsmedicine.org/histmed/images/hmadverse.pdf; Maeder, 1994).

SED 1952: mentioned aplastic anaemia (12 cases) and agranulocytosis. In 1958 Garrod reported an approximate incidence of one case of aplastic anaemia per 400 cases at St Bartholomew's hospital (Garrod, 1958).

SED 1960: the sub-committee of the AMA Research Council–There were 27 certain cases, 30 probable cases and 7 possible cases of agranulocytosis.

US labelling had to include warnings of blood dyscrasias [topical preparations excepted]. Between 1957 and 1961 there were 138 deaths caused by the drug in California. The risk of fatal aplastic anaemia was at least 1:60,000 (Smick et al., 1964) or between 1 in 40,800 and 1 in 24,500 or 13 times the background level (Wallerstein et al., 1969).

Confirmation of causality came when it was shown that reversible marrow suppression could be induced by high dosage (Krakoff et al., 1975; Venning II, 1983). *'Since the risk of serious chloramphenicol toxicity is so small (1:18,000 or probably less) it is of more than historical interest there are still many areas in which the benefits outweigh its risks.'* (Ruef & Blaser, 2000). The use of chloramphenicol eye drops lingered on despite a report in 1955 of a death from bone marrow aplasia resulting from the eye drops (Rosenthal and Blackman, 1965; Doona & Walsh, 1995), but it still remains on the UK market. The estimated risk increased from 1:200,000 in 1951 to 1:20,000 in 1971 a ten-fold increase. Tognoni said that chloramphenicol aplastic anaemia was rare in Southern European countries (Tognoni, 1979). In Sweden there was a steady decline in prescription of chloramphenicol after a warning was given in May 1968 (Böttiger & Westerholm, 1973) Chloramphenicol is possibly carcinogenic to humans (IARC vol 50, 1990).

Restrictions: there was a UK regulatory warning in 1967 (Venning II, 1983) and it was restricted to life threatening infections, particularly those caused by *haemophilus influenzae* and for typhoid fever; also as an ingredient in ear and eye drops (BNF, 1999). Its use was restricted in Germany and Japan (indications restricted) in 1975; Denmark and France in 1978; Philippines in 1982, Egypt in 1983; Netherlands in 1984; Canada and Spain in 1985; Hungary in 1987; Ireland in 1989, because of aplastic anaemia. It remained on the USA and UK markets for Rocky Mountain Spotted fever in the former and for haemophilus influenza infections and typhoid fever in the latter. In Germany its use is restricted to cases of acute attacks of typhoid, paratyphoid or purulent meningitis. It also has strict regulations in countries like Israel and the Netherlands. In the USA the *'detailmen continued to promote the drug as effective for a wide range of uses, resulting in widespread use of the drug for minor infections and an unnecessary toll of serious adverse reactions and death'*. (Waxman, 2003).

Availability: still in wide usage including Indonesia.

Lifespan: 27 years

Delay in recognition: approximately one year before the first papers, but then a delay before it was acknowledged by the AMA.

Delay in regulatory action: 17 years

Time span of restrictions: 22 years

Comment: again if a drug is left on the market for specific indications it is impossible to police the generalised use in poorer countries. The three year delay in recognition stimulated the American Medical Association (AMA) to set up a blood dyscrasia registry, which no longer functions. Chloramphenicol continued to be sanctioned as an eye medication and then in 1955 a case of aplastic anaemia was said to be caused by the eye drops (Rosenthal & Blackman, 1965) and after another paper (Fraunfelder et al., 1982) the sale of the eye drops in the USA dropped by 80% over two years (Doona & Walsh, 1995). Between 1988 and 1995 A survey of in 400 UK general practices found 442,543 patients who had received a prescription for chloramphenicol eye drops and of these there were three cases of serious haematological toxicity, two of which were possibly caused by the drops. The authors said there use seems to be safe (Lancaste et al., 1998). In the USA National Register there were 23 cases and the eye drops were no longer used in the USA (Doona, 1998). The delay by the regulatory authorities revolves around the probable incidence of the ADR. The risk/benefit ratio with such rarities depends on a complex balance of cost, alternative drugs and the different acceptance of risk between rich countries and poor countries.

1949 Phenylbutazone (Butazolidine, Butazone, BTZ)

Marketed in UK in 1951.

Use: rheumatic arthritis, osteoarthritis, ankylosing sponylitis, gout, Reiter's disease, bone pain with Paget's disease and secondary neoplasm, extensive superficial thrombophlebitis, and prolapsed intervertebral disc.

ADR: agranulocytosis, aplastic anaemia, acute interstitial nephritis, thrombocytopenic purpura, hepatic granulomas, hepatitis and cirrhosis, and reactivation of peptic ulcers. 'The problem was predicted from the structural similarity to amidopyrine and other pyrazolones of known toxicity to bone marrow' (Venning II, 1983). The first report of agranulocytosis was in 1952 (Medico-legal, 1952). There were 503 deaths. The first case of aplastic anemia reported in the English press was in 1953 (Leonard, 1953). Thrombocytopenic purpura was first reported in 1952 (Stephens, 1952). There was a high incidence of toxic effects–42% (Nassim & Pilkington, 1953).

SED 1952: neither of the butazones is mentioned.

1955 the 23rd case of death caused by phenylbutazone was reported.

There were 10 deaths from agranulocytosis, 3 from peptic ulcer and gastrointestinal haemorrhage, 3 from exfoliative dermatitis, 2 from renal lesions, and 2 were unclassified. There were single cases reported because of thrombocytopenic purpura, toxic hepatitis, and aplastic anaemia (Mauer, 1955).

In 1957 Venning reported a case of aplastic anaemia due to phenylbutazone. He pointed out that regular white-cell counts are no safeguard against many of its lethal complications (Venning, 1957).

SED 1960: agranulocytosis with loss of all cellular elements (1959).

The estimate of the incidence of death caused by agranulocytosis in the UK was 2.2 per 100,000 with sex ratio in the over 65 years being males/females 1:5 (Inman, 1977). The IAAAS gave a figure of excess risk of 0.2 per million (IAAAS, 1986).

By 1964 there had only been 7 published reports of aplastic anaemia (McCarthy & Chalmers, 1964).

In 1965 The UK regulatory authorities (CSD) issued a warning concerning bone marrow toxicity (Venning II, 1983).

By 1967 Dr PD Fowler of Geigy said in a personal communication to Dr G Venning that the company had received 45 case reports (Venning II, 1983).

In 1977 The Committee on the Safety of Medicines said that they had received reports of 188 deaths from aplastic anaemia or agranulocytosis (aplastic anaemia 233, agranulocytosis 17) with an incidence of 1 in 50,000 patients the risk being greater for older patients (Inman, 1977).

In 1985 Ciba-Geigy's view, according to the authors, was that the drug continued to be valuable for selective use under medical supervision (Herxheimer et al., 1985).

In 1986 the Canadian authorities wrote in a 'Dear Doctor' letter that phenylbutazone should be restricted to use with ankylosing spondylitis and acute gout (Biron, 1986).

Withdrawn: Jordan (1977), Bangladesh (1977), Ethiopia, Netherlands, Chile (1985), Panama, Turkey, Ghana (1989), Sri Lanka (1992), Norway, United Arab Emirates, Armenia (2000), Bahrein and Cyprus. HAI: banned in 12 countries.

Restrictions: restricted in Japan (use only for exacerbation of arthritis, ankylosing spondylitis and acute gout) in 1977; Hungary, Ireland, Tunisia, Argentina, Kuwait, Barbados, Zimbabwe, Spain and Congo in 1984, Greece, Norway, Germany (use not to exceed one week for exacerbation of acute rheumatism or acute gout), Iraq, United Arab Emirates, Paraguay, Hongkong, Oman, New Zealand and Sweden in 1985, Turkey in 1976, Malaysia in 1987, Belgium in 1988, also Australia, Austria, UK (use in ankylosing spondylitis only), Israel, Italy (use not to exceed 10 days) and Philippines. It was restricted to use hospital treatment of ankylosing spondylitis in Finland, UK, Zimbabwe, Kuwait, New Zealand, and South Africa (Herxheimer et al., 1985). HAI: restricted in 26 countries.

Availability: it is still found in many places including Indonesia (numerous combinations with derivatives of amidopyrine and others with derivatives of salicylic acid, some with antacid and another with Carisoprodol. viz) (Informasi Spesialite Obat Indonesia, 2005) and Thailand (HAI, 2008). It is a dangerous drug and should be used only when less toxic alternatives are unavailable (Biscarini, 2000). It was still available in Fiji in 1986 combined with amidopyrine and prednisolone.

Lifespan: 28 years.

Delay in recognition: 25 years.

Delay in regulatory action: 12 years

Time span of withdrawals: 11 years

Comment: Venning said that the magnitude of the problem was underestimated owing to underreporting. (Venning II,1983) Another example of a drug remaining on the market for specific usage, but used for other indications in poor countries. Reactions of this rarity are unlikely to be discovered by a cohort study. Although oxyphenbutazone was taken off the market phenylbutazone, which is almost identical as to its ADRs, remained on the Canadian market (Biron, 1986). It is closely allied to amidopyrine so it was not surprising that it caused agranulocytosis. It needs to be compared with the other pyrazolones: dipyrone, aminopyrine and oxyphenbutazone.

1951 Diamthazole di-Hcl (Dimazol, Asterol)

Use: a topical (powder, ointment and tincture) antifungal (tinea) agent.

ADR: hepatotoxicity, neuropsychiatric and neurotoxic ADRs (Hitch & Raleigh, 1952). Tremor, visual hallucinations, disorientation, nystagmus, ataxia, dysarthria and convulsions (Featherstone, 1952), vomiting, cyanosis, mydriasis and disturbed respiration reported in 1957 (Christen & Jaccottet, 1957; Morton, 1960; Anon, 1957). SED 1960: four infants had convulsions due to the ointment, as well as

tremor, ataxia, hallucinations and changes in behaviour.
SED 1958, SED 1962, SED 1966, SED 1968, SED 1972, SED 1976, SED 1980 and SED 1984: no mention

Withdrawn: in the USA and France in 1977, because of severe neurotoxic reactions, their potential for misuse and the availability of safer alternative products.

Availability: topical preparations of diamazole remain available in some 40 countries (WHO, 2003).

Lifespan: 26 years

Delay in recognition: one year

Delay in regulatory action: 25 years

Comment: the seriousness of the ADRs may have been offset by their rarity. The absorption of the agent will have depended on the amount used, and the area and degree of inflammation.

1951 Arsenate Sodium (Sangart)

Was introduced in France as a tonic. (Na_2HAsO_4), 7 H_2O.

Use: sodium arsenate was formerly used in the treatment of chronic skin diseases, some parasitic diseases, and anaemia (Martindale, 1977).

ADR: dependence on arsenic was reported in 1750 (Lewin, 1928). Arsenic and arsenicals must be considered obsolete in medicine because of their limited therapeutic value, their multiple-system toxicity and their apparent carcinogenic properties (Coulis & Dukes, 2000). Four cases of acute intoxication reported from Paris in 1972 (Fréjaville et al., 1972). BIAM[174]: polyneuritis, proteinuria, hepatitis with cholestasis and sometimes hepatic cirrhosis, and peripheral neuropathy. Arsenic and arsenic compounds are carcinogenic in humans (IARC vol 23, 1980). SED 1952 and SED 1976: arsenic—no mention of abuse. The AFSSAPS[175] is unable to add any more information.

Withdrawn: in France in 1988 because of abuse. A European Court report stated in 1995: every bottle of Sangart mixture is made up, according to the evidence, of distilled water (100 cm^3), syrup (25 cm^3) and 90° alcohol (16 cm^3) to which is added 0.005 g sodium arsenate, 0.02 g sodium nucleinate, 1 g nux vomica, 1.5 g calf liver extract and various flavourings. In its observations, the Commission undertook a detailed review of the very few active substances in the mixtures. For example, it is stated that sodium arsenate is traditionally used in the treatment

---

[174] BIAM = Banque de Données Automatisée sur les Médicaments (http://www.biam2.org/)
[175] AFSSAPS = Agence Française de Sécurité Sanitaire des Produits de Santé

of anaemic conditions, but since each bottle of Sangart mixture contains per 141 cm^3 only 0.005 mg of the substance, any therapeutic effect must be excluded. Sangart lived on in another guise.

Availability: nil

Lifespan: 37 years

Delay in recognition: not known for arsenic and 37 years for this product.

Delay in regulatory action: 238 years

Comment: arsenic was used from the 16th century to improve temporarily the appearance of horses by making their coat shinier. In man it gave cheeks a healthy glow and it was hoped make them stronger, more resistant to infections and able to eat more (Lewin, 1928). Further reading: KK Jain's Drug-induced Neurolgical Disorders. Hogrefe & Huber Publishers 2001, 281–2.

1952 Tetracycline paediatric (Achromycin V)

Use: an antibiotic

ADR: teeth discolouration, temporary inhibition of growth and enamel hypoplasia (Van der Linden, 1965).
SED 1958 and SED 1963: no mention
SED 1966: some discolouration of the teeth

Withdrawn: in Jordan in 1973, Peru in 1974 (restricted), Italy in 1975 (suppositories only), the Philippines and the USA in 1978, Ghana in 1980, Argentina in 1981, Bangladesh and Sudan in 1982, India in 1983, Oman in 1985, Pakistan in 1988, Chile in 1990 (warning), Nepal in 1991, also in Australia, Belgium (warning), New Zealand and Saudi Arabia, United Arab Emirates, Austria and Spain. The doctors were warned not to prescribe the formulations to pregnant women or children under 9 years of age. HAI: banned in 13 countries and restricted in five.

Availability: in the UK allowed in children over the age of 12 years and in the USA in children over 8 years.

Lifespan: 21 years

Delay in recognition: 13 years

Delay in regulatory action: 8 years

Time span of restrictions: 18 years

Comment: an example of restriction of a particular formulation.

1952 Coralgil (MG345, Trimanyl, Koralgil, Diaethiphenum), (4,4' diethylaminoethoxy hexestral dihydrochloride) is closely related to Triparanol (MER-29)

Use: coronary vasodilator and in 1964 as a cholesterol lowering drug.

ADR:'foam cell syndrome' and phospholipidosis' (these diseases are now called 'Non-alcoholic steatohepatitis') found in 1961 (Phillips & Avigan, 1961) leading to liver cirrhosis and death. Estimated 50,000 victims and 250 deaths. Lipidosis had been produced in rats and other experimental animals (Blohm, 1978). The information provided by the drug firm was misleading in several ways: a higher dosage, rarely prescribed in other countries. Periodical suspension was not in the instructions in Japan, but was in other countries; unapproved claims such as 'hypocholesterolemic action' were used, which was not mentioned in the drug insert (Hama, 1980).

SED 1960, SED 1963, SED 1966 and SED 1968: no mention.

Withdrawn: Japan in December 1969

Availability: none

Lifespan: 18 years

Delay in recognition: 18 years

Delay in regulatory action: one month (Nakamura & Kawwamura, 1980)

Comment: possibly it was marketed only in Japan.

1952 Iproniazid (Marsilid)

Was introduced for TB, but it was first introduced for angina and depression in 1957.

Use: a monoamine oxidase inhibitor (MAOI).

ADR: four patients were reported with hepatitis (hepatocellular and sometimes necrosis) in 1954 (Bosworth et al., 1955). In 1955 an interaction between iproniazid and the tyramine in food, especially cheese, which caused hypertensive crises, was recognised, (Ogilvie, 1955). Hepatocellular toxicity and cirrhosis with 20% mortality (Kline, 1958), but the incidence was estimated as under 0.05% (Benaim & Dixon, 1958).

SED 1960: particularly toxic for the liver. Fatalities 15%.

SED 1963: hypertensive crises described.

Robert Temple of the FDA said *'it took 3 years to discover any evidence that it was hepatotoxic and 6 years to recognise that it should be off the market, after hundreds of deaths from liver failure. Given its approximately 10% rate of liver injury, it is not easy to see why discovery of its toxicity took so long'.* (Temple, 1996).

Withdrawn: in the USA in 1959, in Canada in 1964 and in Italy.

Availability: MAOIs retain a place in the treatment of serious depressive illness although there is no international consensus on which compounds should be preferred. Thus, iproniazid remains available in several countries (WHO, 2003).

Lifespan: 7 years

Delay in recognition: 2 years

Delay in regulatory action: 6 years

Time span of withdrawals: 5 years

Comment: it had been known for 50 years that cheese contained tyramine, which was capable of causing a rise in blood pressure. *'there would seem to be no reason why their effects should not have been predicted.'* (Doll, 1969). The interaction with tyramine is a class effect, but autoimmune hepatitis is specific to iproniazid. Further reading: KK Jain's Drug-induced Neurolgical Disorders. Hogrefe & Huber Publishers 2001, 406-414.

1953 Thenalidine (Sandostene)

Introduced in Europe and in 1955 in the USA.

Use: a piperadine anti-histamine

ADR: severe neutropenia and agranulocytosis (Adams & Perry, 1958)). It is to the credit of Sandoz Pharmaceuticals that the drug was immediately withdrawn on 9th July 1958 only four days after the first report (Zolov,1958).

SED 1958: no mention.

SED 1960: agranulocytosis mentioned.

Withdrawn: in the USA in 1958 after 3 cases of agranulocytosis, two of which were fatal (Adams & Perry, 1958); UK in 1961, Canada in 1963, Sweden in 1976, France in 1978 and Cyprus in 1980. Also withdrawn in Australia, Finland, Norway and Venezuela. HAI: banned in 9 countries.

Availability: it is still available in some countries.

Lifespan: 5 years

Delay in recognition: 5 years

Delay by the company: four days

Time span of withdrawals: 22 years

Comment: the prompt action by Sandoz was excellent, but how was it still available in the UK, France, Canada, Sweden and Cyprus?

1954 Diiododiethyltin/isolinoleic acid ester (Stalinon)

Introduced in France.

Use: treatment for staphylococcal infections.

ADR: in 1954 triethyltin was shown to remarkably neurotoxic (Stoner et al., 1955) Cerebral oedema—headache, photophobia, vomiting and drowsiness due to raised intracranial pressure, and death occurring in 4-10 days (Le Quesne, 1981).

The intended dose used for toxicity testing should have been 50 mgm, but due to an error, they used only 3 mgm and the resulting absence of toxicity persuaded them to market a product containing 15 mgm per capsule. The responsible pharmacist was sent to prison for two years and the company held liable (D'Arcy & Griffin, 1986). There were no cases of poisoning for 6–7 months, which, it was suggested, was because organic tin salts have a delayed effect (HP, 1958). It was known that triethyltin was very neurotoxic and Stalinon contained a variable amount of triethyltin as an impurity (Le Quesne, 1981).

Withdrawn: in France in 1957 because 110 patients died out of the 290 patients affected (Le Quesne, 1981).

Availability: Nil

Lifespan: 3 years

Delay in recognition: none

Delay in regulatory action: 3 years

Comment: an error by the pharmaceutical company plus a delayed ADR meant the drug remained on the market too long.

1954 Glutethimide (Doriden)

Use: hypnotic and sedative

ADR: acute glaucoma, dependence and abuse (Sramek & Khajawall, 1982). The first case of dependence was reported in 1957(Rogers, 1958) and of addiction in 1960 (Cohen, 1960).

SED 1960: addiction frequently observed with withdrawal symptoms. Other overdose ADRs were: respiratory depression, hypotension, pulmonary oedema, cerebral oedema, convulsions and sudden apnoea (BMJ Leader, 1976). The mortality from overdosage was 13.9% for glutethimide against 0.7% for barbiturates (Holland et al., 1975).

Withdrawn: its addiction liability and severity of withdrawal symptoms are equal to those of the barbiturates and it is controlled under Schedule III of the 1971 Convention on Psychotropic Substances in UK. Withdrawn in Norway in 1980, Zimbabwe in 1984, Pakistan in 1988, USA and France in 1991. Changed to Schedule II in USA 1955.

Availability: not known

Lifespan: 29 years.

Delay in recognition: 3 years

Delay in regulatory action: 26 years

Time span of withdrawals: 11 years

Comment: wide variation in times to regulatory action probably reflects differing responses to drug dependence.

1955 Oxyphenisatin (Veripaque, Lavema, Noloc, Dialose, Protab)

Introduction first described in 1925. Dialose Plus consisted of: dioctyl sodium sulfosuccinate, carboxymethylcellulose sodium and oxyphenisatin acetate.

Use: a laxative

ADR: chronic active hepatitis and cytolytic hepatitis. Mentioned in Physicians' Desk Reference, 23rd edition 1969 as idiosyncratic jaundice. The first case with a positive rechallenge was in 1970 (McHardy & Balart, 1970; Reynolds et al., 1970). Adequate animal toxicity studies had not been done. *'The sudden recognition of an association between an obvious symptom–jaundice- and compounds such as …oxyphenisatin … which were said to have been widely available for many years, was puzzling. This suggested either a sudden increase in the usage of the drug and, therefore, in the incidence of the reaction leading to its recognition or alternatively, recent changes in formulation affecting toxicity.'* Investigations did not reveal any formulation factor (ADEC, 1972).
SED 1964, SED 1966, SED 1968: no mention.
SED 1984: despite the withdrawal of oxyphenisatin in many areas chronic active hepatitis's occurs from time to time as a result of its continued use.

Withdrawn: in Cuba in 1970; Australia and Japan in 1972; USA in 1973; Norway in 1974; Denmark in 1975; Germany and Italy in 1976; Austria in 1977; the UK and Canada in 1978; France in 1979, which was prompted by a French report of six cases of chronic hepatitis (Delchier et al., 1979); Kuwait in 1980; Belgium in 1981; Mauritius in 1982; Spain, Cyprus, Netherlands, New Zealand and Venezuela and world wide in 1985. Restricted to rectal use. HAI: banned in 20 countries.

Availability: Veripaque still used in Ireland and UK in an enema (BNF, 1999).

Lifespan: 15 years

Delay in recognition: 15 years

Delay in regulatory action: less than one year

Time span of withdrawals: 15 years

Comment: it is curious that that the first country to withdraw the drug was Cuba, which rarely leads the field in this area.

1956 October 1st Thalidomide (Contergan (WG), Distaval (UK), Kevadon (Canada), Softenon (Portugal) introduced (see 1956 AD)

First synthesized in 1954 by Chemie Gruenthal GmbH in West Germany.

Use: a 1956 leaflet said that that the indications were: irritability, weak concentration, stage fright, ejaculation praecox, menstrual tension, postmenopausal symptoms, fear of examination, functional disorders of the stomach and gall bladder, febrile infectious diseases, mild depression, anxiety, hyperthyroidism and tuberculosis (McCredie, 2008). A veritable universal panacea.

ADR: phocomyelia (First case December 25th 1956; Lenz's disclosure on November 18th 1961; McBride's BMJ Letter on December 16th 1961) and peripheral neuritis (First case October 3rd 1959; Florence letter on December 31st 1960; over 300 cases February 15th 1961). Other ADRs: neutropenia, pulmonary embolism, oedema, hypercalcaemia, confusion, nausea, Stevens-Johnson syndrome, toxic epidermal necrosis(TEN), constipation, dizziness, hangover, loss of memory, decrease in blood pressure, purpura and tremor.

Withdrawn: in Germany on November 28th 1961, Australia, Austria, Cyprus, Denmark, Finland, Guinea, Iraq, Jordan, Lebanon, Mozambique, Norway, Portugal, Saudi Arabia, Sudan, Switzerland, Syria, and the UK in 1961; Belgium, Brazil, Ireland, Canada (March), Italy (September), Argentina (March), Spain, Sweden (14th March), Taiwan and India in 1962, in Japan in 1963 (January). Not approved in France, Hungary, Yugoslavia, Venezuela and the USA. Relaunched for treatment of leprosy and multiple myeloma. Due to a delay in obtaining the information and taking effective measures in Japan, an order to stop its distribution and for total recall of the products was not issued until 1962, 9 months after the sale in West Germany had been stopped (Suzuki, 1980). Italy withdrew the drug ten months after it had been withdrawn in West Germany. HAI: banned in 5 countries and restricted in seven.

Availability: for specific indications only: erythema nodosum leprosum, aphthous stomatitis, Bechet's disease, lupus erythematosis, prurigo nodularis. Also used in, but nor so effectively: actinoprurigo, Langerhans cell histiocytosis, cutaneous sarcoidosis, erythema multiforme, graft vs host disease, Jessner's infiltrates, uremic pruritus. Possibly effective in Kaposi's sarcoma, lichen planus, melanoma and pyoderma gangrenosum.

Lifespan: 3 years for original indications.

Delay in recognition: one year

Delay in regulatory action: none

Time span of withdrawals: 2 years

Comment: during the three years after thalidomide was approved in West Germany on 1st October 1957 and before it was submitted to the FDA on 12th September 1960 the first case of polyneuritis was reported to the company on the 3rd October 1959 (Sjöström & Nilsson, 1972), but Dr Burley of the Distillers Company, says that the first possible case of peripheral neuritis was reported on 10th January 1960 and that 6th case on 9th August 1960 and further that the literature was modified to warn of the neuritis in September 1960 (Burley, 1988). One wonders whether this difference was due to the use of different terminology. Sjöström and Nilsson said that by the end of 1960 the company had received over 100 reports of cases of severe polyneuritis. The Florence letter of 31st December 1960 gave the FDA warning of what was to come. The drug had been by rejected by France and East Germany; the latter because of its neurotoxicity, lack of extensive animal tests and clinical investigations and inadequacy of the scientific results that were provided by the company (Shah, 2001). The earlier accounts reported 0.5% of the⁶ cases (Burley, 1988), but on reintroduction that increased to 25% (Knopp et al., 1983) and a further paper suggests 50% (Amelung & Püntmann, 1966). It is, in my opinion, likely that had the company declared all the cases of peripheral neuritis as and when they occurred the drug would have been taken off the market earlier (see 1961).

1956 Mercury Amide Hcl

'precipité blanc' [White precipitate] or Chloramidure de mercure (Crème des 3 fleurs d'orient or Any creme) [Cream from three oriental flowers]

Use: depigmentation of the skin

ADR: mercury poisoning in children, unborn and neonates. This particular drug was not mentioned in SED.

Withdrawn: in Japan in 1969; in France and Oman in 1986; and in Canada in 1997 ('Diana de Beauté' composed of ammoniated mercury, bismuth subnitrate and salicylic acid). It was reformulated with méquinol in France (Vidal, 2008). The AFSSAPS is unable to add any more information. Topical mercuric preparations banned in 8 countries and restricted in eight (HAI, 2008).

Availability: nil

Lifespan: 30 years

Delay in recognition: it had been known for more than a century that mercury was absorbed through the skin.

Delay in regulatory action: 30 years

Comment: it is difficult to know why it was allowed on the market when it was predictable. It is interesting to note that the Japanese despite their pale skins used the drug sufficiently for it to be a problem.

1957 Oxyphenbutazone (Oxazolidin, Tanderil)

Use: antirheumatic and analgesic. One of the active metabolites of phenylbutazone. A pyrazolone derivative.

ADR: aplastic anaemia and agranulocytosis (see phenylbutazone). The incidence of mortality was 3.8 per 100,000 (Inman, 1977). Inman gave the incidence rate as 1 per 45,000 new(assumed) prescriptions of phenylbutazone compared with 1 per 26,500 for oxyphenbutazone (Inman, 1977). The first case of thrombocytopenia was reported in 1961 (Armstrong and Scherbel, 1961). A fatal case of agranulocytosis, thrombocytopenia and hepatic necrosis was described in 1962 (Gaisford, 1962). The risk of developing aplastic anemia with oxyphenbutazone was 1: 124,000 or approximately four times the risk from chance (Wallerstein et al., 1969). SED 1964: granulocytopenia.

Withdrawn: restricted in Japan to acute exacerbations of rheumatoid arthritis and osteoarthritis in 1977; restricted in Austria, Ireland, Kuwait, Barbados, Spain and withdrawn in France, Cyprus, Finland, Tunisia, United Arab Emirates, Zimbabwe, Jordan and Bangladesh in 1984; licence revoked in the UK in 1984, restricted in Germany and the Netherlands and withdrawn in the USA, Canada, Ethiopia, Greece, Sweden, New Zealand and Chile in 1985; withdrawn in Ghana, Oman and Turkey in 1986; withdrawn in Malaysia and Hong Kong in 1987; restricted to prescription only in Belgium in 1988; and withdrawn in Sri Lanka in 1992. Also withdrawn in Bahrain, Congo and Israel and restricted in Italy, South Africa and Hungary. HAI: banned in 21 countries and restricted in eleven.

Availability: still available in Indonesia (Sponderil)

Lifespan: 20 years

Delay in recognition: 5 years

Delay in regulatory action: 15 years

Time span of restrictions: 15 years

Comment: as phenylbutazone and oxyphenbutazone are so similar there is only need for one of them.

1957 Ethchlorvynol (Placidyl, Serenesil, Arvynol)

Introduced in 1957.

Use: a non-barbiturate hypnotic.

ADR: pulmonary oedema, alveolar infiltrates, pleural effusions and dependence after intravenous self-injection (Glauser et al., 1976; Van Swearingen, 1976). Dependency first reported in 1959 (Cahn, 1959).

SED 1960 Ataxia, confusion, disorientation, visual and auditory hallucinations with convulsions on withdrawal.

Withdrawn: restricted in the USA (became a schedule IV drug) and Canada in 1978.

Availability: still killing patients in 1988 (Bailey & Shaw, 1990).

Lifespan: 21 years

Delay in recognition: 19 years

Delay in regulatory action: 2 years.

Comment: abuse had lessened by 1990 but still occurred (Bailey & Shaw, 1990).

1957 Sulfamethoxydiazine (Sulfameter, Durenate, Bayrema)

Use: a long acting sulphonamide antibacterial.

ADR: aplastic anaemia, agranulocytosis and thrombocytopenia (Schwank & Friedlanderova, 1977). Intrahepatic cholestasis (Horák et al., 1984). Stevens-Johnson syndrome (Staudt & Rudert, 1968).
SED 1980, SED 1984, SED 1988: no mention but no longer used in the USA.

Withdrawn: in Germany in 1988.

Availability: not known

Lifespan: 31 years

Delay in recognition: 9 years

Delay in regulatory action: 20 years

Comment: aplastic anaemia, agranulocytosis and thromboctopenias are sulphonamide class effects (Albahary, 1953).

1957 Sulfamethoxypyridazine (Lederkyn, Kynex, Midicel)

Use: long acting sulphonamide and antibacterial agent.

ADR: aplastic anaemia, agranulocytosis and aplastic anaemia (Johnson and Korst, 1961), haemolytic anaemia (Janovsky, 1960) nephrotoxicity, fixed eruption, urticaria, and erythema multiforme (SJS)[176]. Skin reactions had occurred in 11.8% of patients (Lindsay et al., 1958). Of

---

[176] SJS = Stevens-Johnson syndrome.

all the long-acting sulphonamides it is the most likely to cause Stevens-Johnson syndrome and caused at least eight deaths (Leader BMJ, 1964). Also reported thrombocytopenia, interstitial myocarditis and hepatitis (Melvin & Howie, 1961).

SED 1960: of 672 patients 2.2% had rashes. There were two cases of thrombocytopenia. Fatal myocarditis and toxic psychosis.

SED 1963: agranulocytopenia, thromboctopenias and pancytopenia. It is not proven that it is more toxic than the others.

Withdrawn: an FDA warning that it could cause Stevens-Johnson syndrome was given in 1968 after a report of a large number of cases (Carroll et al., 1966). It was withdrawn in Canada in 1978, UK and Sweden in 1984; France, UK and United Arab Emirates in 1986, Pakistan in 1988, also Argentina. Commercial manufacture of the drug has been discontinued by at least one major manufacturer but supplies can still be obtained on special request, particularly for patients with dermatitis herpetiformis in which condition it has been claimed to be beneficial (WHO, 2003).

Availability: not known

Lifespan: 21 years

Delay in recognition: 4 years

Delay in regulatory action: 17 years.

Time span of withdrawals: 10 years

Comment: aplastic anaemia, agranulocytosis and thrombocytopenia are sulphonamide class effects (Albahary, 1953).

1957 Phenformin, Phenylethylbiguanide (Dibotin, Diphod)

Marketed in the UK in 1969.

Use: an antidiabetic drug (a biguanide).

ADR: lactic acidosis.A study in 1959 showed that an early diguanide (phenethyldiguanide) caused lactic acidosis in 10% of patients and that it could be fatal (Walker and Linton, 1959). The first paper was 'phenformin acidosis' published in 1962 (Gottlieb, 1962). Several papers were published in 1963, one a report from a conference saying that '*It is possible that Phenformin may add to the excess lactic acid*'. (Danowski et al., 1963)*; 'another reported the death of two patients.'* (Bernier et al., 1963). A study of 330 cases of lactic acidosis showed that 86% had had phenformin, 9% buformin and 5% metformin (Ching et al., 2008; Luft, 1978). FDA office estimated that 4 in 1000 users died from lactic acidosis (The Poh, 1985).

The frequency of lactic acidosis was estimated as 1 per 1110 patient-years (Stang, 1998). In 1960 it was found that the blood lactate and plasma hydrazine levels were raised at rest and this was exaggerated on exercise (BMJ, 1960).

SED 1963: blood lactic acid raised.

A paper published in 1978 (Bergmanet al., 1978) showed more cases of lactic acidosis with phenformin than with metformin. This paper led to the withdrawal in Sweden. The sale of Phenformin in the United States went up after there was a threat that the drug would be withdrawn from the market (Lunde, 1980). Official warnings were sent out in the UK (1976), Ireland (1977), USA (1977), Germany (1977), Sweden (1970) Netherlands (1975)(Griffin & D'Arcy, 1981). The relative risk calculated from the French data (1968-1977) was 0.016 for metformin and 0.23 for phenformin (SED, 1980). There were 47 fatal reports in the UK between 1964 and 1980 and the rate per million general-practitioner prescriptions 1975–9 was 2.2 (Venning I, 1983).

Withdrawn: from Turkey in 1970, USA, Canada, Switzerland, Norway, New Zealand, Singapore and Brazil in 1977, Denmark, Finland, Italy, but still reported as widely used in 1979, Germany, Sweden and Thailand in 1978, Cyprus, Ethiopia, Ireland, and Yemen in 1979, Kuwait in 1980, France and UK in 1982, Hongkong in 1985, India in 2003, also in Mauritius, Israel, Netherlands, Saudi Arabia, Austria, Cyprus, Yemen and Venezuela. The withdrawal in the USA had been prompted by a petition from The Health Research Group and it is the only drug that the FDA has ever declared to be an 'imminent hazard' (Wysowski & Swartz, 2005). HAI: banned in 24 countries and restricted in four.

Availability: in China, Brazil, Italy (1997) and Spain.

Lifespan: 13 years

Delay in recognition: 2 years

Delay in regulatory action: varied between 11 years in Turkey and in India 46 years.

Time span of withdrawals: 33 years

Comment: a class ADR, which could have been foreseen. Griffin and D'Arcy quoted Phenformin, in an article on 'information lag', saying it was one of the worst examples. The 'information lag' was defined as the time between the first substantial mention of a given ADR in the literature and the time the warning was issued. The first mention being 1968, well established by 1973 and the first warning given in August

1976 in the Current Problems Series, which would give the lag to be 8 years. If we take the Gottlieb paper to be the first then the lag is 14 years. Griffin and D'Arcy do not put forward any reasons why there was so large a delay. This was a Pharmacovigilance failure.

1957 Carisoprodol (Soma, Sanoma, Somadril, Carisoma) N-isopropylmeprobamate

Use: muscle pain, lower back pain, rheumatoid arthritis, arthritis deformans, spondylosis, myositis and tension headache.

ADR: psychomotor dependence was reported in 1969 (Raffel et al., 1969). Dependence and abuse. The first report of intoxication was in 1969 (Goldberg, 1969). First case of dependence on Carisoprodol (Morse & Chua, 1978). Found to cause 'heavy psychomotor impairment' which manifested as a traffic problem. Patients who filled a prescription for carisoprodol had almost four times higher risk of being involved in a traffic accident (Bramness et al., 2007). Carisoprodol was recognised as drug of abuse in 2002 (Bailey & Briggs, 2002). It is metabolised to meprobamate, which is also addictive. It causes a withdrawal syndrome (Reeves & Parker, 2003). It could also cause: extreme weakness, transient quadriplegia, dizziness, ataxia, temporary loss of vision, diplopia, mydriasis, dysarthria, agitation, euphoria, confusion and disorientation (www.fda.gov/medwatch/safety/2006/jun06.htm).
SED 1972, SED 1976, SED 1984, SED 1988, SED 1992 and SED 1996: no mention.
SED 1988 its toxicity is low.

Withdrawn: the FDA made it a Schedule IV drug in July 2002 and warned of idiosyncratic and allergic reactions on 6th June 2006. Norway withdrew the combination product containing paracetamol, caffeine in 1996 and the company withdrew the monotherapy in May 2007. Sweden withdrew carisoprodol in June 2008. Withdrawn by the European Union in November 2007 (Bramness et al., 2008).

Availability: prior to EU edict–Spain, Sweden, Denmark, Norway, Finland, Czech Republic, Greece, Hungary, Iceland, Italy, Slovak Republic, and UK.

Lifespan: 50 years

Delay in recognition: 12 years

Delay in regulatory action: 5 years

Time span of withdrawals: < one year

Comment: there seems to be a reluctance to withdraw drugs of abuse until they become a social problem.

1958 Bunamiodyl (Orabilex, Boniodyl)

Introduced in Holland.

 Use: cholecystographic contrast medium

 ADR: two cases of renal failure (Rene & Mellenkoff, 1959). March 1961 six cases developed renal dysfunction out of 593 patients (Blythe & Woods, 1961). Renal tubular necrosis (Malt et al., 1963) One hundred died of renal failure in the USA (Schreiner, 1966).

 SED 1966: number of cases of acute renal failure.

 Withdrawn: in January 1964 it became a schedule IV drug in many US states. Withdrawn in Canada 1963 and not approved in Sweden in 1964. Withdrawn worldwide by manufacturer in 1984. ' *Despite the occurrence or 28 cases of renal damage following Bunamiodyl and the withdrawal of the drug by the FDA the evidence is not conclusive that the agent is more toxic than those previously used.'* (Harrow & Sloane, 1965). Buniamiodyl was withdrawn worldwide by the manufacturer in 1984.

 Availability: Belgium, Netherlands, UK, Germany and Switzerland.

 Lifespan: 5 years

 Delay in recognition: ≤ one year

 Delay in regulatory action: 4 years

 Time span of withdrawals: 21 years

 Comment: congressional hearings conducted as early as 1964 exposed FDA's lack of knowledge of important information linking the use of Orabilex (bunamiodyl sodium), (www.thefreelibrary.com/Turning+the+tables+on+drug+companies%3B+exposing+deficiencies+in+FDA...-a014940642).

1958 Buformin (Silubin, Sindiatil)

 Use: an anti-diabetic drug (a biguanide).

 ADR: lactic acidosis. First mention of lactic acidosis was in 1978 (Depperman et al., 1978).

 Withdrawn: in 1978 in Germany, Austria and Italy (restricted dosage), and in Belgium and Ireland in 1979, because of lactic acidosis.

 SED 1980: the relative risk calculated from the Swiss data (1972–1977) was 0.07 for metformin, 0.31 for buformin and 0.40 for phenformin. Phenformin and Buformin are more lipophilic that metformin.

 Availability: still available in some countries–Czechoslovakia, Hungary, Spain and Japan.

Lifespan: 20 years

Delay in recognition: less than one year.

Delay in regulatory action: none

Time span of withdrawals: one year

Comment: an example of a class ADR with differing incidences of the ADR in one class member.

1958 Cupric bis-quinolone sulfate/triethylamine (Cuproxane)

Use: Vidal 1964 – anti-inflammatory, analgesic and anti-infective used for rheumatism and furunculosis resistant to antibiotics contained copper 9% and triméthylamine 18%.

ADR: neuromuscular problems, metallic taste, sore throat, dysphagia, epigastric pain, vomiting, diarrhoea, limb, chest and abdominal cramps and circulatory collapse. No mention in SED.

Withdrawn: in France in 1978

Availability: none

Lifespan: 20 years

Delay in recognition: unable to find any relevant papers. The AFSSAPS is unable to add any more information.

Delay in regulatory action: ?

Comment: probably only licensed in France.

1959 Danthron (Chrysazin , Dantron, Fructimer, Dorbanex, Codalax)

Use: an anthraquinolone laxative (a bacterial mutagen).

ADR: the results of two chronic toxicity studies in rats, (Four out of 12 developed adenocarcinoma of the large bowel) (Mori et al., 1985) and mice (four out of 17 developed hepatocellular carcinomas) (Mori et al., 1986), have shown that administration of high doses is associated with the development of intestinal and liver tumours (Patel et al., 1989; WHO, 2003). Animal intestinal carcinogenicity (Anonymous, 1990). There is sufficient evidence for the carcinogenicity of dantron in experimental animals (IARC vol 50, 1990).

SED 1984: no mention

SED 1992: bacterial mutagens seem capable of inducing intestinal tumour in animals.

Withdrawn: in the USA, Norway, Denmark, Japan, and France in 1987; in Spain in 1988, but reintroduced with restricted indications in 1989 in Canada and Germany (1986) and then withdrawn in 1998. Norway in 1997, In the UK its use was restricted to geriatric medicine and analgesic-induced constipation in the terminally ill in 1987 and then restricted just to the terminally ill in 2000 (BNF, 1999), but mentioned as available on the NHS without any caveats in 1992. HAI: banned in 6 countries and restricted in one.

Availability: in Ireland, UK, New Zealand, Canada, Brazil, France, Chile, Mexico and South Africa (Martindale). In the UK it is restricted to geriatrics, terminally ill patients and patients with heart failure or coronary thrombosis (BNF, 1999).

Lifespan: 28 years

Delay in recognition: 26 years

Delay in regulatory action: 2 years

Time span of withdrawals: 11 years

Comment: reasonably anticipated to be a human carcinogen. A class effect.

1959 Triparanol (MER-29)

'The approval letter to Merrell stated that no review of the drug's efficacy had been undertaken'...'Associate Commissioner John Harvey would conclude that his agency's conditional approval of MER/29 in April 1960 was mistaken.'(Waxman, 2003). Prior to approval it had been said that before we release this drug for general distribution... the company should submit results of well controlled extensive clinical studies in which the individuals have received the drug for periods of years.

Use: cholesterol lowering drug blocked the last step in cholesterol biosynthesis in animals and man (Steinberg et al., 1961).

ADR: cataracts, impotency and baldness.

SED 1960: no mention

SED 1963: withdrawn – hair loss, abnormal liver function tests, exfoliative dermatitis and leucopenia.

Withdrawn: USA 1962

Availability: nil

Lifespan: three years

Delay in recognition: despite the fact that both subacute and chronic toxicity studies in animals (rats and dogs) showed clear evidence of toxicity in doses dangerously close to those proposed for use in humans (approximately 4 mgm/kg/day) the application was approved in April 1960. Subsequently 40 mgm/kg/day in rats produced cataracts within 3 months and 20–40 mgm/kg/day caused cataracts in dogs in 3-4 months (Nestor, 1975). Cataracts were first reported in patients in

April 1962 (Kirby, 1962). The FDA had been tipped off to investigate the manufacturer's records. The manufacturers, William S Merrill, had failed to reveal the fact that they had found that it had produced cataracts in both rats and dogs (JAMA July 1962). Damages were paid to the injured patients and the company paid the maximum fine.

Delay in regulatory action: the drug should not have been approved for human use.

Comment: the evidence was ignored by the company. MER/29 had some similarities with Coralgil.

Nialamide (Niamid)

Use: a monoamine oxidase inhibitor. Antidepressant.

ADR: cytolytic hepatitis (Hammer et al., 1969) and drug interaction with food (tyramine) causing hypertensive crises was recognised in 1959 (Davies, 1959).

SED 1960 and SED 1963: no mention

SED 1966: hypertensive crises have been reported.

Withdrawn: in Canada in 1963, the USA and Japan in 1974, UK in 1978, India in 1983, in France in 1987, and Norway in 1995, also in Cuba, Denmark, Saudi Arabia, Thailand and Venezuela. HAI: banned in 7 countries.

Availability: in Belgium (Martindale)

Lifespan: 4 years

Delay in recognition: 10 years for hepatitis

Delay in regulatory action: 4 years

Time span of withdrawals: 32 years

Comment: a class ADR + a specific ADR. All MAOIs interact with tyramine.

Analysis

Delay in recognition (Time to first case)

There were several factors that hindered the early recognition of new ADRs.

1. The diagnostic techniques had not been developed:
    a) Abuse liability testing in animals: chloral hydrate, phenobarbitone, datura, sodium arsenate and glutethimide.
    b) Carcinogenicity testing in animals: chloroform, piperazine, phenolpthalein, thorium dioxide, methapyrilene, diethylstilboestrol and dantron.
    c) Laboratory testing had not been developed: phenacetin, amidopyrine, dipyrone, pyrithyldione, chloramphenicol, phenylbutazone, oxyphenbutazone, thenalidine, sulfamethoxydiazine and sulfamethoxypyrazine.
    d) The disease entity had not been discovered: SMON, Reye's syndrome, SIDS and tetracycline tooth problem.
2. Failure to carry out known precautionary studies: dinitrophenol, diiododiethyltin, phenformin and buformin.
3. A clear symptom complex was known but the association with the drug was not recognised: bismuth insoluble salts, mercury amide Hcl and thalidomide.
4. Prior to 1960 there were no spontaneous reporting systems, other than the American Medical Association's registry for cases of drug-induced blood dyscrasias instigated in 1952.

There was frequently more than one factor that was responsible for the ADR with some of these drugs. These are dealt with in detail below....

Delay in regulatory[177] action (Time from first case to first regulatory action)

After the first case had produced a hypothesis one would expect, these days, that further investigation would take place. This might be a prospective epidemiological investigation (clinical trial, cohort study) or a retrospective investigation (inspection of spontaneous reports, case control studies, cohort studies). Pharmaceutical companies have often undertaken their own cohort study, but without a control group and these have not resulted in published accounts of the ADRs found. In the USA the FDA, when it has decided that a change in product information is required, will request the action from the manufacturer. In most situations, drugs are voluntarily withdrawn by the market authorization holder (Wysowski et al., 2005).

---

[177] Regulatory = An official body, not an individual, which had the power to take some action.

Prior to 1960, other than the AMA registry, the only other body that took action was the BMA in 1877 when it set up the committee for the investigation of the chloroform deaths. The only other source of new ADR data was the publication in books and journals of interesting cases, but the journals have always been more reluctant to publish reports of ADRs that have already appeared in print rather than new original reports.

Table 12. Number of drugs withdrawn by country

[major pharmaceutical research countries in italics (Ballance et al., 1992)]

Number of withdrawals	Countries
34	*USA*
31	*France*
22	*Italy*
21	*Germany*
20	*UK*
19	Canada
19	*Japan*
18	Sweden
15	Denmark, Spain
14	Norway
13	Australia, *Belgium*
12	Oman,
11	Austria, Ireland, *Netherlands*, Saudi Arabia, Philippines, Greece
10	Brazil, Argentina, Bangladesh, New Zealand
9	Kuwait, India, Thailand, *Switzerland*, Venezuela, Malaysia
8	Turkey, Cyprus, Israel, Kuwait, Hongkong
7	Bahrain, Egypt, Ethiopia, Finland, Mauritius, Yemen, Zimbabwe
6	Singapore, Chile, Cuba, Domenica, United Arab Emirates
5	Ghana, Sri Lanka, Pakistan, Panama, Nepal, South Africa
4	Jordan, Nigeria, Sudan, EU,
3	Hungary, Tunisia, Congo, Iraq, Armenia, Syria, Worldwide
2	Romania, Rwanda, Peru, Morocco, Barbados, Columbia, Taiwan, Korea,
1	Zambia, Libya, Mexico, Lebanon, Surinam, Lithuania, Poland, Paraguay, Guinea, Portugal, Honduras, Korea, Mozambique, Viet Nam
nil	Bulgaria, Belize, Jamaica, Indonesia, Iran, Iceland, Chad, Brunei, Tanzania, USSR, Costa Rica

One mustn't jump to too many conclusions from such fragile data since a country, which approved a toxic drug and then withdrew it counts higher then one that refused to approve it because of its lack of safety. Again we do not know how many of the 50 drugs were approved in each country, e.g. if Chad did not approve of any of the drugs then it should be no surprise that they did not ban any of them. It is surprising to find Canada so high on the list and Belgium, the Netherlands and Switzerland so low. First country to withdraw: *France* and **USA** 10, Japan 8, **Canada** 7, **Germany** 6, **UK, Norway** and *Italy* 3, **Denmark** and Turkey 2 , **Australia**, *Austria*, *Brazil*, Cuba, *Domenica*, Egypt, *Spain,* **Finland,** Hongkong, Malaysia, *Panama*, Singapore, **Sweden** and Yemen 1. Those in italics have more than 50% Roman Catholics. Those in bold have less than 50% Roman Catholics. Griffin and Weber suggested that there was inverse relationship between the percentage of Catholics in a country and the rate of spontaneous adverse reaction reporting (Griffin & Weber, 1986), based on the hypothesis that Catholics tend to accept 'authority' more easily and that Catholic members of the medical profession are more paternalistic. In this survey there seems not to be a religious bias as far as withdrawing drugs is concerned.

Curiosities

Bismuth: Egypt and Japan were the first to withdraw it, but the problem first struck Australia and France.

Phenacetin: First noted in watchmakers in Switzerland, but withdrawn first in Finland because of neuropathy.

Phenolpthalein: Norway and Yemen, but carcinogenicity found in the USA.

Thiomersal: First withdrawn in Malaysia in 1995, but it became controversial in the mid 1990s when it was suggested that it caused autism and the USA undertook extensive research and although the findings were negative advocated stopping its use in vaccines.

Phenylbutazone: First withdrawn in Jordan and Bangladesh, but first reports in UK.

Tetracycline Paediatric: First withdrawn in Jordan and Peru.

Oxyphenisatin: First withdrawn in Cuba at the time of the first confirmed report.

Phenformin: First withdrawn in Turkey, but problem known for eleven years.

Withdrawal times (lifespan) from first approval to withdrawal or restriction

Figure 9. Withdrawal times (lifespan) from first approval/mention to withdrawal or restriction

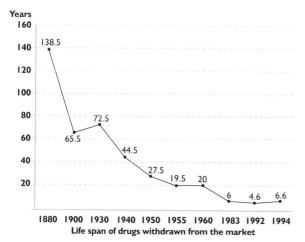

0–1880 median = 138.5 years (4 drugs) range 100–458 years

1880–1900 median = 65.5 years (6 Drugs) range 36–100 years

1900–1930 median = 72.5 years (6 drugs) range 27–83 years

1930–1940 median = 44.5 years (4 drugs) range 5–65 years

1940–1950 median = 27.5 years (6 drugs) range 22–57 years

1950–1955 median = 19.5 years (8 drugs) range 3–37 years

1955–1960 median = 20 years (15 drugs) range 3–50 years

A study of withdrawals in the UK and the US, between 1964 and 1983, had a median time of 6 years (24 drugs) range 1–80 years (Bakke et al., 1984).

A survey of withdrawals in the UK and the US, between 1971 and 1992, had a median time of 4.6 years (23 drugs) range 4 months–13 years (Abraham & Davis, 2005).

In the 1970s the average drug lifespan was 12.3 years, which dropped to 6.6 years in the 1980s and dropped further in the 1990s to 2.6 years (Armer & Morris, 2004).

A study of withdrawals in the UK, US and Spain, between 1974 and 1993, had a median time of 5 years (29 drugs) range 0–17 years (Bakke et al., 1995).

There is a steady decline in withdrawal times until 1960/1964 when there is a sudden plateauing at 5 /6 years, presumably as a result of the response to the Thalidomide disaster. One of the factors may have been that as the number of drugs increased the number of alternatives increased allowing the more easy banning of a doubtful drug.

Reasons for differing dates for drug withdrawals in different countries

1. Marketing. Pharmaceutical companies rarely market a drug simultaneously throughout the world, but choose to start either in their own country or in the most profitable market. Another factor may be the different approaches of the main licensing authorities. The differences between the US and UK regulatory authorities in the development of their drug regulations is explored in 'Science, Politics and the Pharmaceutical Industry' by John Abraham, UCL Press and between the US and Germany in 'Regulation of the Pharmaceutical Industry' by John Abraham and Helen Lawton Smith, Palgrave Macmillan.

2. Countries needs and capabilities. Inevitably new drugs are more expensive than the alternatives, the knowledge of the safety of a drug

improves, usually, with the passage of time, the medical problems vary from country to country, the experience and expertise of the regulatory authorities varies greatly between countries, the degree of corruption also varies between countries.

3. Country idiosyncrasies. It is not known why Japan was specifically hit by SMON. The annual rate/per million/years for agranulocytosis 2.9 in Ulm Germany; 1.6 in Israel and 0.6 in Budapest Hungary (IAAAS, 1986) and the reason for this difference is not known.

Countries that were the first to take regulatory action

France and the USA were the first on 10 occasions, Japan on 8 occasions, Canada on 7 occasions, Germany on 6 occasions, the UK, Norway and Italy on 3 occasions and Denmark and Turkey on 2 occasions. Those which were only first on one occasion were: Australia, Austria, Brazil, Cuba, Domenica, Egypt, Finland, Hongkong, Malaysia, Panama, Singapore, Spain, Sweden and Yemen. Possibly those that were the first on only one occasion were those authorities that had a single enthusiastic expert.

Availability in some countries after withdrawal in others.

There are several reasons why a drug might remain in some countries despite withdrawal in other countries:

1. The ADR frequency may be different, e.g. SMON in Japan.
2. A poor country may allow a cheap, but toxic drug, to remain if the alternatives are too expensive for the bulk of the population, i.e. different countries will have different 'toxic thresholds'.
3. Pharmaceutical company pressure.
4. Patients may be unaware of the adverse effect of drugs because of differences in labelling.
5. *'Analysis of the pharmaceutical section indicates that a country's capacity to restrict dangerous drugs depends heavily on its wealth, as illustrated by the strong correlation of restrictions with per capita gross national product (r = 0.65, n = 162, P < 0.001).'* (Menkes, 1997).
6. *'Poor countries with notable restrictions (including Bangladesh and Ethiopia) lack administrative machinery to police them.'* (Menkes, 1997).

Delay

The time between the first report of an ADR and the drug's removal from the market varies with the type of ADR. Type 'A' ADRs tend to be common and dose-related and therefore likely to be discovered during clinical trials or shortly after marketing. On the other hand type 'B' ADRs are rare and, therefore, unlikely to be discovered during clinical trials. There are numerous factors, which influence the time to withdrawal:

1. Incidence rate: type 'A' reactions discovered early; type 'B' discovered late.
2. Strength of evidence: the strongest evidence is from clinical trials, then cohort studies, case-control studies, case series and finally case reports. The main source of information for the restriction/withdrawal of drugs are case reports (Venning III, 1983; Arnaiz, 2001; Clarke, 2006).
3. Failure to follow-up initial signals (Loke et al., 2006).
4. Causality: if we wait for certainty too many people die, if we act on probability some people will be deprived of help.
5. Alternative treatments: e.g. streptomycin was less ototoxic than di-hydro-streptomycin. The marketing of a new and safer drug for the same indication may alter the balance of benefit/risk.
6. Efficacy: drugs can be marketed if they are more active than placebo, even if they are inferior to those already on the market. The inefficacy of old treatments meant many suffered ADRs unnecessarily, e.g. bleeding.
7. Number of persons who take the drug: this combined with the incidence gives an approximate proportion of patients who suffered the ADR. Aggressive marketing of a new drug allows a large number of patients to be treated within the first few years of marketing and therefore there will be an increased likelihood that any type 'B' ADRs will be discovered early.
8. Availability of databases: none available prior to 1960?
9. Establishment of a clinical entity: erythema multiforme 1866, Stevens-Johnson syndrome 1922, aplastic anaemia 1888, arterial hypertension 1893, agranulocytosis 1922, acrodynia 1830, and Reye's syndrome 1962.
10. Countries in which it is marketed: The more developed countries in which the drug is marketed the more likely the ADR will be discovered early. If only marketed in a single country discovery is likely to be delayed. Different countries are likely to have different 'toxic thresholds' (Bakke et al., 1984).
11. Reaction of manufacturer: if a company initiates a prospective safety study, it will be difficult for a regulatory authority to take decisive action before the study has reached a conclusion, e.g. amidopyrine and Hoechst in 1980.
12. Cost of treatment: cheap toxic drugs have remained on the market despite the availability of safer more expensive drugs.

13. Extrapolation from animals to humans:
    a. carcinogenicity, e.g. chloral hydrate, phenolphthalein, methapyrilene, dantron and chloroform
    b. other, e.g. chloroform fatalities.
14. Class effects allowing potential predictability: pyrazolones/pyrazolidines, e.g. amidopyrine, dipyrone, butazolidines; MAO inhibitors, e.g. iproniazid and nialamide; biguanides, e.g. buformin and phenformin.
15. Chronicity of ADR: e.g. phenacetin where the study started in 1968 and the result published in 1991 (Dubach et al., 1991); 38 years after the hypothesis was first mooted.
16. Under reporting of ADRs: Prior to 1960 there were no centres for the reception of suspected ADRs?
17. Even the most advanced countries, from the regulatory point of view, were hampered by insufficient regulations, inadequate science, absence of databases and few experts. *'Before 1938 it would be difficult to say that drug development had any plan or requirements at all, although certainly some effective agents emerged and some facts about them were discovered. But there were few of the drugs we now consider effective and there were real disasters.'* (Temple, 1996).
18. Variation in the incidence of the ADR due to poorly known factors, e.g. analgesic nephropathy was greater in Glasgow perhaps because most of the factories making phenacetin were sited there. Similarly in Belgium, most cases were found in the county of Antwerp where the factories were sited. The incidence varied considerably from country to country: Australia 20%, Belgium 18.4%, Switzerland 17.5%, USA 7-10%, Germany 5%, Scandinavia 3.4%, Canada 2.5% France 1.6%, UK 1.2% Italy 1.0% (Vanherweghem & Even–Adin, 1982).
19. Although only one ADR might be named as the reason for withdrawal of a drug from the market the regulatory authorities would also have been influenced by the other ADRs attributed to the drug.
20. Date when the drug was introduced. Over the time span of this book there have been many changes in the attitude of patients and regulators towards the adverse effects of drugs. It is only post 1960 that research into why drugs are withdrawn from the market has been undertaken. Information concerning the reasons(s) why a drug has been removed from a specific market are difficult to obtain, e.g. Health Canada did not maintain a comprehensive list of drugs that had been removed from Canada because of safety concerns, nor did it have a database that would allow the construction of such a list. For sixteen out of the 41

products removed from the Canadian market between 1963 and 2004 there was no definite information about why they were removed from the Canadian market, although they were withdrawn in either the UK or the US (or both) because of safety concerns (Lexchin, 2005).

Grouping of drugs withdrawn

Metals: antimony, mercury (+ Mercurothiolate), bismuth, arsenic, tin and copper.

Addictive drugs: chloral, phenobarbitone, glutethimide, ethchlorvynol, datura and sodium arsenate.

Analgesics/anti-inflammatory drugs: Aspirin, amidopyrine, Phenacetin, metamizole, phenylbutazone and cincophen.

Laxatives: phenolphthalein, oxyphenisatin and dantron.

Hypnotics: pyrithyldione, thalidomide and chloral hydrate

Antihistamines: methapyrilene, oxomemazine and thenalidine.

Anti–diabetic drugs: Phenformin and Buformin.

Monoamine oxidases: iproniazid and nialamide.

Antibiotics/antibacterials: chloramphenicol, tetracycline, clioquinol, sulfathiazole, sulfamethoxydiazine, sulfamethoxypyridazine and di-hydro-streptomycin.

Others: thorium, diethylstilboestrol, piperazine, diamthazole,c chloroform, triparanol and urethane.

Chemical classification

Inorganic drugs: mercury, antimony, bismuth and arsenate sodium. These were first used between 3000 BC (arsenic)and 1753 AD (bismuth). The use of metals ran parallel to the use of herbs and was boosted by Paracelsus.

Aliphatic organic drugs: urethane, chloroform, chloral hydrate, carisoprodol, urethane, Stalinon, pyrithyldione, buformin and ethchlorvynol. There is a strange anomaly in that ether was first mentioned in 1275 and again in 1546 when it was made by equal parts of thrice rectified spirit of wine (ethanol) and oil of vitriol (sulphuric acid) in contact for two months and then it was distilled. How was it that there was a gap of over 500 years before the next synthesis was made? These drugs are organic drugs lacking a benzene ring and the first (urea) was synthesised in 1923. Chloral hydrate was synthesized in1832.

Aromatic organic drugs: Phenacetin, piperazine, amidopyrine, clioquinol, Aspirin, phenobarbitone, dipyrone, dinitrophenol, promethazine, diethylstilboestrol, sulfathiazole, sulphamethoxypyridazine, dihydrostreptomycin, chloramphenicol, phenylbutazone, tetracycline paediatric, iproniazid, thenalidine, glutethimide, oxyphenbutazone, cincophen, phenolphthalein, oxyphenisatin, thenalidine, triparanol, methapyrilene, danthron, thiomersal, bunamiodyl, cupric bis-quinolone sulphate, diamthazole and phenformin. These drugs all contain a benzene ring. Benzene was first isolated in 1836.

Grouping by type of ADR

Agranulocytosis/Aplastic anaemia: amidopyrine, dipyrone, cincophen,pyrithyldione, sulfathiazole, chloramphenicol, phenylbutazone, thenalidine, sulfamethoxydiazine, sulfamethoxypyridazine and urethane. For further references, see Hart PW in 'Blood dyscrasias due to drugs and other agents.' Girdwood RH, 1973. The term 'agranulocytosis was proposed by Schultz in 1922 and has been defined as a neutrophil count of less than 0.2 x 109/1. *'It appears unlikely that agranulocytosis occurred in any considerable numbers before the year 1922, for, if it had, expert clinicians of the preceding period would certainly have described it* '(Kracke & Parker, 1935). Aplastic anaemia was first described by Paul Ehrlich in 1888. It is defined as peripheral pancytopenia occurring in the presence of a hypoplastic bone marrow with replacement of normal haemopoiesis by fat cells. Haematological ADRs account for 10% of worldwide withdrawals (Smith, 2006).

Carcinogenicity (Drug introduced–found to be carcinogenic): thorium (1928–1933), diethylstilboestrol (1938–1938), urethane (1894–1943), Phenacetin (1902 - 1974), chloroform (1831–1976), methapyrilene (1947–1980), danthron (1959–1985), chloral hydrate (1869–1986) and phenolphthalein (1902–1997).

Carcinogenicity testing in animals started about 1918 when Yamagiva and Ichikawa applied coal tar experimentally to rabbits' ears and produced skin carcinomas (Yamagiva & Ichikawa, 1918). In the 1920s it was proposed that cancer might be the result of a somatic mutation and from this the study of classical carcinogens through in vitro and in vivo approaches showed that they yielded mutants in certain organisms. In 1961 at the National Cancer Institute, the Bioassay Program started to test chemicals for carcinogenicity. These bioassays lasted for 24 months in rats and approximately 20 months in mice, the results of which were published over the next 10 years (Weisburger, 1999). Some drugs bind covalently with DNA resulting in mutagenicity and Dr Ames developed a short–term mutagenicity test using *Salmonella typhimurium* in 1970. In Japan over 700 chemicals were tested for mutagenicity and there was a good correlation between mutagenicity and carcinogenicity, e.g. among 167 kinds of compounds with mutagenic activity 146 (87%) were carcinogens. Phenacetin was shown to be mutagenic in 1974 and carcinogenic in 1978 illustrating the longer time needed to show carcinogenicity (Kawachi, 1980). As evidence that already in the 1930's experimental evidence of carcinogenicity obtained in long-term animal tests was held as predictive of a similar effects in humans (Tomatis, 2006). '*Most of the early withdrawals, i.e., before 1970, were related to reports of side-effects in patients. Since 1970, however, a number of drugs have been discontinued in light of benign or malignant tumours that appear after chronic exposure in animals. After 1980 all drug discontinuations have been in association with data from clinical use.*' (Bakke et al., 1984). The National Cancer Institute's Bioassay program in 1961 either did not test or tested but not found a problem with: phenacetin, chloroform, methapyrilene, danthron, chloral hydrate and phenolpthalein. The knowledge that diethylstilboestrol was carcinogenic did not stop its development.

The IARC has placed drugs into four groups:

Group 1   Carcinogenic to humans, e.g. arsenic, thorium and diethylstilboestrol.

Group 2. a) Probable carcinogenic to humans, e.g. chloramphenicol, urethane and phenacetin.

b) Possible carcinogenic to humans, e.g. antimony trioxide, chloroform, dantron, phenobarbital and phenolphthalein.

Group 3. Unclassifiable, e.g. antimony trisulphide, chloral hydrate, mercury and its inorganic compounds, oxyphenbutazone and phenylbutazone.

Group 4. Probably not carcinogenic to humans. None.

Carcinogenicity accounts for 6% of worldwide withdrawals (Smith & O'Donnell, 2006).

There were 165 chemicals 'known not to be teratogenic in man', but only 28% were negative in all species tested and 41% were positive in more than one animal species (Lasagna, 1990).

Dependence (habituation, abuse, addiction):opium, morphine, henbane, phenobarbitone, glutethimide, chloroform, chloral hydrate, datura stramonium, arsenate sodium and ethchlorvynol.

These terms have come into use over the last 50 years and may be used differently. The word 'habituation' was used by Lewin in the context *'even in chloral drinkers' causes no habituation to the effects of the drug'*. 'Addiction', a term used by Lewin in 1881, implies physiologic and somatic withdrawal symptoms whilst in habituation the withdrawal symptoms are psychological (Cohen, 1960). In 1957, while not explicitly saying that 'drug abuse' was synonymous with 'addiction', the committee first attempted to clarify existing definitions of addiction and habituation as had been in common parlance since at least 1931: Drug addiction is a state of periodic or chronic intoxication produced by the repeated consumption of a drug (natural or synthetic). Its characteristics include: (i) an overpowering desire or need (compulsion) to continue taking the drug and to obtain it by any means; (ii) a tendency to increase the dose; (iii) a psychic (psychological) and generally a physical dependence on the effects of the drug; and (iv) detrimental effects. Drug habituation (habit) is a condition resulting from the repeated consumption of a drug. Its characteristics include (i) a desire (but not a compulsion) to continue taking the drug for the sense of improved well-being which it engenders; (ii) little or no tendency to increase the dose; (iii) some degree of psychic dependence on the effect of the drug, but absence of physical dependence and hence of an abstinence syndrome [withdrawal], and (iv) detrimental effects, if any, primarily on the individual. In 1964, a new WHO committee found these definitions to be inadequate, and suggested using the blanket term 'drug dependence': on the individual and on society. (en.wikipedia.org/wiki/Drug_addiction). Accessed 5th June 2008. There are several animal tests for abuse potential.

Addiction is a noun which was first used in 1906 in reference to opium, but it was used in 1779 with reference to tobacco. The first use of the adjective 'addict' (with the meaning of 'delivered, devoted') was in 1529 and comes from Latin addictus, pp. of addicere ('deliver, yield, devote,' from ad-, 'to' + dicere, say). WHO defines 'drug abuse' as persistent or sporadic excessive drug use inconsistent with or unrelated to acceptable medical practice (WHO, 2002).

Lactic acidosis: Buformin and Phenformin.

This is a biguanide class effect which is shared with metformin, but which has a much lower incidence and has not been withdrawn (Enia et al., 1997). There were two earlier diguanides which produced lactic acidosis: phenethyldiguanide in 1958 (Walker & Linton, 1959) and Compound 2254RP (para-aminobenzene sulphonamide-isopropyl thiadazol) which was originally used for typhoid fever, but was found to cause fatal hypoglycaemia. This should have been a warning for future diguanides.

Hepatotoxicity: cincophen, sulfathiazole, diamthazole, oxyphenisatin, iproniazid and nialamide.

Since most cases of hepatotoxicity, if caught in time, are reversible they do not have the same consequences as blood dyscrasias or neurological ADRs. *'in many cases a compound found to be hepatotoxic in an animal species will be tested in man for definite assessment of its hepatotoxic potential.'* (Ballet, 1997). Type 'B' liver reactions are relatively rare and therefore are not picked up until many patients have been treated. *'given that the idiosyncratic risk for liver damage lies between 1/10,000 and 1/100,000 exposures for most drugs'.* (Andrade & Lucena, 2001).

Neurotoxicity: thalidomide, bismuth, clioquinol, piperazine, Stalinon and diamthazole. Neurological adverse effects ~~are~~ may well not be reversible on stopping the drug.

Drugs whose manufacturers were found culpable: thalidomide, Coralgil, clioquinol, Stalinon and triparanol

Actions taken by a regulatory authority will depend on:
The level of suspicion
The severity of the reaction
Other ADRs attributed to the drug
The severity of the disease for which the drug is used
The availability of alternative drugs
The incidence of the reaction
The overall cost/benefit ratio
The possibility to detect who is predisposed (Westerholm, 1980).

There are also other courses open to a regulator other than allow on the market or remove from the market:
Restrict the indications, e.g. chloramphenicol (resistant infections); butazolidines (acute rheumatism, ankylosing spondylitis and acute gout).
Warnings of adverse effects (Black box warnings). An American study found that 0.7% of patients received a prescription violating a black box warning (Lasser et al., 2006).
Restrictions on dose and dosage forms.
Restrictions on prescriptions, i.e. over-the-counter v prescription only.

Demand monitoring of all patients, e.g. penicillamine and urine testing; clozapine and neutropenia.

Restrict the type of patients who can be prescribed the drug, e.g. aspirin and Reyes's syndrome; thalidomide and pregnancy.

Restriction to named patients (tiabendazole and strongyloidiasis). The process of subjectively estimating whether the possible outcomes are favourable or unfavourable, weight these by the probability that each outcome will occur and intuitively choose the option with the heaviest weighted score. This is known as 'subjective expected utility theory'. This is the application of logic to a problem, but this is only part of the decision process.

There remains the illogical approach, which probably always plays a part.

There are many unethical factors, which come into play:

Political corruption

Pressure from the Pharmaceutical industry

Pressure from patient groups, which are frequently financed by the pharmaceutical industry.

There are also well known cognitive biases, which are likely to influence decision making (Greenhalgh et al., 2004).

An example of a drug with important ADRs that was allowed to stay on the market

In 1928 Sedormid, allyl-isopropyl-acetyl carbamide (urea), was marketed in Germany by Hoffman-La Roche as a hypnotic, and was first shown to cause thrombocytopenic haemorrhagic purpura in 1931. The first paper published on this ADR was in 1934 (Loewy, 1934), but it wasn't until after July 1938 that it was mentioned on the packet (Loewy, 1938). It had been said in 1936 that *'There was no reason for prescribing drug with this alarming potentiality'*, but elsewhere that it was *'practically non-toxic'*. In 1958 it was said to be *'almost completely discontinued'* and in 1963 it was said to be *'too toxic for general use'*. (Leader, 1963). Hoffman-La Roche introduced Librium in 1960 and probably lost interest in marketing Sedormid. By 1969 Sedormid was *'no longer available'*. It was last sold in Mexico in 1975 (Roche, 2009). In 1992 BIAM said that the ADR was *'certain, very rare'*. From 1993 until 2006 a few cases of fixed drug eruption were published in the Japanese press indicating that it was still available. In 2003 there were 57 OTC drugs containing the drug on sale in Japan. It is strange that several Japanese companies started incorporating Sedormid in analgesic tablets with such analgesic drugs as paracetamol, Phenacetin, isopropylantipyrine and Ibuprofen from about 1992. It is perhaps even stranger that there were no further reports of purpura and that fixed drug eruptions, not previously reported with Sedormid despite 65 years on the market, started occurring. Sedormid is a good example of a drug with an important ADR that was not restricted or removed from the market but was allowed to wither in a competitive market.

Discussion

The many factors involved in a decision to remove a drug from the market make it unlikely that there will be any pattern to the regulatory authorities' decisions. However, it is clear that those countries with an active pharmaceutical research industry will tend to be those who first perceive a problem with toxicity and who will be the most likely to remove a drug from the market. There was a steady decrease in the lifespan of the drugs over the years, probably due to improving technology leading to improved pharmacovigilance and the increasing availability of alternative drugs.

The problem remains as to how to follow up hypotheses generated by substantiated individual cases. Clinical trials tend to be unethical, unless the ADR is not serious and is reversible, and prospective studies require time during which more patients will be exposed to a possible danger. Cohort studies without control groups are very poor at discovering new ADRs.

The 50 drugs examined here include three where there is an unknown factor: insoluble bismuth salts, Clioquinol and Phenacetin.

In several cases the decision whether to withdraw a drug has hung on the incidence of a very rare adverse effect, e.g. agranulocytosis and hepatotoxicity and in this case, different studies tend not to replicate the same frequency. Different regulatory authorities will interpret these incidences according to how relevant they consider it is to extrapolate the findings to their own situation. Carcinogenicity has depended, in most cases, on extrapolating from animal studies without waiting for corroboration in humans. The exceptions to this have been diethylstilboestrol and thorium, where, despite evidence in animals, the drugs were not withdrawn.

The most common form of toxicity requiring withdrawal from the market is hepatotoxicity and animal studies are not very effective in predicting the human response as far as idiosyncratic reactions are concerned. The serious haematological ADRs are so rare that discovery is late and require large studies in order to reveal them. Most drugs having central effects are candidates for drug dependency, but there is rarely a specific time when a new drug's addictive powers reach a threshold when action has to be taken. Neurological tissue is very unforgiving and once damaged may never be repaired, so although fairly rare they are important because of their potential irreversibility.

Dr Judith Jones, speaking of the 'epidemic' of drug withdrawals in 1989 said that such withdrawals suggested several possibilities:

1. A greater awareness of risks of the medications, some of which were established drugs for some time (debendox, phenformin and oxyphenbutazone).
2. A growing ability to study and characterize the risks of the agents.
3. A growing risk averseness on the part of the media and consumer public.
4. A lower threshold and/or facilitated means for regulatory action.
5. A greater awareness and reporting of events relating to health risk, including adverse effects of chemical and drugs, in the media (Jones, 1990).

Until the mid-nineteenth century herbs, whose adverse effects had been known for centuries, gave way to the synthetic drugs as the main armamentarium of the prescriber and with this flood of new drugs came their new problems. The response was slow but steady until an acceleration of new drugs in the 1950s when thalidomide arrived and pharmacovigilance changed forever.

Part 4. Discussion

The development of the pharmacovigilance process

It seems that every substance on this planet has been used as a medicine at some time and in some place and the results depended largely on how much they took of each substance. We have to presume that the earliest humans could distinguish between poisonous and non-poisonous berries, etc. and were aware that, in the majority of cases, the amount that they took of them influenced the results. i.e. they knew of type A reactions. The first published evidence that they also knew of type B reactions was in 49 BC when Titus Lucretius Carus wrote ' *What is food to one to some becomes fierce poison*'. This was explained in 1657 by Culpepper and his colleagues '*One and the same plant, is sometimes salutary to one man but noxious and death to another, by reason of the peculiar constitution of the individuum*' and 8 years later by Nedham '*The very same remedy which saved a man's life to-day may in the same disease, at a different time, kill another tomorrow*'. This adds the sense of personal idiosyncrasy, rather than that it is a fault of the dose of the drug. It wasn't until 1786 that Leigh gave a healthy volunteer increasing doses of a drug and notes the increasing severity of the reaction and then 7 years later a self-experimenter Crumpe records the results of a reaction every 5 minutes, thereby giving a temporal dimension to the reaction. Self-experimentation was first recorded as occurring in 2500 BC when Emperor Shen-nung was reputed to have tasted seventy kinds of toxic substances in a single day. No doubt many healers followed and still follow his example, but did not record their results. However, common sense must have caused them to try drugs in animals before using them in man and Rhazes in 865 AD tried proposed remedies first in animals. In 1680 Wepfer added a moral twist by saying '*My sin will be less, if I explore the effects of poison in animals in order to be of benefit to me*'. The first rules for the testing of drugs were given by Avicenna in 980 AD when he said that the drug must be free from any extraneous accidental quality. That it must be used on a simple, not a composite, disease and the drug must be tested with two contrary types of diseases, because sometimes a drug cures one disease by its essential qualities and another by its accidental ones. His next rule was that the quality of the drug must correspond to the strength of the disease, by which he presumably meant that the cost-benefit ratio must be favourable. The problem of distinguishing the disease from the action of the drugs was summed as 'the time of action must be observed, so that essence and action are not confused. He was well aware of the risks of anecdotal reports when he said "*The effect of the drug must be seen to occur constantly or in many cases, for if this did not happen, then it only constitutes an accidental effect*'. It was in Holland in 1662 that the first randomised clinical trial was proposed based on the occurrence of adverse events whilst comparing two drugs–'*see how many funerals both us shall have*'. The first mention of training physicians in regard to pharmacovigilance comes in 1800 when Lucas, writing on education of surgeon-apothecaries, says '*A practitioner versed in chemistry, may not only be better apprised of the noxious effects of some remedies, but be more quick-sighted in opportunely counteracting their pernicious effects*'.

Carus had, many years before in 49 BC, pointed out a problem with relying on the results from testing in animals when he said '*fierce poison is the Hellebore to us, but puts the fat on goats and quails*' and Avicenna had added that experimentation must be done with the human body, for testing a drug on a lion or a horse might not prove anything about its effect on man. Similarly Woodville in 1790 said '*Henbane is poisonous to birds and dogs; but horses, cows, goats and swine it does not affect*'. This truth was rammed home with Thalidomide. It is quite common even these days that drugs go on the market with too high a dose (Bashaw, 1992). Yet, in 1689 Wills gave the general rule, particularly where active medicines are employed to begin with small doses and gradually increase them to the extent the constitution will bear. Moyse in 1676 pointed out that with mercury it sometimes excites the salivation in delicate persons indicating that he realised that different constitutions required different treatment. Pechey was more precise when he wrote in 1694 concerning Hellebore '*the root ought not be given to old men, women, or children, or to such as are weakly, and costive in the body*'. Continued use of a drug may cause delayed effects. In 1752 James said of mercury '*For the miners and others employed about it, though of the strongest constitutions imaginable, seldom remain four years in that state, but are seized with trembles and palsies and die miserable*'. On the other hand 40 years earlier Pomet had written of morphia '*Custom will bring people to*

bear great doses of it, but at first every one must begin with very small ones'
illustrating that tolerance to some drugs occurs. The idea of titrating the
dose until there was a satisfactory conclusion might seem admirable but in
some cases the appearance of side effects was linked to a 'satisfactory' dose,
e.g. salivation washed out the evil of syphilis and Withering said that at
first he thought it was necessary to bring on sickness to ensure that digitalis
produced the correct diuretic effect. Quinine dosage was increased until
there was singing in the ears. It was suggested that the dose of salicylate
in rheumatism should be increased daily, or every second day, until any
unpleasant side-effect, such as vomiting, deafness, tinnitus or a tendency
to delirium is observed (Lees, 1909). The principle of increasing the doseage
until an adverse reaction occurred must have been common with drugs/herbs
with a low therapeutic index. Even now the idea that side effects indicate
that a drug is working correctly lingers on.

We have seen that ever since 865 AD rulers have fought against
adulteration and still do so today. The apothecaries added their voice.
Healers tended to work alone only joining together as a trade union when
their livelihood was threatened by competition from quacks selling cheaper
adulterated drugs. In 1316 The Guild of Pepperers wrote a code for quality
control and 10 years later in 1332 the College of Medicine of Paris made
certain that all apothecaries had a standard textbook. A hundred years
later, in 1423 the Commonality of Physicians and Surgeons of London
are inspecting the wares in apothecaries' shops. In 1540 King Henry VIII
appointed four inspectors of apothecaries' wares, drugs and stuffs. One of
the earliest examples of a drug being taken off the market because of an
ADR was when a University faculty, the Paris Faculty of Physicians, in 1566
forbade the sale of antimony because it was a dangerous poison that should
not be taken internally. In 1747 the Apothecaries of the Cities of London
and Westminster petitioned the English House of Commons to strengthen
the law against 'practitioners dispensing drugs of dubious quality; an early
example of the pharmaceutical industry trying to influence the government.
A paper in 1779 on *'Quackery, and the most effectual means of checking its
dangerous progress'* suggested having a public board to judge new drugs
before being allowed to be sold or advertised; the first step towards having
a committee for the safety of medicines. About the same time in France,
1778, the Société Royale de Médicine became the only competent authority
for the authorisation of new drugs. This would seem to be the first example
of the licensing of drugs. The medical societies became interested in the

serious ADRs and in 1832 the Royal Medical and Chirurgical Society
set up a committee to enquire into the problems with chloroform, but it
wasn't until 1877 that the BMA put this into action and it was 1880 before
the McKendrick report was published. In 1914 in the UK there was a
recommendation that all medicines should be registered after considering
their quality, safety and efficacy; but the publication coincided with outbreak
of the First World War and it was shelved. In the US a bill to expand
government authority including performing safety tests was drafted but
nothing happened until 1938, when after the Elixir of Sulphonamide disaster
in 1937, the Federal Food, Drug and Cosmetics Act was passed, which meant
that they controlled the marketing of a new drug. In 1941 the UK Pharmacy
and Medicines Act legislated against 'secret remedies'.

2. Factors influencing the occurrence, recognition, reporting and publication of Adverse Drug Reactions Occurrence

1) Numbers: The world population was much smaller and so there were fewer people to be affected.

Table 13. The world population over time

Year	8000 BC	1000 BC	500 BC	100 AD	1000	1750	1800	1850	1900	1950
World Population (100,000s)	8	50	100	200+	310	791	978	1,262	1,650	2,518

(wikipedia.org)

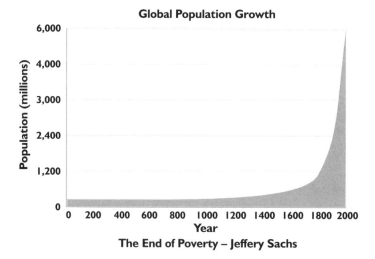

The End of Poverty – Jeffery Sachs

2) The life expectancy of the population was much shorter and therefore a patient's first illness was often their last and they did not live to experience more illnesses and more treatments and more adverse effects. The sudden increase in life expectancy post 1900 has disproportionately increased the drug consumption because of the increase in age–related diseases. The dates in the table are fallible as different criteria have been used in each case, e.g in 1950 the life expectancy in Asia and Africa was c40 years and Eastern Europe had 10 years less in life expectancy than Western Europe.

Table 14. Life expectancy over time

Humans life expectancy	4500 – 3500 BC	2300– 1900 BC	Classical Greece	Rome 30 BC– 330 AD	Time of Christ	1540– 1800 (UK)	1900 Developed countries	1950 Western Europe	2005 (Europe)
Years from birth	34	26	28	25	21	37	42	68	Men: 76 Women: 82

3) Cost: Only a small proportion of the world's population could and can afford to go to doctors/healers and afford herbs/drugs. The agricultural labourers and others who were illiterate would have had to rely on their homemade herbal mixtures gathered from the local fields. Most of their herbs would have been without an active principle and therefore innocuous. Most of their ADRs would come from mistakenly eating a poisonous herb. If their illness failed to abate they would probably consult the local 'healer' or 'wise women' who, although probably still illiterate, would have acquired more knowledge from past experience. It would have been the literate middle classes, e.g. farmers, who would have been able to consult an apothecary or physician who may have had access to the literature derived from the ancients. The apothecaries and physicians were likely to have a greater range of medicines available including many with active principles with their inherent risks of ADRs. The number of people with access to active medicines is likely to have risen proportionate to their income. Again we see a sudden surge, this time in incomes around the start of the beginning of the 19th century.

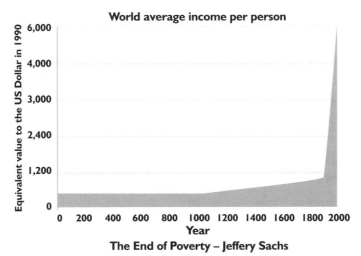

World average income per person

The End of Poverty – Jeffery Sachs

4) There was less risk of having an ADR because most medicines were mild herbs, many without any activity at all and had few adverse effects compared with our present day synthetic drugs. The drugs, which might affect the cause of illnesses, were very few, e.g. cinchona bark, mercury. The sudden increase in the availability of synthetic drugs in the early 20th century meant there would have been an exponential rise in the numbers of ADRs.

3. Recognition

There are several factors that need to be considered before a diagnosis of a drug-induced reaction can be made. Of the various factors that need to be considered and the one that patients will use is the time to onset of the adverse effect. The shorter the time between taking the drug and the adverse events the more likely that the patient/doctor will consider the herb/drug as the cause.

For the doctor the most important factor will be the alternative diagnoses. Even in Hippocrates' days there were 'epidemics of jaundice' which later was called 'catarrhal jaundice' or 'acute yellow atrophy' and probably today would be recognised as viral hepatitis (A, B, etc). The latter was not recognised prior to 1937 and the many cases during World War II stimulated further research. In Hippocrates' works he gives individual case histories and from these we can appreciate his thorough examination of the patient, first by interrogation and then by observation. All the body secretions and excretions were examined. We know, from Laennec, that Hippocrates listened to the lungs by placing his ear on the chest (Laennec, 1819) and that

396

the latter believed that it fell out of use until the 19th century. I have found no record of Hippocrates using palpation of the abdomen. In 1707 Floyer introduced timing of the pulse rate by a pulse-watch, but the importance of the pulse had been known since 2,500 BC and Herophilus (c330–260 BC) of Chalcedon had used a water clock for timing the pulse in 280 BC. The first measurement of blood pressure by Stephen Hale in a horse required opening an artery and over the next few years various improvements were discovered, which could be used in man for routine usage[178].Although the mercury thermometer was invented in 1714 it wasn't until 1865 that the small, efficient clinical thermometer came into practice. Auenbrugger started using chest percussion for diagnosis in 1761, but it only came into popular usage in 1808. The discovery that heating urine could cause it to coagulate, because of the presence of albumin was a great advancement for the diagnosis of renal disease (Blackall, 1813), but why had this not been noted earlier? In 1816 Laennec introduced the stethoscope. The introduction of the opthalmoscope in 1850, the Lauder-Brunton auriscope in 1862, followed by the discovery of X rays in 1895 expanded the diagnostic possibilities for physicians. The next year saw the Riva-Rocci mercury sphygomometer, the forerunner of our present machine, come onto the market. The new century started with the invention of the ECG in 1901 and the gastroscope in 1932 (Walker, 1990). Blood dyscrasias could, in theory, have been recognised after the discovery of the microscope by Leeuwenhoek in 1673 since he saw blood films in which absence of white cells would have been noticeable, but it wasn't until 1888 that aplastic anaemia was recognised and 1927 before agranulocytosis was discovered, so drug induced dyscrasias are a fairly new phenomenon. Most of the early 'doctors' were untrained; others had served apprenticeships of varying qualities. Only a few physicians were university trained. In the UK prior to the mid 19th century physicians did not physically examine patients, but did feel the pulse and examine the urine (Loudon, 1986). Only a few physicians or healers would publish books. The translation of symptoms and signs into their specific pathological causes only evolved as medical science advanced. It can be difficult to translate old diagnoses into modern terms, e.g. cardiac depression? cardiac failure. The first mention of individual variation in susceptibility to drugs was in 49 BC and had not advanced much further by 1874. It wasn't until Pirquet recognised allergy in 1907 that real progress was made. Only those with access to publications would be able to learn from distant experts, so that it would require a certain level

---

[178] Blood pressure measurement see http://www.bloodpressurehistory.com/dates.html, Accessed 15th August 2009.

of education and wealth. It wasn't until 1862, with a thesis on drug induced skin reactions, that the diagnosis of ADRs was discussed. Liver function tests were mentioned in 1916 in respect of salavarsan, but these were very limited and it wasn't until the 1970s that transaminases were used.The fact that a particular advance had been published did not mean that its use immediately became widespread. Some years might pass before the medical elite accepted a new idea sufficiently to mention it in a standard textbook. It would take even longer before new advances were used routinely in general practice. In 1960 few general practices in the UK would have had an ECG.

4. Reporting

There would always have been reluctance for patients to report adverse events to their healer/physician since there is an implication of blame. The side effects of a drug might have been accepted as showing that the drug was working. The salivation with mercury was taken as showing that the evil was being washed out and therefore the dose was increased until the required amount of salivation was occurring. People who accepted that human excrement[179] dried and powdered and then puffed into the eyes was a reasonable treatment for conjunctivitis might not have been very discerning. Many of the writers comments have been whether the drug was safe or could it kill, rather than mentioning temporary inconveniences. When death was all about them patients may have been more stoical and accepted adverse effects more willingly. Now we have effective drugs most of our illnesses can be cured and we live to have more side effects from the next treatment for the next illness, but one can see from the life expectancy figures ~~below~~ that for our ancestors their first illness was often their last, as most medicines were to relieve symptoms rather than cure illnesses. It is apparent that from the earliest times writers have experimented upon themselves and since they almost certainly did not have the ailment for which the drug was appropriate the assessment of any reaction would not have been confused by alternative diagnoses. However, since they were only experimenting upon themselves only the most common ADR would have been discovered by this means.

Terminology: The meaning of words changes with passage of time, semantic shift, and many new specific terms have appeared. There was no standardization of language, such as MEDRA[180] or its equivalent, so foreign languages need to be translated and their every day language interpreted.

5. Publication

1) Prior to 1750 the literature was confined to generalisations befitting

their educational purpose and it was only when medical journals
appeared that individual case histories were published frequently.

2) The herbals, dispensatories and pharmacopoeias covered such a large
number of medicines that it would not have been feasible to mention
anything but the most serious adverse effects.

3) The early authors would not have treated enough patients to pick up a
sufficient number of rare ADRs to have made a generalisation.

4) The steady increase in the number of medical journals published meant
that there was a greater opportunity to be published.

The ever increasing availability of ever increasing numbers of powerful
drugs to an increasingly rich and sophisticated and ever increasing
population of patients has produced and will continue to produce an
exponentially increasing number and variety of ADRs. The number of
reported serious adverse events from drug treatment more than doubled
in the United States from 1998 to 2005, rising from 34,966 to 89,842 and
the number of deaths relating to drugs nearly tripled from 5,519 to 15,107
(Moore, 2007).

Conclusion

The memory of past events should influence future actions. However,
pharmaceutical companies still minimise the adverse effects of their drugs
and, with many of the prescribers, put profits before the welfare of the
patients. So-called 'Complementary medicine' is riddled with quackery. The
adulteration of drugs is still widespread, especially in traditional Chinese
medicines. The predators flount the laws and regulations, and exploit their
many loopholes.

References

Ackernecht EH. A short survey of drug therapy prior to 1900. In 'Safeguarding the public. Historical aspects of medicinal drug control'. JB Blake ed. The John Hopkins Press, Baltimore, 1970.

Ackerknecht EH. Therapeutics. From the primitive to the 20th century. 1973.

ADEC (Australian Drug Evaluation Committee) Sub-acute myelo-optic neuropathy and the halogenated hydroquinolones. Med J Aust 1971; 2: 1090-1091.

ADEC Adverse effects of bismuth subgallate. A further report from the Australian Drug Evaluation Committee. Med J Aust 1974; 2: 664–666.

Aery Lancelot. The symptoms, nature, causes of the essera, or nettle rash, to which are added some general observations on the causes and cure of cutaneous diseases. 1774.

Adverse effects of Aspirin: Guidebook for Medicine, Reference and Research. Abbe Pub. Assn. of Washington DC; 1st edition (April 1984) (Paperback).

Abenheim L, Moore N. and Bégaud B. The role of Pharmacoepidemiology in Pharmacovigilance. Pharmacoepidemiol Drug Saf 1999; 8(S1): S1–S7.

Abraham JJ. Some account of the history of the treatment of syphilis. Br J Ven Dis 1948 December; 24(4): 153–60.

Abraham J and Davis C. A comparative analysis of drug safety withdrawals in the UK and the US (1971–1992): Implications for current regulatory thinking and policy. Soc Sci Med 2005; 61: 881–892.

Abraham J and Lawton Smith H. Regulation of the Pharmaceutical Industry. Palgrave Macmillan, 2003; p22.

Abraham J and Lewis G. Regulating Medicines in Europe, competition, expertise and public health. Routledge, 2000.

Abraham J. Science, Politics and the Pharmaceutical Industry, controversy and bias in drug regulation, UCL Press Ltd. 1995.

Abramowitz EW. Historical points of interest on the mode of action and ill effects of mercury. Bull N Y Acad Med 1934; 695–705.

Adams DA and Perry S. Agranulocytosis associated with Thenalidine (Sandostene) Tartrate Therapy. JAMA (July) 1958; 167:1207–1210.

ADEC Australian Drug Evaluation Committee. Med J Aust May 13th 1972; 1051–1053.

Alleyne James. A new English dispensatory, in four parts. Containing, I. A more accurate account of the simple medicines, ... IV. A rational account of the operation of medicines. To which are added, the quantities of the middle syllables of the Latin names, ... By James Alleyne, M.D. London, 1733. Based on information from English Short Title Catalogue. Eighteenth Century Collections Online. Gale Group. http://0-galenet.galegroup.com.libsys.wellcome.ac.uk/servlet/ECCO

Almuete VI (Millenium 2000 Series Pharmacy: 'A Look Back at the First 1000 Years and a Vision for the Future' from Medscape Pharmacotherapy).

Altman LK. Who Goes First? The Story of Self-experimentation in Medicine. New York: Randon House. 1986.

Alvarez-Del-Castillo MA, Alvarez-Prechous A, Garcia-Sabina A, Arca-Pineiro A and Pardina-Anon MC. Hepatic toxicity produced by cinchophen, Analysis of five cases. Gastroentero Hepatol 1991; 14(10): 546–549.

Amery W. Post-marketing drug safety management: A Pharmaceutical Industry perspective. Int J Risk Safety Med. 1994; 5: 91–104.

Anderson DG and Jewell M. The absorption, excretion, and toxicity of streptomycin in man. New Engl J Med 1945; 233(17): 489–491.

Andrade RJ and Lucena MI. Is drug-induced hepatotoxicity unavoidable? Rev Esp Enferm Dig (Madrid) 2001; 93(1): 51–53.

Angervall L, Bengtsson U, Zetterlund CG and Zsigmond M. Renal pelvic carcinoma in a Swedish district and abuse of a phenacetin-containing drug. Br J Urol 1969; 41: 401–5.

Anonymous. Review of The London Dispensatory. Medical Tracts. 1745.

Anomymous. Abuse of Chloral hydrate. Quart J Inebriety January 1880; 4: 53-54.

Anonymous. Round the Fountain, In St Bartholomew's Hospital Medical Journal, 1923.

Anonymous. Dantron (chrysazin; 1,8-dihydroxyanthraquinon). IARC Monographs on the Evaluation of Carcinogenic Risks to Humans 1990; 50:265–75.

Anonymous. Diamthazole dihydrochloride. JAMA May 1957; 18164(3): 281–2.

Anon. The dangers of Thorotrast. Lancet 1938; 1: 36.

Anon. Is Thorotrast safe? BMJ 1938; 1: 903.

Armer RE and Morris ID. Trends in early drug safety. Drug News Perspect 2004; 17(2) 143–148.

Armstrong FB and Scherbel AL. Review of toxicity of oxyphenbutazone. Report of a case of thrombocytopenic purpura. JAMA 1961 Feb 18th: 614–5.

Arnaiz JA, Carné X, Riba N, Codina C, Ribas J and Trilla A. The use of evidence in pharmacovigilance. Case reports as the reference for drug withdrawals. Eur J Clin Pharmacol 2001; 57: 89–91.

*Arztl Forsch 1956; 9: 364.

Astruc John. A treatise of the venereal disease, In six books; containing an account of the original, propagation, and contagion of this distemper in general. London, 1737.

Atkins MJ. Who discovered inhalational anaesthetics? Pharml Med 1995; 9: 33–43.

Aw TC and Vale JA. Poisoning from metals. Oxford Textbook of Medicine, 3rd edition, 1996; 1111.

Awsiter John ' Extracts from an essay on the effects of opium considered as a poison and with the most rational method of cure deduced from experience' *The Medical Museum* 1763–1764.

Backer M. Historical note on the concept of arterial hypertension. *Yale J Biol Med* 1944; 16(6): 613–618.

Bailey DN and Shaw RF. Ethchlorvynol ingestion in San Diego county: a 14-year review of cases with blood concentrations and findings. *J Anal Toxicol* 1990; 14(6): 348–352.

Bailey DN and Briggs JR. Carisoprodol: an unrecognised drug of abuse. *Am J Clin Pathol* 2002; 117: 396–400.

Baker BJ, Armelagos GJ, Becker MJ, Brothwell D, Drusini A,Geise MC, Kelley MA,Moritoto I, Morris AG, Nurse GT,Powell ML, Rothschild BM, Saunders SR. The Origin and Antiquity of Syphilis: Paleopathological Diagnosis and Interpretation [and Comments and Reply] *Current Anthropology*, 1988; 29(5): 703–737.

Bakke OM, Wardell WM and Lasagna L. Drug discontinuations in the United Kingdom and the United States. 1964–1983; Issues of safety. *Clin Pharmacol Ther* 1984; 35(5): 559–567.

Bakke OM, Manochia M, De Abajo F, Kaitin KI and Lasagna L. Drug safety discontinuations in the United Kingdom, the United States, and Spain from 1974–through 1993: A regulatory perspective. *Clin Pharmacol Ther* 1995; 58: 108–17.

Ballance R, Pogany J and Forster H. The World's Pharmaceutical Industries. United Nations Industrial Development Organisation 1992.

Balz E*. Salicylsäure, salicylsaures Natron und Thymol in ihrem Einfluss auf Krankenheiten [Salicylic acid, sodium salicylate and thymol in their influence on diseases]. *Archiv. Fur Heilkunde*, 1877; XVIII: 63.

Banister John, 1540-1610. 'An antidotarie chyrurgicall containing great varietie and choice of all sorts of medicines that commonly fal into the chyrurgions vse: partlie taken out of authors, olde and new, printed or written: partlie obtained by free gifte of sundrie worthie men of this profession within this land' 1589.

Baohua H & Xingjun K. On the connotation of 'Shennong tastes all kinds of herbs and encounters seventy kinds of toxic substances in a single day'. *Zhonghua yishi zazhi*, Beijing 1980; 32(4): 218–222.

Barber G. Country Doctor. The Boydell Press, Ipswich, 1974.

Barclay GJ. and Russel-White, C. J. Excavations in the ceremonial complex of the fourth to the second millennium BC at Balfarg/Balbirnie, Glenrothes, Fife. *Proceedings of the Society of Antiquaries of Scotland* 1993; 123: 43–210.

Barnett AH, Jones FW and Williams ER. Acute poisoning with Potter's Asthma Remedy. *BMJ* 1977; 2: 1635.

Barros E. Amebas Y Mas Amebas. *Semana Med* 1935; 42: 907.

Barsky AJ, Saintfort R, Rogers MP and Borus J. F. Nonspecific medication side effects and the nocebo phenomenon. *JAMA* 2002; 287: 622–627.

Bashaw ED. Application of clinical pharmacological tools to facilitate drug development. In DIA Conference, Methods and Examples for Assessing Benefit/Risk and Safety for New Drug Application, 20–21 July 1992.

Bayes Thomas. *Phil Trans R Soc London* 1763; 53: 370–418.

Bégaud B. Dictionnaire de Pharmaco-epidemiologie. ARME-Pharma-covigilance Editions. Bordeuax, 1995.

Belloni C and Rizzoni G. Neurotoxic side effects of piperazine. *Lancet* Aug 12 1967; 2(7511): 369.

Belloste Augustin, 'An essay on mercury'. *Tract*, 1721 and 1733; 117.

Belluci G. Storia della anestesiologia. 1982; Piccin Editor Padova.

Benaim S and Dixon MF. Jaundice associated with administration of iproniazid. *BMJ* 1958; 395104: 1068–1070.

Berenguier J 'Des éruptions provoquée par l'ingestion des médicaments' Thèse pour le Doctorat en Médicine, 59 pages, Paris, 1874.

Bergman U, Boman G and Wiholm B-E. Epidemiology of adverse drug reactions to phenformin and metformin. *BMJ* 1976; 2: 464.

Berman A. Drug control in nineteenth-century France: Antecedents and directions. In 'Safeguarding the public. Historical aspects of medicinal drug control'. JB Blake Ed. The John Hopkins Press. Baltimore, 1970 .

Berniers GM, Miller M and Springate CS. Lactic acid and phenformin hydrochloride. *JAMA* 1963; 184(1): 43–46.

Bertagnini C. Sulle alterazioni che alcuni acidi subiscono nell'organismo animale.

Il Nuovo Cimento. Marson, G. Pasero, 1855; 1: 363-72.

Besle A, Bussel B, Chapelle JG and Scherrer P. Myoclonic encephalopathy due to bismuth poisoning. *Ann Méd Psychol*. April 1975; 11(4): 493–8.

Bethel RG. Abuse of asthma cigarettes. *BMJ* September 30th 1978; 2(6142):959.

Bidstrup PL. Toxicity of Mercury and its compounds. Elsevier Publishing Company. 1964.

Bigham M and Copes R. Thiomersal in vaccines. *Drug Saf* 2005; 28(2): 89–101.

Bignall JR and Crofton J. Antihistamine drugs in treatment of nausea and vomiting due to streptomycin. *BMJ* 1949; 1:13–14.

Biron P. Withdrawal of oxyphenbutazone: What about phenylbutazone?. *CMAJ* 1986; 134: 1119–1120.

Blackall J. Observations on the nature and cure of dropsies on the presence of the coagulable part of the blood in dropsical urine; to which is added an appendix, containing several cases of angina pectoris with dissections. London for Longman, Hurst, Rees, Orme, and Brown 1813.

Blackburne W. Account of the effects of a large dose of Emetic Tartar with remarks. Communicated to Dr SF Simmon by Wm Blackburne. *Lond Medic Journ* 1788.

Blake FC et al. Agranulocytic angina. *Yale J Biol Med* 1935; 7: 465.

Blohm TR. Drug-induced lipidosis: biochemical interpretations. *Pharmacol Rev* 1978; 30(4): 593-603.

Blythe WB and Woods JW. Acute renal insufficiency after gallbladder dye. *New Eng J Med* 1961; 264: 1045.

Boardman WW. Rapidly developing cataracts after dinitrophenol. *Calif West Med* 1935; 43(2): 118-9.

Boerhaave H. Boerhaave's aphorisms: concerning the knowledge and cure of diseases. Translated from the latest edition printed in Latin at Leyden, 1728 with useful observations and explanations. London. 1735.

Boerhaave H. Treatise on the powers of medicines, Translated from the most correct Latin edition. London: J Wilcox and J Hedges, 1740.

BMJ leader. Glutethimide – an unsafe alternative to barbiturate hypnotics. *BMJ* 12th June 1976.

BMJ leader. A carcinogenic method of treatment. *BMJ* 1935; 1(3873): 652–656.

BNF, British National Formulary, British Medical Association and the Royal Pharmaceutical Society of Great Britain 1999; 37th edition.

Bohn S J. Agranulocytosis angina following ingestion of dinitrophenol. *JAMA* 1934; 103: 249.

Bonser GM. Cancer hazards of the pharmacy. *BMJ* 1967.

Borghi C and Canti D. 'Tollerabilita di un farmaco valutazione clinica' by Orginizzazione Editorale Medico Farmaceutica, 1986.

Bostock J and Riley HT. The Natural History. Pliny the Elder. London. Taylor and Francis, Red Lion Court, Fleet Street. 1855.

Bosworth DM, Fielding JW, Demarest L and Bonaquist M. Toxicity to Iproniazid (Marsilid) as it affects osseous tuberculosis. *Sea View Hospital Bulletin* 1955; 15: 134.

Bottered. Ancestors of the West. University of Chicago Press, 2000.

Böttiger LE and Westerholm B. Drug-induced blood dyscrasias in Sweden. *BMJ* 1973; 3: 339–343.

Bouvet M. Histoire de la pharmacia en France des origins à nos jours. Paris. Edition Occitania.1937.

Boyle Robert. Medicinal experiments; or, A collection of choice remedies, for the most part simple and easily prepared. 1692. Reproduction of original in Henry E Huntington and Art Gallery Library Wing. Wellcome Library, London.

Boyle R. Some considerations touching the usefulness of experimental natural philosophy, 1663.

Boylston A. Zabdiel Boylston's evaluation of innoculation against smallpox. *J R Soc Med* 2008; 101: 476-477.

Boylston AW. Did clinical science begin in 1767? The James Lind Library (www.jameslindlibrary.org) accessed 2nd February 2009 © Arthur Boylston, 2008.

Bradley Henry, surgeon. A treatise on mercury, shewing the danger of taking it crude for all manner of disorders, ... with some remarks on The antient physician's legacy. The second edition. To which are added, a reply to the remarks on the Treatise of the use and abuse of mercury, in the fourth edition of Dr. Dover's Antient physician's legacy.

... London, 1733. Based on information from English Short Title Catalogue. Eighteenth Century Collections Online. Gale Group. http://0-galenet.galegroup.com.libsys.wellcome.ac.uk/servlet/ECCO

Bramness JG, Skurtveit S, Mørland J and Engeland A. The risk of traffic accidents after prescription of carisoprodol. *Accid Anal Prev* 2007; 39: 1050-5.

Brest Vincent. An analytical inquiry into the specifick property of mercury. relating to the cure of venereal diseases, when well apply'd and skilfully managed. ... By Vincent Brest, London, 1732. Based on information from English Short Title Catalogue. Eighteenth Century Collections Online. Gale Group. http://0-galenet.galegroup.com.libsys.wellcome.ac.uk/servlet/ECCO

Brochin. *Gazette des Hôpt.* 1877; 226.

Brookes R. (Richard). An introduction to physic and surgery. Containing I. Medicinal institutions, X. An explanation of the terms of art, ... By R. Brookes, M.D. London, 1754. Based on information from English Short Title Catalogue. Eighteenth Century Collections Online. Gale Group. http://0-galenet.galegroup.com.libsys.wellcome.ac.uk/servlet/ECCO

Brown HA and Hinshaw HC. Toxic reactions of streptomycin on the eighth nerve apparatus. *Proc Mayo Clin* 1946; 21: 347 353.

Buckell M, Hunter D, Milton R and Perry KMA. Chronic mercury poisoning. *Br J Ind Med* 1946 April; 3(2): 55- 63.

Buggs CW, Pilling MA, Bronstein B and Hirsgfeld JW. Absorbtion, distribution, and excretion of streptomycin in man. *J Clin Invest* 1946 Jan; 25(1): 94–102.

Bull JP (1951). A study of the history and principles of clinical therapeutic trials. MD Thesis, University of Cambridge..

Bulletin Med Soc. Emulation. *Bull de la Soc Méd d'Em.* 1818.

Burba J. Cinchona Bark, James Ford Bell Library, University of Minnesota. 2007.

Butlletí groc, 9: 6, 1996. La Fundació Institut Català de Farmacologia (FICF).

Cabot RC and Cabot HC. Case records of the Massachusetts General Hospital, Case 11231. *Boston Medical and Surgical Journal*. 1925; 192: 1122–6.

Cahn CH. Intoxication by ethchlorvynol (Placidyl). Report of four cases. Canadian Cases. *Can Med Assoc J* Nov 1 1959; 81: 733–4.

Camac CNB. Intramuscular and intravenous injections of antimony in trypanosomiasis. *Am J Med Sc* 1911; 142: 218–20.

Capasso L. 5,300 years ago, the Ice man used natural laxatives and antibiotics. *Lancet*, 1998; 352: 1864.

Cahill H. 'Every person naturally seeks to know': An exhibition of books on ancient Greek science and medicine from the Foyle Special Collections Library'. Information Services System. King's College, London. 2005.

Carr Suzanne. Entoptic Phenomena, MA Dissertation 1995.

Carroll OM, Bryan PA and Robinson RJ. Stevens-Johnson syndrome associated with long-acting sulfonamides *JAMA* 1966; 195: 691.

Carter AJ. Dwale: an anaesthetic from old England. *BMJ* 1999; 319: 1623-1626.

Cartwright S. The origins of medicine; assessment and implications of the Eurasian evidence from the Upper Palaeolithic to the Bronze Age, http://www.oxford-homeopathy.org.uk/PDF/the-origins-of-medicine.pdf. Accessed 25th February 2008.

Cartwright T. An hospitall for the diseased wherein are to bee founde moste excellent and approued medicines, as well emplasters of speciall vertue, as also notable potions or drinkes, and other comfortable receptes, bothe for the restitution and the preseruation of bodily healthe: very necessary for this tyme of common plague and immortalitie, and for other tymes when occasion shall require: with a newe addition/ gathered by TC. 1579. Early English books online. Wellcome Library.

Cawthorne T and Ranger D. Toxic effect of Streptomycin upon balance and hearing. *BMJ* 1957 June 22nd; 1444–1446.

Cerf R. Les ictères au cincophen. Lyon University thesis.

Chadwick J and Mann WNV. The Medical works of Hippocrates, Blackwell Scientific Publications, Oxford.

Chapman & Tweddle. A new herball by William Turner; edited by George T.L. Chapman, Marilyn N. Tweddle; with indexes compiled by Frank McCombie Cambridge; New York: Cambridge University Press, 1995.

Chase JS. Return of the vestibular function following Streptomycin toxemia. *Calif Med* 1951; 74(3): 185–187.

Chatterjee SS and Thakre NW. Fiedler's myocarditis: report of a fatal case following the intramuscular injection of streptomycin. *Tubercle* 1958; 39(4): 240-1.

Chemin E. Richard Pearson Strong and the Iatrogenic Plague Disaster in Bilibid Prison, Manila, 1906. *Rev Infect Dis* 1989; 2: 996–1004.

Chemin E. Ross defends Haffkine: the aftermath of the vaccine-associated Mulkowal Disaster of 1902. *J History Med* 1991; 46: 201–218.

Ching CK, Lai CK, Poon WT, Wong ENP, Yan WW, Chan AYW and Mak AWL. Hazards posed by a banned drug—phenformin is still hanging around medical practice. *Hong Kong Med J* 2008; 14: 50–4.

Christen JP and Jaccottet M. Convulsant poisoning in children; Meta and Asterol. *Rev Méd Suisse-Romande* 1957; 77(9): 657-78.

Christoffel T and Teret SP. Epidemiology and the law : Courts and confidence intervals. *Am J Public Health* 1991; 81(12): 1661–1666.

Cilliers L and Retief FP. (University of the Free State) Poisons, poisoning and the drug trade in ancient Rome. 2000. http://209.85.129.104/search?q=cache: Qt-t0Z_jIZQJ:academic.sun.ac.za/as/journals/akro/Akro45/cil-et2.pdf+helle bore+convulsions&hl=en&ct=clnk&cd=22&gl=uk. Accessed 25th February 2008.

City of Glasgow 'Supplementary abstracts to charters in volume 2: 1578-1606' Charters and Documents relating to the City of Glasgow 1175-1649: Part 1 (1897), pp. 28-55. URL: http://www.british-history.ac.uk/report.asp?compid=47928. Date accessed: 22 April 2007.

Clarke A, Deeks JJ and Shakir SAW. An assessment of the publicly disseminated evidence of safety used in decisions to withdraw medicinal products from the UK and US markets. *Drug Saf* 2006; 29(2): 175-181.

Clutton Joseph . A true and candid relation of the good and bad effects of Joshua Ward's pill and drop… By Joseph Clutton. London, 1736. Based on information from English Short Title Catalogue. Eighteenth Century Collections Online. Gale Group. http//0-galenet.galegroup.com.libsys.wellcome.ac.uk/servlet/ECCO

Cohen M. Primary Glutethimide addiction. *N Y State J Med* 1960; 60: 280.

Colebrook L and Purdie AW. Treatment of a 100 cases of purperal fever by Sulphonamide. *Lancet* 27th November 1937; 1237–1242.

Coke F. Asthma and anaphylaxis. *BMJ* 1921 12th March; 372–376.

Combes B, Damon A and Gottfried E. Piperazine (antepar) neurotoxicity; report of a case probably due to renal insufficiency. *N Engl J Med* Feb 2 1956; 254(5): 223-5.

Consolidated List of Products - Whose Consumption and/or Sale Have Been Banned, Withdrawn, Severely Restricted or Not Approved by Governments, Eight Issue–Pharmaceuticals (http://www.who.int/medicinedocs/en/d/Js4902e.4.1.82)

Cooper A. Cases from the early note-books of the late Sir Astley Cooper. *Prov Med Surg J* 1841 Oct 23rd; 3(4): 67–8.

Coste JF. An account of some experiments with opium in the cure of venereal disease. *London Medical Journal* 1788; 9:7–27.

Courcy C. The basic principles of medicine in the primitive mind. A lecture given at the Welcome Historical Medical Library on 12th July 1996.

Cozanitis DA. One hundred years of barbiturates and their saint. *J R Soc Med* 2004; 97: 594–598.

Crockett R. Death following the inhalation of a mixture of ether and chloroform. *Am J Med Sci*. July 1857; 284–285.

Crofton J. The MRC randomised trial of streptomycin and its legacy: a view from the clinical front line. *J R Soc Med* 2006; 99: 531–533.

Crofton J. Desensitisation to streptomycin and PAS. *BMJ* 1953; 2: 1014–1017.

Crofton J. Personal communication. 2009.

Crumpe, Samuel. An inquiry into the nature and properties of opium; wherein its component principles, mode of operation, and use or abuse in particular diseases, are experimentally investigated; and the opinions of former authors on these points impartially examined. By Samuel Crumpe, … London, 1793. Based on information from English Short Title Catalogue. Eighteenth Century Collections Online. Gale Group. http://0-galenet.galegroup.com.libsys.wellcome.ac.uk/servlet/ECCO

Cullen W. Treatise of the Materia Medica. Edinburgh, 1789; 2: 64.

Cullen W. The Edinburgh practice of physic and surgery, preceded by an abstract of the theory of medicine and the nosology of Dr Cullen. Printed for G Kirasley 1800.

Cupp MJ. Toxicology and clinical pharmacology of herbal products. Totowa NJ: Humana Press, 2nd edition, 2000.

Current Practice. Today's Drugs. Drugs of addiction – 1 *BMJ* 1964 24th October; 1055-6; Drugs of addiction – 2 *BMJ* 31st October; 119- 20.

Cutting WC, Meartens HG and Tainter ML. Action and use of Dinitrophenol. Promising metabolic application. *JAMA* 1933; 10: 193.

D'Arcy PF & Griffin JP. (ed) 1986 Iatrogenic diseases, 3rd edition. Oxford University Press.

Dahlgren S. Thorotrast tumoren. Literaturüberblick und Bericht darüber [Thorotrast tumours: review of literature and report thereon]. *Acta Path Microbiol Scand*. 1961; 53: 147.

Dameshek W and Colmes A. Aminopyrine hypersensitivity, with particular reference to effect of drugs in production of agranulocytosis .*J Clin Invest* 1936; 15:85–97.

Danowski TS et al. Lactic acid in diabetes mellitus. *JAMA* 1963;184(1): 169.

Dauriol M. Nouveau procede pour plonger dans la stupeur les maladies qui doivent subir une operation. *Journal de medicine et Chirurgie de Toulouse*. 1847; 10: 178.

David NA, Johnstone HG, Reed AC and Leake CD. The treatment of amebiasis with iodochlorhydroxyquinolone. *JAMA* 1933; 100: 1658.

Davies EB. J *Soc Ciénc Méd Lisb* 1959; 123: 163.

Debue-Barazer C. Le médicament 1803-1940. Histoire et art pharmaceutique. *Ordre Pharmacien*. March 2003. www.ordre.pharmacien.fr/upload/Syntheses/164.pdf Accessed 2nd June 2008.

De Craen AJ M, Kaptchuk TJ, Tijssen JGP and Kleijnen J. Placebos and placebo effects in medicine: historical overview.*J R Soc Med*. 1999:92: 511–515.

Delchier JC, Métreau JM, Lévy VG, Opolon P and Dhumeaux D. L'oxyphénisatine, laxatif responsable d'hepatites chroniques et de cirrhoses… toujours commercialisé en France. *Nouv*

Presse Méd 1979; 8: 37, 2955- 2958.

Depperman D, Heidland A, Ritz E and Hörl W. Lactic acidosis–a possible complication in buformin-treated diabetes. Klin Wochenschr. September 1st 1978; 56(17): 843–53.

Dieckmann WJ, Davis ME, Rynkiewicz LM and Pottinger RE. Does the administration of diethylstilboestrol during pregnancy have therapeutic value? Am J Obstet Gynecol 1953; 66: 1062–81.

Diethelm O. On bromide intoxication. J Nerv Ment Dis 1930;71:151-165.

Dinitrophenol. Not acceptable for new and non-official remedies. Report of the Council of Pharmacy and Chemistry. JAMA July 6 1935; 105: 31.

Dioscorides Pedanius, of Anazarbos 'De Materis Medica: being an herbal with many other medicinal materials: written in Greek in the first century of the Common Era: a new indexed version in modern English by TA Osbaldeston and RPA Wood, Johannesburg: IBIDIS, 2000.

Dioscorides, De noxiis venenis. Cap. xxiii. Venetiis, 1516; p 124.

Direcks A, Figueroa S, Mintzes B and Banta D. DES European Study: DES Action the Netherlands in the European Commission Programme ' Europe against Cancer' Utrecht: DES Action the Netherlands. 1991:13, 25.

Discombe G. Agranulocytosis caused by amidopyrine. An avoidable cause of death. BMJ June 14th 1952;1270–1273.

Doll R. Recognition of unwanted drug effects. BMJ 1969; 2: 69-70.

Doona M and Walsh JB. Use of chloramphenicol as topical eye medication: time to cry halt?. BMJ 1995; 310: 1218 –9.

Doona M. Topical choramphenicol is an outmoded treatment. BMJ 1998; 316: 1903.

Douglas John. A dissertation on the venereal disease. Wherein the safety, and surprising good effects of our method (when managed with judgement not only in all the stages of this distemper… will be further confirm'd by many rare and remarkable cases. London, 1737 Based on information from English Short Title Catalogue. Eighteenth Century Collections Online. Gale Group. http://0-galenet.galegroup.com. libsys.wellcome.ac.uk/servlet/ECCO

Dover, Thomas. The ancient physician's legacy to his country, being what he has collected in forty-nine years practice: ... By Thomas Dovar [sic], M.D. ... London, 1733. Based on information from English Short Title Catalogue. Eighteenth Century Collections Online. Gale Group. http://0-galenet.galegroup.com.libsys. wellcome.ac.uk/servlet/ECCO

Dragstedt CA and Gerauer-Fuelnegg E. Studies in anaphylaxis. Am J Physiol 1932; 102: 512–526.

Draves AH and Walker SE: Analysis of the hypericin and pseudohypericin content of commercially available St. John's wort preparations. Canadian J Clin Pharmacol 10:114–118, 2003 [PMID: 14506510]

Drugs and Narcotics in History. Edited by Roy Porter and Mikuáš Teich. Cambridge University Press, 1995.

Dtsch Med Wschr. 1959; 104: 166.

Dubach UC, Rosner B and Stürmer T. An epidemiologic study of abuse of analgesic drugs. N Engl J Med 1991; 324 (3): 155–160.

Duffin J and René P. 'Anti-moine; Anti-biotique': The public fortunes of the secret properties of antimony potassium tartrate (Tartar emetic). J Hist Med Allied Sci 1991; 46: 440–456.

Dykes MH. Postoperative hepatic dysfunction in perspective. 1970. Int Anesthesiol Clin. 1998; 36(4): 155–62.

Earles MP. Studies in the development of experimental pharmacy in the eighteenth and early nineteenth century. October 1961, University College London PhD thesis.

Ebers G. The papyrus Ebers: the greatest Egyptian medical document. Translated by B Ebell, Munksgaard & Oxford University Press. 1937.

Editorial. Dipyrone hearing by the German Drug Authority. Lancet Sept 27th 1986.

Edwards JE and McQuay HJ. Dipyrone and agranulocytosis: what is the risk? Lancet 2002; 360: Nov 9th.

Elek SR, McNair JD and Griffith GC. Veratrum viride–hypotensive and cardiac effects of intravenous use. Calif Med 1953; 79(4): 300–305.

Engelmann F. Berlin. Klin. Wochenschr. 1870; p 647.

Enia G, Garozzo M and Zoccali C. Lactic acidosis induced by phenformin is still a public health problem in Italy. BMJ 1997; 315: 1466–7.

Erlich P. Ueber einen Fall Anämie mit Bemerkungen über regenerative Veränderungen des Knochenmarks [On a case of anaemia with comments on regenerative changes to the bone marrow]. Charité-Ann 1888: 13: 301–309.

Ernst E and Resch K.L. Concepts of true and perceived placebo effects. BMJ 1995; 311: 551–3.

Ersley A J, and Wintrobe MM. Detection and prevention of drug-induced blood dyscrasias. JAMA 1962; 181: 114, 37.

Esbach and Bérard. Ictère hémolytique mortel après traitement prolongé par l'atophan. Bull Soc Méd Hôpital Paris 1937; 21 Mai: 717.

Esunge PM. From blood pressure to hypertension: the history of research. J R Soc Med 1991; 84(10): 621.

Etkin NL. 'Side effects': cultural constructions and reinterpretations of western pharmaceuticals. Med Anthropol Q 1992; 6(2): 99–113.

Euripides. The Bacchae and other plays. Translated by Philip Velacott. Penguin Classics, 1972.

Evans GM and Gaisford WF. Treatment of pneumonia with 2-(p- aminobenzene sulphonamido) pyridine. Lancet July 2nd 1938; 14–19.

FPHRCP (Faculty of Public Health Royal College of Physicians). A chronology of state medicine, public health welfare and related services in Britain 1066–1990. Compiled by MD Warren 2000.

Fabre, Traité des maladies vénériennes, 1765.

Fabry von Hilden W. Von der Fürtrefflichkeit und Nutz der Anatomie [On the excellence and use of anatomy], H.R. Sauerländer & Co. Aarau, Leipzig. 1936.

Fanconi, Botsztejn and Schenker. Réaction d'hypersensibilité à la médication mercurielle dans l'enfance avec une consideration particulière de la maladie du calomel. Clinique Infantile de Zurich. Helv Paed Acta 1947; Suppl.2.

Farber SM and Eagle HR. Streptomycin therapy of tuberculosis. Calif Med 1948; 69(1): 6–11.

Farrington RF, Hull-Smith H, Bunn PA, and McDermott W. Streptomycin toxicity- reactions to highly purified drug on long-continued administration to human subjects. JAMA 1947; 134: 679.

FDA Modernisation Act of 1997, section 503A (a) Proposed list of agents not to be compounded due to withdrawal for safety/efficacy concerns. (http://www.ijpc.com/chart.html) accessed on 30th April 2002.

FDA. List of drug products that have been withdrawn or removed from the market for reasons of safety or effectiveness. 21 CFR Part 216, 1999.

Featherstone WH. Convulsions following use of Astérol dihydrochloride. Report of a case. JAMA 1952; 150: 1006.

Feinman SE. Beneficial and Toxic Effects of Aspirin. Edited by S E Feinman. CRC Press. 1994.

Feldman WH and Hinshaw HC. Streptomycin: a valuable anti-tuberculosis agent. BMJ 1948 January 17th; 87–92.

Fernel J. De luis venereae curatione perfectissma liber. Antwerp, 1579.

Fiks AP. Self-experimenters: Sources for study. West Port: Praeger Publishers. 2003

Finney DJ. The design and logic of a monitor of drug use. J Chron Dis 1965; 18: 77-98.

Flückner FA and Hanbury D. Pharmacographia; A history of the principal drugs of vegetable origins met with in Great Britain and British India. Second ed. London, MacMillan. and Co, 1879, pp 567–571.

Foster RHK. Standardisation of safety margin. J Pharmacol Experimental Therap 1939; 65: 1–18.

Fouassier Eric. Le cadre général de la loi du 21 germinal An XI. March 2003.

Fowler EP and Seligman E. Otic complications of streptomycin therapy. JAMA 1947; 133(2): 87–91.

Fowler T. Medical reports of the effects of arsenic, in the cure of agues, remitting fevers, and periodic headachs. Together with a letter from Dr Arnold of Leicester, and another from Dr Withering. London 1786, Eighteenth century collections Online, Gale Group.

Francis. The effects of mercury in its natural state and on its abuse in certain diseases. The Medical and Physical Journal 1815; 207.

Fraunfelder FT, Bagby GC, Kelly DJ, Abrams SM, Degnan TJ and Vinciguerra V. Fatal aplastic anaemia following topical administration of ophthalmic chloramphenicol. Am J Ophthlmol 1982; 93: 356–60.

Freie HMP. Antipyretic analgesics. Meyler's 'Side Effects of Drugs'. 14th edition. Eds. Dukes MNG and Aronson JK. Levier, 2000.

Freind John. The history of physick; from the time of Galen, to the beginning of the sixteenth century. Chiefly with regard to practice. In a discourse written to Doctor Mead. By J. Freind, M.D. Part I. Containing all the Greek writers. The second edition, corrected London, 1725. Eighteenth Century Collections Online. Gale Group.

Fréjaville J-P, Bescol J, Leclerk J-P, Guillam L, Crabie P, Conso F, Gervais P and Gaultier M. Intoxication aiguë par les dérivés arsenicaux; (à propos de 4 observations personelles); troubles de l'hémostase; étude ultramicroscopique du foie et du rein. Ann Méd Interne 1972; 123(8–9): 713–722.

Feund* Deuts Med Irchnechr. April 27th 1905.

Frobenius WG. An account of a Spiritus Vini Aetherus. Philos Trans R Soc Lond. 1730.

Fung M, Thornton A, Mybeck K, Hsiao-Hui J, Hornbuckle K and Muniz E. Evaluation of the characteristics of safety withdrawal of prescription drugs from worldwide pharmaceutical markets – 1960–1999. Drug Inf J 2001; 35: 293–317.

Gaisford W. Fatality after oxyphenbutazone in Still's disease. BMJ 1962; 2(5318): 1517.

Garrod EP. The production of bone marrow aplasia by chloramphenicol. In 'Sensitivity Reactions to Drugs' CIOMS Symposium, Ed. ML Rosenheim and R Moulter, Blackwell Science Publications, Oxford.

Garth S. The Dispensary. A Poem. Printer John Nutt, 1699.

Gauchet. Bulletin Génér De Therap. 1871; LXXXX: P 373.

Gazz Int Med Chir 1954; 59: 159.

Geiling EMK and Cannon PR. Pathological effects of elixir of sulfanilamide. (diethylene glycol) poisoning. JAMA 1938; 111: 919–926.

George MH, Moore T, Kilburn S, Olson GR and DeAngelo AB. Carcinogenicity of chloral hydrate administered in drinking water to the male F344/N rat and male B6C3F1 mouse. Toxicol Pathol 2000; 28(4): 610–8.

Gharpure K, Sharma S, Thawani V. Pharmacovigilance: Is it possible if bannable medicines are available over the counter? Indian J Pharmacol June 2005; 37(3): 191–191.

Giertz H, Hahn H and Lange A. Toxicity of phenothiazines. Klin Wschr 1954; 39-40: 983–4.

Giusti RM, Iwamoto K and Hatch EE. Diethylstilboestrol revisited: a review of the long term health effects. Ann Int Med 1995; 122(10): 778–88.

Glasgow JFT. Reye's Syndrome; The case for a causal link. Drug Saf. 2006; 29(12): 1111-1121.

Glauser FI, Smith WH and Caldwell A. Ethchlorvynol (Placidyl) induced pulmonary oedema. Ann Intern Med 1976: 84: 46–48.

Goldberg A. Development of drug regulating authorities. Br J clin Pharmac. 1986; 22: 67s–70s.

Goldberg D. Carisoprodol toxicity. Mil Mede 1969; 134: 597–601.

Goltdammer Several cases of collapse after 5G doses. Berl. Klin. Wochenschr 1876, p 47.

Good, John Mason. The history of medicine, so far as it relates to the profession of the apothecary, From the earliest Accounts to the present Period: the evils to which the profession and the public have been of late Years equally exposed; and the means which have been devised to remedy them. Published at the request of the Committee of the General Pharmceutic Association of Great Britain. By John Mason Good, Fellow of the Medical Society of London, Member of the Corporation of Surgeons, and Author of the ``dissertation on the Diseases of Prisons and Poor houses.'' The second edition. To which are prefixed, observations on a tract, entitled Murepsologia; And published in Answer to the former Edition. London, 1796. Eighteenth Century Collections Online. Gale. The Wellcome Trust. 24 Dec. 2009 http://0-ind.galegroup.com.libsys.wellcome.ac.uk/ecco/infomark.do?&contentSet=ECCOArticles&type=multipage&tabID=T001&prodId=ECCO&docId=CW

Goodall C. The Royal College of Physicians of London. London, 1684.

Goodall EW. Hypersensitivity. Proc RSM 1912; 5(Section Epid. State med) 203–214.

Gordon J. A contribution to the study of piperazine. BMJ June 16th 1894; 1291–1294.

Gottlieb A, Duberstein J and Geller A. Phenformin acidosis. New Eng J Med 1962: 18: 806–9.

Gottlieb R. The effect of colloidal thorium on the blood picture. *Can Med Assoc J* 1933; 28(5): 496-497.

Gøtzsche PC. Non-steroidal anti-inflammatory drugs. *BMJ* 2000; 320: 1058–1061.

Gould GM & Pyle WL. Anomalies and Curiosities of Medicine. Pyle Publisher: The World Wide School. November 1997 Published from: Seattle, Washington, USA.

Goulding R. Wellcome Witness to Twentieth Century Medicine, vol.1, Wellcome Trust, 1997, p116.

Graham JDP and Parker WA. The toxic manifestations of sodium salicylate therapy. *Quart J Med* 1948; 41: 153-163.

Granger GA. Use of Thorotrast. *BMJ* 1967; ii: 112.

Grant Alexander. Observations on the use of opium in diseases supposed to be owing to morbid irritability. By Alexander Grant, ... London, 1785. Based on information from English Short Title Catalogue. Eighteenth Century Collections Online. Gale Group. http://0-galenet.galegroup.com. libsys.wellcome.ac.uk/servlet/ECCO

Grawitz P. Nuevas orientaciones en la terapeutica de las amebiasis. *Semana Med* 1935; 42: 525.

Green FHK. Clinical evaluations of remedies in Britain. *Lancet* 27th November 1954; 1085–1091.

Green FHK. Clinical evaluations of remedies in Britain. *Brit Med Bull* 1944; 2: 58–60.

Greenhalgh T. Drug marketing in the third world: beneath the cosmetic reforms. *Lancet* 1986; June 7th: 1318–1320.

Greenhalgh T, Kostopoulou O and Harries C. Making decisions about benefits and harms of medicines. *BMJ* 2004; 329: 47–50.

Griffin JP. Venetian treacle and the foundation of medicines regulation. *Br J Clin Pharm* 2004; 58(3): 317–325.

Griffin JP and Weber JCP. Voluntary systems of adverse reaction reporting– Part II. *Adv Drug React Ac Pois Rev* 1986; 1: 23–55.

Griffin JP and D'Arcy JP. Adverse drug reactions–the information lag. In Side Effects of Drug Annual V, 1981

Grollman A. Pharmacology and Therapeutics. Lea & Febiger, Philadelphia, 1951.

Grootheest Kees van. The Dawn of Pharmacovigilance. *Int J Pharm Med* 2003; 17 (5-6): 195-200.

Gruner OC. A Treatise on the Canon of Medicine of Avicenna. Luzee & Co. London, 1930.

Grünpeck, Joseph. Tractatus de Pestilentiali Scorra sive Mala de Franzos: Originem Remediaqu[ue] Eiusdem Continens. Nuremberg: Kaspar Hochfeder, 1496 or 1497.

Guglielmo da Brescia, Canon 1.4 Padua, Biblioteca Universitaria, MS al numero provisorio 202, fo. 121v: 'Item si possumus uti via securiori non debemus uti farmacia sed possumus uti via securiori ad evacuationem humorum ut bono regimine et fricationibus et resolventibus et medicinis non dando medicinas fortes.... Item si possumus uti via securiori non debemus uti periculosiori, sed via securior est flobotomia... apparet per Galenum] secunduo regiminis, dicit enim quod flobotomia est via secura evacuanda farmacia autem periculosa...,' as quoted in Nancy Siraisi, Taddeo Alderotti: 254, note 38.) Excellentisimi (1508),

Guibert V. Histoiren naturelle et médicale des nouveaux médicaments introduit dans la thérapeutique depuis 1830 jusqu'a nos jours. Librairie Médicale de H. Manceaux. 1865.

Haggenstoss AH, Feldman WH and Hinshaw HC. Streptomycin in miliary tuberculosis. *Am Rev Tuberc* 1947; 55: 54–75.

Hahnemann S. Organen der reaktionellen Heikunde [Organs of reactional therapy] Dresden: Arnold, 1810. [Organon de l'art de guérir, Dresden 1824].

Hahnemann S. Materia Medica Pura. 1825.

Halls Dalle JF. Discussion on blood-letting. *Proc R Soc Med* 1927 April 7th; 1569.

Hama R. Transmission of drug information to physicians and drug-induced suffering. In: Soda T Ed. Drug Induced Suffering, Excerpta Medica, 1980, 142–150.

Hamburger F and M E. Ueber die biologisch nachweisbaren Veränderungen des menschlichen Blutes nach den Seruminjektion [On the biologically demonstrable changes to human blood after serum injection]. *Wein Klinn Wschr* 1903; 16:445–7.

Hamilton AL (1816). Dissertatio Medica Inauguralis De Synocho Castrensi. Edinburgh: J Ballantyne.

Hamilton Archibald. The effects of semen hyoscami albi. Philosophical Society of Edinburgh. Essays and observations, physical and literary. Vol. II, Edinburgh, 1756.

Hamilton J. Observations on the utility and administration of purgative medicines in several diseases. Edinburgh: J Simpson. 1806.

Hammer W. Holmberg G. Sjoqvist F and Wiklund PE. Drug interaction: lethal interaction between nialamide and blue-veined cheese. *Lakartidningen.* Dec 15 1969; 66: Suppl IV: 20.

Hancher L. Regulating for competition: government, law and the pharmaceutical industry in the United Kingdom and France, 4. PhD thesis. University of Amsterdam.

Handersen HE. Gilbertus Anglicus. Medicine of the thirteenth century. The Cleveland Medical Library Association. 1918.

Hardman W. 'Ehrlich-Hata' or '606'. *BMJ* 1911; 1: 54–55.

Harris Thomas, surgeon. A treatise on the force and energy of crude mercury. ... By Thomas Harris, ... London, 1734. Based on information from English Short Title Catalogue. Eighteenth Century Collections Online. Gale Group. http://0-galenet.galegroup.com.libsys. wellcome.ac.uk/servlet/ECCO

Harrow BR, and Sloane JA. Acute renal failure following oral cholecystography, a unique nephrographic effect. *Am J Med Sci* 1965; 249: 26.

Haselkorn T, Whittemore AS, Udaltsova N and Friedman GD. Short-term choral hydrate administration and cancer in humans. *Drug Saf* 2006; 29(1): 67–77.

Hauben M and Aronson JK. Defining 'signal' and its subtypes in pharmacovigilance based on a systematic review of previous definitions. *Drug Saf* 2009(2); 2: 99–110.

Hayes AW. Principles and Methods of Toxicology. CRC Press. 2001.

Haygarth J. Of the Imagination, as a Cause and as a Case of Disorders of the Body; Exemplified by Fictitious Tractors and Epidemical Convulsions. Bath: Crutwell, 1801.

Heberden W. Antiohpiaka, an essay on Mithridatium and Theriaca. *Medical Tracts* 1745.

Hedenmalm K and Spiget O. Agranulocytosis and other blood dyscrasia associated with dipyrone (metamizole). *Eur J Clin Pharmacol* 2002; 58: 265–274.

Heilman DH, Heilman FR, Hinshaw HL, Nichols DR and Herrell WE. Streptomycin: absorbtion, diffusion, excretion and toxicity. *Am J Med Sci* 1945; 1: 554–559.

Heinlein. Urticaria in Folge der Darreichung von salicylsaurem Natron [Consequences of administration of sodium salicylate]. *Aerztl. Intelligenzblatt.* April 1878.

Herbst AL, Scully RE. Adenocarcinoma of the vagina in adolescence. A report of seven cases including 6 clear cell carcinomas (so-called mesnephromas) *Cancer* 1970; 25: 745–57.

Herbst AI, Vilfelder H and Posakanzer DC. Association of maternal stilboestrol therapy and tumour appearance in young women. *N Engl J Med* 1971; 284: 878.

Herbst AL, Kurman RJ and Poskanzer DC. Clear-cell adenocarcinoma of the genital tract in young females. Registry Report. *N Engl J Med* 1972; 287: 1259–64.

Herisham Y and Taustein V. The antibiotics and the peripheral nerves. *Contin Neurol* (Basel) 1971; 33: 146.

Herxheimer A, Collier J, Rawlins MD, Schönhöfer P, Medawar C, Melrose D, Bannenberg W and Beardshaw V. Butazones under fire. *Lancet* March 9th 1985; 580.

Herxheimer K and Krause D. "Ueber eine bei Syphilitischen vorkommende Quecksilberreaktion". *Deutsch Med Wochenschr* 1902; 28: 895–7.

Hettig RA and Adcock JD. Studies on the toxicity of streptomycin for man: A preliminary report. *Science* 1946; 103(2673): 355–357.

Hill DR and Ryan ET. Management of travellers' diarrhoea. *BMJ* 2008; 337: 863–7.

Hinshaw HC, Feldman WH and Pfuetze KH. Treatment of tuberculosis with streptomycin. *JAMA* 1946; 132(13): 778–782.

Hinshaw HC and Feldman WH. *Proc Mayo Clin* 1945; 20: 313-317.

Hodel C and Bass R. Are newer scientific concepts in regulatory toxicology used timely and appropriately? *Toxicol Lett* 1992; 64/65: 149–155.

Hoffman AM, Butt EM and Hickey NG. Neutropenia following amidopyrine. *JAMA* 1934; 102: 1213.

Holland J, Massie MJ, Grant C and Plumb MM. Drugs ingested in suicide attempts and fatal outcome. *N Y State J Med* 1975; 75: 2343.

Holley HL and Koffler IA. Veratrum viride in treatment of hypertension. *Amer Prac* 1950; 1(8): 840–844.

Holmyard EJ. Medieval Arabic pharmacology. *JRSM* 1935;29:99-108.

Home Francis. Clinical experiments, histories, and dissections. By Francis Home, M.D. Edinburgh, 1780. Based on information from English Short Title Catalogue. Eighteenth Century Collections Online. Gale Group. http://0-galenet.galegroup.com.libsys.wellcome.ac.uk/servlet/ECCO

Homer. The Odysseys of Homer, translated by George Chapman. Published by JR Smith. 1857.

Hong FF. History of medicine in China. When medicine took an alternative path. *McGill J Med* 2004; 8(1): 79–84.

Hooper Robert. A compendious medical dictionary. Containing an explanation of the terms in anatomy, physiology, surgery, materia medica, chemistry, and practice of physic. Collected from the most approved authors by R. Hooper, M.D. ... London, 1798. Based on information from English Short Title Catalogue. Eighteenth Century Collections Online. Gale Group. http://0-galenet.galegroup.com.libsys.wellcome.ac.uk/servlet/ECCO

Horák J, Mertl L and Hrabal P. Severe liver injuries due to sulfamethazole-trimethoprim and sulfamethoxydiazine. *Hepatogastroenterology* 1984; 31(5): 199–200.

Howard John. A treatise on the medical properties of mercury. By John Howard, surgeon. London, 1782. Based on information from English Short Title Catalogue. Eighteenth Century Collections Online. Gale Group. http://0-galenet.galegroup.com.libsys.wellcome.ac.uk/servlet/ECCO

HP. 'Stalinon': A therapeutic disaster. *BMJ* March 1st 1958; 515.

Hróbjartsson A, Gøtzsche PC and Glund C. The controlled clinical trial turns 100 years: Fibiger's trial of serum treatment of diphtheria. *BMJ* 1998; 317:1243–1245.

Hubbard WH. Public health in Norway 1603-2003. *Med Hist* 2006; 50(1): 113–117.

Huchard H. Traité clinique des maladies du coeur et des vaisseaux. 1893.

Huette M. On the activity of bromide of potassium . *The British and Foreign Medico-chirurgical Review.* 1850; VI: July–October, 555–6 Quoting the Gazette Médicale.

Huffman MA, Gotoh S, Izutsu D, Koshimizu K and Kalunde MS. (Further observations on the use of the medicinal plant, Vernonia amygdalina (Del) by a wild chimpanzee, its possible effect on parasite load, and its phytochemistry. African Study Monographs 1993; 14(4): 227–240.

Huffman MA. Self-medicative behaviour in the African great apes: An evolutionary perspective into the origins of human traditional medicine. *Bioscience* 2001; 51: Issue 8:651–662.

Huffman MA. The medicinal use of plants by chimpanzees in the wild, primate research at Institute, Kyoto University, Japan, http://jinrui.zool.kyoto-u.ac.jp/CHIMPP/CHIMPP.html. 1996 Accessed 25th February 2008.

Huguley CM. Agranulocytosis induced by dipyrone, a hazardous antipyretic and analgesic. *JAMA* 1964; 189: 162–165.

Hutchinson R and Hunter D. Clinical methods. Cassell and Company Ltd., 1951.

Hutchinson R and Rainy H. Clinical methods, Cassell and Company Ltd., 1902.

Hummel AW. The printed herbal of 1249 A.D. *Isis,* 1941; 33(4): 439–442.

Hunter M. Boyle versus the Galenists: a suppressed critique of seventeenth-century medical practice and its significance. *Med Hist* 1997; 41:322–361.

Huxtable RJ. The harmful potential of herbal and other plant products. *Drug Saf* 1990; 5 (Suppl.1):126–136.

Hyman HT. A critical evaluation of the results of routine conservative treatment of syphilis. *Bull New York Acad Med* 1941; 17(6): 467–487.

Ibáñez L, Ballarin E, Pérez E, Vidal X, Capellà D and Laporte JR. Agranulocytosis induced by pyrithyldione, a sedative drug. *Eur J Clin Pharmacol* Jan 2000; 55; 761–4.

Ibáñez L, Vidal X, Ballarín E and Laporte J-R. Population-based drug-induced agranulocytosis. *Arch Int Med* 2005; 165.

Imerman SS and Imerman CP. Dinitophenol poisoning. *JAMA* 1936; 106(13): 1085–1087.

Inman PM , Gordon B and Trinder P. Mercury absorption and psoriasis. *BMJ* 1956 November 24th; 1202 1206

Inman WH. Study of fatal bone marrow depression with special reference to phenylbutazone and oxyphenbutazone. *BMJ* 1977; 1: 1500–1505.

International Agranulocytosis and Aplastic Anaemia Study. Risks of agranulocytosis and aplastic anaemia, A first report of their relation to drug use with special reference to analgesics. *JAMA* 1986; 256; 1749–1757.

J Belge Radiol 1956; 29: 607.

Jack WR. Wheeler's Handbook of Medicine. 5th edition E & S Livingstone, 1916.

Jaffe AM, Gephardt D and Courtemanche L. Poisoning due to ingestion of Veratrum viride (false hellebore). *J Emerg Med* 1990; 8:161–7.

Jain KK. Drug-induced neurological disorders. Hogrefe & Huber Publishers. 2nd edition, 2001.

James R. (Robert). Pharmacopœia universalis: or, a new universal English dispensatory ... By R. James, M.D. ... The second edition. With very large and useful additions, and improvements London, 1752. Based on information from English Short Title Catalogue. Eighteenth Century Collections Online. Gale Group. http://0-galenet.galegroup. com.libsys.wellcome.ac.uk/servlet/ECCO

Janovsky RC. Fatal thrombocytopenic purpura after administration of sulfamethoxypyridazine. *JAMA* 1960; 172: 155.

Jarisch A. "Therepeutische Versuche bei Syphilis". *Wien Med Wochenschr* 1895; 45: 721–42.

Jisaka M, Ohigashi H, Takegawa H, Hirota M, Irie R, Huffman MA and Koshimizu K. Steroid glucosides from Vernonia amygdalina, a possible chimpanzee medicinal plant. *Phytochemistry* 1993; 34(2): 409–413.

Johnson WM and Korst DR. Pancytopenia associated with sulfamethoxypyridazine administration. *JAMA* 1961; 175: 967.

Johnstone F. Acute mercury poisoning: report of twenty-one cases with suggestions for treatment. *Can Med Assoc J* 1931 April; 500–507.

Jones J. In Idiosyncratic adverse drug reactions: impact on drug development and clinical use after marketing. *Excerpta Medica*, Amsterdam–New York Oxford 1990; 78.

Jones CE. A Pharmacopoeia Empirica of 1748. *Bull Med Libr Assoc* 1957; 45(2): 220-237.

Jörg ME and Aguirre JA. Late effects of 'Thorium' used in radiological investigations. *BMJ* 1934; 1(3818): E37–E40.

Jovic P. The first witness of separation of medicine and pharmacy. Sci Soc for the hist of Serbian Health Culture. 283 www.bium.univ.paris5.fr/ISHM/abstract

Kahn A and Blum D. Phenothiazines and Sudden Infant Death syndrome. *Pediatrics* 1982; 70(1): 75-8.

Kahn A and Blum D. Possible role of phenothiazines in Sudden Infant Death. *Lancet* 1979; 1: 364.

Kalinowski SZ, Lloyd TW and Moyes EN. Complications in the chemotherapy of tuberculosis. *Am Rev Resp Dis* 1961; 82: 391 –371.

Kassel D. Les spécialités pharmaceutiques d'aujoud'hui sont nées dans les officines d'hier. Histoire et art pharmaceutique. www.ordere.pharmacien.fr. accessed 22nd November 2008.

Katahira K. SMON probably occurred in 1938 in Japan. *JAMA* 1976; 236(8): 919.

Kaufman DW, Kelly JP, Jurgelon JM, Anderson T, Issaragrisil S, Wiholm B-E, Young NS, Leaverton P, Levy M, and Shapiro S. Drugs in the aetiology of agranulocytosis and aplastic anaemia. *Eur J Haematol* 1996; 57(suppl): 23–30.

Kawachi T. Mutagenicity test for monitoring drugs to prevent DNA damage. In: Soda T ed. Drug-Induced Suffering, 1980; 56–61.

Kebler LT, Morgan F and Rupp P. The harmful effects of acetanilide, antipyrin and phenacetin. US Department of Agriculture, Bulletin 126, 1909.

Keefer CS, Blake FG, Lockwood JS, Long PH, Marshall EK and Wood WB. Streptomycin in the treatment of infections. A report on a thousand cases. *JAMA* 1946; 132: 70–77.

Kelly J. Health for sale: mountebanks, doctors, printers and the supply of medication in eighteenth-century Ireland. *Proceedings of the Royal Irish Academy* 2008;108C:75–113.

Kennedy WP. The nocebo reaction. *Med World* 1961; 95: 203-205.

Kereković M and Curković M. Olfactoxicity of streptomycin. *Int Rhinol (Leiden)* 1971; 9: 97–8.

Kerr CE, Milne I and Kaptchuk TJ. William Cullen and a missing mind-body link in the early history of placebos. *J R Soc Med* 2008; 101: 89–92.

Ketham J. de. The Fasciculus Medicinae of Johannes de Ketham, Alemanus : facsimile of the first (Venetian) edition of 1491. With English translation by Luke Demaitre; commentary by Karl Sudhoff; trans. and adapted by Charles Singer. (Birmingham, Ala.): The Classics of Medicine Library, 1988.

Key George. A dissertation on the effects of mercury on human bodies, in the cure of the venereal disease, London, 1747.

Kingcade GF, Saxton GD, Morse Pwand and Mathisen AK. Streptomycin in the treatment of tuberculosis. *Can Med Assoc J* 1948; 59: 105–112.

King S. A Fylde Country Practice. Medicine and Society in Lancashire, circa 1760–1840. Centre for North-West Regional Studies at the University of Lancashire. 2001. p45.

King's American Dispensatory 1898 www.henriettesherbal.com

King, *Vierteljahrschr Dermatologie und Syphilis*, 1879; p370.

Kitchener S, Malekottodjary N and McClelland GR. Adverse effects from placebo-treated healthy volunteers. *Br J Clin Pharm* 1996; 41: 473P.

Kono R. Subacute myelo-optic-neuropathy. A new neurological disease prevailing in Japan. *Jpn J Med Sci Biol* 1971; 24: 195-216.

Kotslas BA. Scopolamine and the murder of King Hamlet. *Arch Otolaryngol Head Neck Surg.* 2002; 128: 847–849.

Koutsaimanis DG and Wardener HE de. Phenacetin nephropathy, with particular reference to the effect of surgery. *BMJ* 1970; 4(5728): 131–4.

Kracke RR and Parker FP. The relationship of drug therapy to agranulocytosis. *JAMA* 1935; 105: 960–966.

Kracke RR. Agranulocytosis: Its classification; cases and comments illustrating the granulopenic trend from 8000 blood counts in the South. Ann. Internal Med. 6: ... *Am J Clin Pathol* 1931; 1: 385.

Krakoff IH, Karnofsky DA and Burchenal JH. Effects of large doses of chloramphenicol on human subjects. *N Engl J Med* 1975; 253: 7-10.

Kuborn M. Poisoning by strammonium and by hyoscyamus. *BMJ* 1866; 1: 522–526.

Kühn B. The annual museum. *BMJ* 1894 August 25th; 2(1756): 414–423.

Kushimoto H and Aoki T. Toxic erythema with gene raised follicular pustules caused by streptomycin. *Arch Dermatol* 1981; 17: 444.

Lacassagne A. Apparition des adenocarcinomes mammaires chez des souris males traités par une substance œstrogène synthetique. *C R Séances Soc Biol.* 1938; 129 : 641–3.

Lambin and Gerard. *Rev Belge des Sci Med* 1931; 3: 891.

Lancaster T, Swart AM and Jick H. Risk of serious haematological toxicity with use of chloramphenicol eye drops in a British general practice database. *BMJ* 1998; 316: 667.

Larrick GP. How the Food and Drug Administration evaluates New Drug Applications. Appendix A, In 'Clinical Testing of New Drugs' Ed AD Herrick and M Cattell, Revere Publishing Company, Inc 1965.

Larsen K, Moller CE. A renal lesion caused by abuse of phenacetin. *Acta Med Scand* 1959; 164: 53–71

Lasser KE, Seger DL, Yu DT, Karson AS, Fiskio JM, Seger AC, Shah NR, Gandhi TK, Rothschild JM and Bates DW. Adherence to black box warnings for prescription medications in outpatients. *Ann Intern Med* 2006; 166(3): 338–344.

Latham R. The shorter Pepys. Folio Society 1985.

Laughlin S and Jackson R. A brief history of drug reactions. *Clin Dermatol* 1986;4(1): 1–14.

Launay C, Fabiani P, Grenet P, Hadenour A, Solignac and Strauss, Un nouveau cas d'acrodynia avec presence de mercure dans les urines. *Arch Fr Péd* 28th Juin 1949;7: 21.

Le Clerc D. Histoire de la Médicine. Amsterdam, G Gallet, 1702; XVI: 188.

Le Quesne PM. Toxic substances and the nervous system: the role of clinical observation. *J Neurol Neurosurger Psychiatry* 1981; 44 :1–8.

Leader. Datura preparations banned in France. *New Sci* (22 August 1992).

Leader. Dipyrone hearing by the German drug authorities. *Lancet* September 27th 1986.

Leader. Streptomycin in tuberculosis. *BMJ* 1947; 2(4516): 136–138.

Leader. Today's drugs. *BMJ* 1963;1:107-8.

Leake CD. The pharmacologic evaluation of new drugs. *JAMA* 1929; 93(21): 1632–36.

Lechat P. Periodical re-evaluation of the undesirable side effects of old drugs. An important mission of drug surveillance. *Nouv Presse Méd.* 1974; 3(24): 1571–3.

Lee MR. Solanaceae IV. Atropa belladonna. Deadly Nightshade. *J R Coll Physician Edin* 2007; 37: 77–94.

Leech DJ and Hunter W. An inquiry regarding the importance of ill-effects following the use of antipyrin, antifebrin,and phenacetin conducted by the Therapeutic Committee of the British Medical Association. *BMJ* 1894; January 13: 85–90.

Lees DB. The effective treatment of acute or subacute rheumatism. *Proc R Soc Med* 1909; 2: 34–48.

Lenyer AR, Lockie M and Becker CF. Acute yellow atrophy following cincophen administration. *New Eng J Med* 1947; 236: 500–4.

Lenz W. Lecture at 1992 UNITH Congress http://www.Thalidomide.ca/history.html

Leonard JC. Toxic effects of phenylbutazone with special reference to disorders of the blood. *BMJ* 1953; 1: 1311.

Leroux Henri. Découvert de la salicine, *J Chem Med* 1830; 6: 341.

Leung AY. Chinese medicinals. In Janick J and Simon LE. Advances in New Crops. Timber Press, Portland OR. USA., 1990. http://www.hort.purdue.edu/newcrop/proceedings1990/V1-499.html#INTRODUCTION. Accessed 26th February 2008.

Lev Efraim and Zohar Amar. Practical Materia Medica of the Medieval Eastern Mediterranean According to the Cairo Genizah . Leiden: Brill, 2008.

Levey M. Medieval Arabic toxicology: The book on poisons of Ibn Wahshiya and its relation to early Indian and Greek texts. *Transactions of the American Philosophical Society*: New Series; 1966; 56: pt 7.

Levi C. Cristo si è fermato a Eboli. Einaudi Tascabile 1945.

Levy AG. Heart irregularities resulting from the inhalation of low percentages of chloroform vapour, and the relationship to ventricular fibrillation. *Heart* 1911; 3: 99.

Levy M. Epidemiological evaluation of rare side-effects of mild analgesics. *Br J Clin Pharmacol* 1980; 10(suppl 2): 396s–399s.

Lévy-Valenai J. La Médicine et les médicins Français au XVII siècle. Paris Bailiere, 1933

Lewin DL. Les Paradis Artificiels. Translated by DF Gidon. Payot Paris, 1928.

Lewin L. Untoward Effects of Drugs, A Pharmacological and Clinical manual. Translated by JJ Muheron, George S Davis, Detroit, Michigan 1883.

Lewin R. Stone Age Psychedelia, *New Sci* 8th June 1991, p30.

Lewis A. Why does the Committee on Safety of Medicines do what it does? *BMJ* July 28th 1979; 2(6184): 274.

Lewis CN, Putnam LE, Hendricks FD, Kerland I and Welch H. Chloramphenicol (Chloromycetin) in relation to blood dyscrasias with observations on other drugs. A special survey. *Antibiot. & Chemother* 1952; 2(12): 601–609.

Lewis T and Grant RT. Vascular reactions of the skin to injury . II The liberation of a histamine-like substance in injured skin; the underlying cause of factitious urticaria and of wheals by burning and observations upon the nervous control of certain skin reactions. *Heart* 1924; 11: 209–65.

Lexchin J. Drug withdrawals from the Canadian market for safety reasons, 1963–2004. *Can Med Assoc J* March 15th 2005; 172(6); doi:10.1503/cmaj.045021.

Lietava J. 'Medicinal plants in a Middle Paleolithic grave Shanidar IV?' Science, 190 (28): 880. In: *J Ethnopharmacol* 1992; 35(3): 263-6. ISSN: 0378–8741) (18).

LijinskyW, Reuber MD and Blackwell BN 198. Liver tumors induced in rats by oral administration of the antihistaminic methapyrilene hydrochloride. *Science* 1980; 209: 817–819).

List of banned products, which failed to record in other countries, cited in the book: Banned Products – UN. They are present in the Brazilian market. (http://www.uol.com.br/idec/lista.doc) Accessed December 2001.

Liu Yanchi. The Essential book of traditional Chinese medicine. Volume 2 Clinical practice, Columbia University Press. 1988.

Lloyd J U. May 23rd. History of the Vegetable Drugs of the U.S.P. 1911: P105. www.swsbm.com/manualsother/USP_Drug_History_Lloyd.pdf accessed 2nd June 2008.

Loewy F. Thrombocytopenic purpura from Sedormid. *BMJ* August 6th 1938: 320.

Loewy F. Thrombocytopenic haemorrhagic purpura due to idiosyncrasy towards the hypnotic Sedormid: allergotoxic effect. *Lancet* 1934; 223: 845–6.

Loke YK, Price D and Aronson JK. Case reports of suspected adverse drug reactions- systemic literature survey of follow-up. *BMJ* 2006; 332: 335–339.

London physician. The modern quack; or, the physical impostor, detected. In three parts. ... With a supplement, displaying the present set of pretenders to clap-curing, ... To which ... a catalogue is annexed of all the members of the Royal College of Physicians, ... By a London physician. London, 1718. Based on information from English Short Title Catalogue. Eighteenth Century Collections Online. Gale Group. http://0-galenet.galegroup.com.libsys.wellcome.ac.uk/servlet/ECCO

López-Muñoz F, Álamo C and García-G P. Psychotrophic drugs in the Cervantine texts. *J R Soc Med.* 2008; 101: 226–234. DOI 10,1258/krsm.2008.070269.

Loudon I. Medical Care and the General Practitioner 1750–1850. Clarendon Press, Oxford, 1986; p19.

Loudon I. The use of historical controls and concurrent controls to assess the effects of sulphonamides, 1936–1945. *J R Soc Med* 2008;101: 148–155.

Louis PCA. Recherche sur les effets de la saignée dans plusieurs maladies inflammatoires. *Archives générales de Médecine* 1828; 18: 321–336.

Louis-Courvoisier M. An 18th century controlled trial prompted by a potential shortage of hospital beds. *J R Soc Med* 2007; 100(10): 481-482; doi: 10.1258/jrsm.100.10.481.

Lucey HC. The therapeutic and reaction effects of Kharsivan. *BMJ* 1916; 1: 614–616.

Luft D, Schmülling RM and Eggstein M. Lactic acidosis in biguanide-treated diabetics: a review of 330 cases. *Diabetologia* 1978;14: 75–87.

Lunde PKM. Drug and product selection - an essential part of the therapeutic benefit/risk ratio strategy? In: Soda T Ed. Drug-Induced Sufferings: Excerpta Medica, 1980: 129–136.

MacCallum RI. Antimony in medical history: an account of the medical uses of antimony and its compounds since early times to the present. Pentland Press Edinburgh 1999.

MacGregor AB. The search for a chemical cure for cancer. *Med Hist* 1966 October; 10(4): 374-385.

Madison FW and Squier TL. The etiology of primary granulocytopenia (agranulocytic angina) *JAMA* 1934; 102: 755–9.

Maeder T. Adverse Reactions. New York: William Morrow 1994.

Maehle A-H. Opium: explanations of an ambiguous drug in drugs on trial: experiential pharmacology and therapeutic innovation in the eighteenth century. *Clio Medica* 1999; 53, Rodopi.

Magendie F. Lectures on blood. Philadelphia. Haswell, Barrington and Haswell, 1839.

MacMahon B. More on Bendectin. *JAMA* 1981; 246: 371–2.

Making Medicines – A brief history of Pharmacy and Pharmaceuticals. Ed. Stuart Anderson. Pharmaceutical Press. 2005.

Malon De M. Preserver of the blood: or bleeding demonstrated to be always pernicious, and often mortal. London: Wilson & Nicol, 1774.

Malt RA, Olken HG and Goade WJ. Renal tubular necrosis after oral cholecystography. *Arch Surg* 1963; 87: 743.

Manigand G. Accidents neurologiques des médicaments. *Thérapie* 1982; 37: 113-141.

Mann R. Modern Drug Use. An enquiry on historical principles, MTP Press Ltd. 1984.

Maoshing Ni (translator) The essential text of Chinese health and healing. The Yellow Emperors Classic of Medicine. Shambala Publications, Boston.

Mapother ED. Piperazine and other eliminents in the treatment and prevention of gout. *Practitioner* October 1894.

Marson P and Pasero G. Il contibuto Italiano alla storia dei salicilati. *Reumatismo* 2006; 58(1): 66–75.

Marten J. A treatise of the Venereal Disease. 7th edition, 1711.

Martinet L. A manual of pathology containing the symptoms, diagnosis and morbid characters of diseases, together with an exposition of the different methods of examination applicable to the affections of the head, chest and abdomen. Translated with notes and Additions by Jones Quain. 2nd ed. London: W Simpkin and R Marshall, 1827.

Martinez-L J, Letona L, Barbolla L, Frieyro E, Bouza E, Gilsanz F and Fernández MN. Immune haemolytic anaemia and renal failure induced by streptomycin. *Br J Haematol* 1977; 35: 561.

Masheter HC. The Debendox saga. *BMJ* 1985; 291: 1580.

Mathias A. Mercurial disease: an inquiry into the history and nature of the disease produced in the human. London: Becket & Ponder, 1810

Mattioli PA. Dioscorides. De materia medica. Translated by Pietro Andrea Mattioli. Venice: Bascarini, 1544; 443 pp.

Mauer EF. The Toxic Effects of Pheny Ibutazone(Butazolidin), review of the literature and report of the twenty-third death following its use. *New Engl J Med*; 253(10): 404–410.

Mayanagi M. Pharmacotherapy and Chinese hygienic concepts as seen in the Xiao Pin Fang of medieval China. Proceedings of the 12th International Symposium on the Comparative History of Medicine. 1987 Susono-shi, Shizuoka, Japan.

Maywood Robert. An essay, on the operation of mercury, in the human body; in which, the manner how salivation is produced, by that medicine, is attempted to be explained: interspersed with observations on the treatment of the venereal disease. By Robert Maywood, ... London, 1787. Based on information from English Short Title Catalogue. Eighteenth Century Collections Online. Gale Group. http://0-galenet.galegroup.com.libsys.wellcome.ac.uk/servlet/ECCO

McCarthy DD and Chalmers TM. Hematological complications of phenylbutazone therapy: review of the literature and report of two cases' *Canad Med Ass J* 1964; 90: 1061–1067.

McConaghey RMS. The dawn of state medicine in Britain. *Pro Roy Soc Med.* 1967; 60: 483–487.

McCredie J. Chapter 2 in 'Beyond Thalidomide. Birth defects explained'. RSM Press. 2008.

McDermott W. Toxicity of streptomycin. *Am J Med* 1947; 2: 491–500.

McEwen J. Adverse reactions–a personal view of their history. *Int J Pharm Med* 1999; 13: 269–277.

410

McHardy G and Balart LA. Jaundice and oxyphenisatin. *JAMA* 1970; 211(1): 83–85.

McKenna T. Food of the Gods, Bantam Books, New York, 1992.

Mead Richard. A mechanical account of poisons in several essays. By Richard Mead, M.D. ... The second edition, revised, with additions London, 1708. Based on information from English Short Title Catalogue. Eighteenth Century Collections Online. Gale Group. http://0-galenet.galegroup.com.libsys.wellcome.ac.uk/servlet/ECCO

Meade TW. Subacute myelo-optic neuropathy and clioquinol. *Brit J Prev Soc Med* 1975; 29: 157–169.

Medawar C. Power and Dependence, Social Audit on the safety of drugs, Social Audit Ltd. 1992.

Medical Research Council. Streptomycin treatment of pulmonary tuberculosis. *BMJ* 1948; ii: 769–782.

Medico-legal. Deaths due to Butazolodin. *BMJ* 1952; 2: 1427.

Mellin GW and Katzenstein M. The saga of thalidomide. Neuropathy to embyopathy, with case reports of congenital anomalies. *New Engl J Med* 1962; 267(23): 1184–1193.

Menkes DB. Hazardous drugs in developing countries. *BMJ* 1997; 315: 1557–1558.

Menninger WC. Skin eruptions with phenobarbital (Luminal). *JAMA* 1928; July 7th: 14–18.

Merlin MD. On the Trail of the Ancient Opium Poppy. (1984) London, AUP.

Meyrick William. The new family herbal; or, domestic physician: ... By William Meyrick, surgeon. Birmingham, 1789. Based on information from English Short Title Catalogue. Eighteenth Century Collections Online. Gale Group. http://0-galenet.galegroup.com.libsys.wellcome.ac.uk/servlet/ECCO

Mez-Mangold L. A history of Drugs, 1971; p83. F Hoffman-La Roche and Co., Basle.

MHRA, Safety of Herbal Medicinal Products, 2002. http://www.mhra.gov.uk/home/idcplg?IdcService=GET_FILE&dID=665&noSaveAs=0&Rendition=WEB.

Mialhe L. Die Recepturkunst [On the art of formulation], übers. [transl.] Von Biefel. Breslau, 1852; 239.

Michaelis F. On the efficacy of opium in the cure of venereal disease. *Medical Communications* 1784; 1: XXIII p 307.

Miller CG and Carpenter R. Neurotoxic side effects of piperazine. *Lancet* Apr 22nd 1967; 1(7495):895-6.

Milne I and Chalmers I (2002). Hamilton's report of a controlled trial of bloodletting, 1816. The James Lind Library (www.jameslindlibrary.org). Accessed Monday 2 February 2009. © Iain Milne, 2002.

Milot SHB, Els J, Neustadt ND, Oliff HS, Oppel M, Rapp C, Webb D and Von Bingen H. Hildegard von Bingen's Physica. *Healing Arts*, Rochester, Vermont (1998).

Minkenhet JE. Lange Kuren. *Ned Tijdschr Geneeskd* 1950; 94: 2129.

Molitor H. Pharmacology of streptomycin. *Bull N Y Acad Med* 1947; 23: 196–206.

Moore TJ. Serious adverse drug events reported to the Food and Drug Administration, 1998-2005. *Arch Int Med* 2007; 167: 1752–9.

Morabia A. Piere-Charles-Alexandre Louis and the evaluation of bloodletting. *J R Soc Med* 2006; 99: 158–160.

Morano RA. Drug abuse involving stramonium alkaloids. *Med Leg Bull* 1972 Jan; 21(1): 1-6.

Morgan AA. Agranulocytosis caused by cincophen. *BMJ* July 3rd 1954; 2: 4878.

Mori H, Sugie S, Niwa K, Takahashi M and Kawai H . Induction of intestinal tumours in rats by Chrysazin. *Br J Cancer* 1985; 52: 781–783.

Mori H, Sugie S, Niwa K, Yoshimi N, Tanaba T and Hiron I. Carcinogenicity of Chrysazin in large intestine and liver of mice. *Jpn J Cancer Res (Gann)* 1986; 77: 871-876.

Morrow PA. The etiology and pathogenesis of drug eruptions. *J Cutaneous and Venerial Diseases*. 1885:3: 104–110 and 130–135.

Morse RM and Chua L. Carisoprodol dependence: a case report. *Am J Drug Alcohol Abuse* 1978; 5(4): 527-30.

Morton HG and Durham NC. Atropine intoxication, its manifestations in infants and children. *J Pediatrics*. 1939; 14: 755–760.

Morton K. Convulsions following diamthazole (Asterol). *Am J Dis Child* Jan 1960; 99:109.

Morton LT. A medical bibliography (Garrison and Morton) an annotated check-list of texts illustrating the history of medicine. 3rd edition, Andre Deutsch. 1970, p 28.

Moshe Maor. Organizational reputations and the observability of public warnings in 10 pharmaceutical markets. In The Israel National Institute for Health Policy Research 'Patients, Physicians and Pharma'. Workshop Report. Ed. H Halkin and O Tal. April 2006; Haifa.

Motherby George. A New Medical Dictionary, or, general repository of physic containing an explanation of the terms and description of the various particulars ' 2nd edition. London 1785.

MRC. Streptomycin in Tuberculosis Trials Committee. Streptomycin treatment of pulmonary tuberculosis. *BMJ*; 1948; ii: 769–782.

MRC. At National Archives: FD1/6769, FD1/7943, FD1/3157/20, FD1/3157/21, FD1/6775c, FD1/3157/12b pt3, FD1/6758, FD1/3157/12b pt3, FD1/6763 and FD1 6764. 2009.

Nachmann R, Javid J, and Krauss S. Streptomycin induced haemolytic anaemia. *Arch Int Med* 1962; 110: 187.

Nakamura S and Kawamura M. The Coralgil trial in Japan and its future problems. In; Drug-induced sufferings Medical, pharmaceutical and legal aspects' Ed. T Soda Excerpta medica International Congress series 513.

Nasser M and Tibi A. Ibn Hindu and the science of medicine. *J R Soc Med* 2007; 100: 55–56.

Nassim JR and Pilkington T. Toxic effects of phenylbutazone. *BMJ* 1953; June 13th: 1310–1311.

National Audit office (NAO) Safety, quality, efficacy: regulating medicines in the UK. 2003; 20: 3.13–3.16.

Nations Health. *Am J Public Health* October 1934; 24(10): 1045–1053.

Nencini Paolo, 'The rules of drug taking: wine and poppy derivatives in the Ancient World. VIII. Lack of evidence of opium addiction' *Subst Use Misuse* 1997; 32(11): 1581–6. PMID 9336867.

Nestor JG. Results of the failure to perform adequate preclinical studies before administering new drugs to humans. *S Afr Med J/SA Medtese Tydskrif* 1975; 49, 287–290.

Nettleship AH, Henshaw PS and Meyer HL. Induction of pulmonary tumors in mice with ethyl carbamate. *J Natl Cancer Inst* 1943; 4: 309–319.

Nettleton T. A letter from Dr Nettleton, physician at Halifax in Yorkshire, to Dr Whitaker, concerning the innoculation of the smallpox. *Philos R Soc London* 1724; 32: 35–48.

411

Newman BA. Phenolphthalein intoxication. *JAMA* 1933; 101(10): 761.

Newman C. Physical signs in the London hospitals. *Med Hist.* 1958; 2: 195–201.

News *BMJ* 2007;334:1132, doi: 10.1136/bmj.39227.457037.4E

Neyman J. Statistics Servant of All Sciences. *Science* 1955; 122(3166): 401–406.

Nicholls AG. Nicolas de Blegny and the first medical periodical. *Can Med Assoc J* 1934 August; 198–202.

Nichols DR and Herrell WE. Streptomycin its clinical uses and limitations. *JAMA* 1946; 132: 200–206.

Nutton V. Roman medicine, 250 BC to AD 200. In The Western Medical Tradition 800 BC to AD 1800. Conrad LI, Neve M, Nutton V, Porter R and Wear A. Cambridge University Press,1995.

Oakley GP. The neurotoxicity of the halogenated hydroxyquinolines. In: Soda T Ed. Drug-Induced Sufferings. 1980: 90–96.

O'Carroll RE, Masterton G, Dougall N, Ebmeier KP, Goodwin GM. The neuropsychiatric sequelae of mercury poisoning: The Mad Hatter's disease revisited. *Br J Psychiatry* 1995; 167:95–98.

Ödergård S and Löfroth .The Swedish Lex Maria–patient injuries and historical perspective. In Swedish. *Nordisk Medicin* 1996; III, 352–355.

Oeppen J and Vaupel JW. Broken limits to life expectancy. *Science* 2002; 296: 1029–30.

Ogilvie CM. The treatment of pulmonary tuberculosis with iproniazid (1-isonicotinyl-2-isopropyl hydrazine) and isoniazid (isonicotinyl hydrazine). *Quart J Med* New series xxiv, 1955; 94: 175–186.

Oke WS. Mercurial ptyalism and erethism. *Association Medical Journal* 1856; November 8th: 952-954.

Orlowski JP, Hanhan UA. and Fiallos MR. Is aspirin a cause of Reye's syndrome? A case against'. *Drug Saf* 2002: 25 (4) 225–2321.

Orlowski JP, Hanhan U and Fiallos M. The authors' reply. *Drug Saf* 2005; 27(1): 73–4.

Orme M L'E. The Debendox saga. *BMJ* 1985; 291: 918–9.

Ormerod FC. Tuberculosis of the upper air passages. In Modern Trends in Diseases of the Ear, Nose and Throat. Ed. Maxwell Ellis, Butterworths & Co. 1954.

O'Shea JG. 'Two minutes with Venus, two years with mercury'–mercury as an antisyphilitic chemotherapeutic agent. *J R Soc Med* 1990; 83:392–395.

P.O. Box 144345 Austin, TX 78714 – 4345 512.926.4900 Fax: 512.926.2345 www.herbalgram.org. Accessed 25th February 2008.

Palmlund I, Apfel R, Buitendijk S, Cabau A and Forsberg J-G. Effects of diethylstilboestrol (DES) medication during pregnancy: report from a symposium at the 10th International Congress of ISPOG. *J Psychosomatic Obst & Gynae* 1993; 14(1): 71–89.

Parascandola JL. Diet and die with excess alpha dinitrophenol. *Drug Intell Clin Pharm* 1977; 11: 439.

Paris J. Pharmacologia; or the history of medicinal substances,with a view to establish the art of prescribing and of composing extemporaneous formulae upon fixed and serendipitous principles. London: WPhillips, 1820

Parsons AC. Piperazine neurotoxicity: 'worm wobble.' *BMJ* December 25th 1971; 4(5790): 792.

Parsons L and Kimball T. Fatalities due to cinchophen. *Calif West Med* October 1931; 35(4): 307–308.

Penn RG. 'The State control of medicines: the first 3000 years. *Br J Clin Pharmacol* 1979; 8: 293-305.

Petersen FJ. The Materia Medica and Clinical Therapeutics, 1905.

Pfister JA. Behavioral Strategies for Coping with Poisonous Plants. Presented in 'Grazing Behaviour of Livestock and Wildlife.'1999. Idaho Forest, Wildlife & Range Exp. Sta. Bull. #70, Univ. of Idaho, Moscow, ID. Editors: KL Launchbaugh, KD Sanders, JC Mosley.

Phillips WA and Avigan J. *Proc Soc Exp Biol Med* 1963; 112: 233–6.

Physicians' Health Study Research Group. Final report on the aspirin component of the ongoing Physicians' Health Study Reseach Group. *NEJM* 1989; 321(3): 129–35.

Pilpoul P. La quarelle de l'antimoine (Essai historique) Paris. Librairie Louis Annette 1928.

Pirquet von Cesenatico CP. Klinische Studien uber Vakznation und vakzinale Allergie Leipzig F. Deuticke, 1907.

Pirquet C and Schick B. Die Serumkrankheit. *Wien, F. Deuticke*, 1905.

Pirquet C. Klinische Studien über Vakzination und vakzinale Allergie. *Münch Med Wochenschr*, 1906, 53, 1457-1458.

Plaitakis A and Duvoisin RC. Homer's moly identified as Galanthus nivalis L: physiologic antidote to strammonium poisoning. *Clin Neuropharmacy* 1983; 6(1): 1–5.

Poelman S. Foxgloves, woody beans, and old hag. Nothing new under the sun. Proceedings of the 11th annual History of Medicine. Faculty of Medicine, University of Calgary. 2002.

Polatin P and Horwitz W. Clinical evaluation of new sedative hypnotic in psychiatric conditions. *Br J Psych* 1947; xciv: 108.

Pomet Pierre. A compleat history of druggs, written in French by Monsieur Pomet, ... to which is added what is further observable on the same subject, from Messrs. Lemery, and Tournefort, divided into three classes, vegetable, animal and mineral; ... illustrated with above four hundred copper cutts ... Done into English from the originals. ... Vol. 1. London, 1712. 2 vols. Based on information from English Short Title Catalogue. Eighteenth Century Collections Online. Gale Group. http://0-galenet.galegroup.com.libsys. wellcome.ac.uk/servlet/ECCO

Prescott L. Phenacetin nephropathy. *BMJ* 1970; 4(5733): 493.

Presse Méd 1956; 64: 175.

Prien RF. A brief history of the New Clinical Drug Evaluation Unit meeting. How it began. *Psychopharmacology Bulletin* 1995; 31(1): 3–5.

Prieto CC, Pol EN, Eiras AB, Iglesias LC, Becerra EP and Zúñiga VL. Hepatitis tóxica por cincofeno: descripción de tres enfermos. Os médicos são avisados a prescreverem esta droga somente a adultos e não por mais de uma semana *Med Clin (Barc)* Jun 15 1991; 97(3): 104-6. De modo geral as autoridades regulatórias nacionais consideram que produtos mais novos são alternativas mais seguras para a maior parte dos pacientes, portanto tem sido retirado do mercado e restrito a pacientes que não respondem a outras drogas. [Toxic hepatitis due to cincophen: description of three patients. Doctors are advised to prescribe this drug for adults only, and not for longer than a week *Med Clin (Barc)* Jun 15 1991; 97(3): 104–6. Generally, the national regulatory authorities consider that more recent products are safer alternatives for the majority of patients, and therefore it (cincophen) has been withdrawn from the market and restricted to patients who do not respond to other drugs.]

Pringle J. 'The effects of hyoscyamus albus, or white henbane'. *Philosl Trans R Soc Lond* Vol. 47, (1751–52).

Prioreschi Plinio. A History of Medicine. Horatio Press, 1996.

Quétel C. The history of Syphilis. Polity Press 1992 Translated by Braddock J and Pike P. Accessed 2nd February 2009. http://www.dahsm.medschool.ucsf.edu/history/DiseasePDF/6_Quetel.pdf

Quincy John. Pharmacopœia officinalis & extemporanea. Or, a complete English dispensatory, in four parts. By John Quincy, M.D.... The sixth edition, much enlarged and corrected London, 1726. Based on information from English Short Title Catalogue. Eighteenth Century Collections Online. Gale Group.http://0-galenet.galegroup.com.libsys.wellcome.ac.uk/servlet/ECCO

Raffel S, Swink R, Lampton T. The influence of chorphenesin carbamate and carisoprodol on psychological test score. *Curr Ther Res* 1969; 11: 553–60.

Rainsford KD. Aspirin and Related Drugs. Routledge. UK. 2004.

Rawlins MD and Jefferys DB. United Kingdom product licence applications involving new actice substances, 1987-1989: their fate after appeals. *Br J Clin Pharmacol* 1993; 35: 599–602.

Rayoux J. Dissertatis Epistolarius de Cicuta, strammoniuio, hyoscyamus et aconito' *London Medical Journal* volume 1, 293.

Reeves RR and Parker JD. Somatic dysfunction during carisoprodol cessation: evidence for a carisoprodol withdrawal syndrome. *J Am Osteopath Assoc* 2003; 103: 75–80.

Rene RM and Mellenkoff SM. Renal insufficiency after oral administration of a double dose of cholecystographic medium–report of two cases. *New Engl J Med* 1959; 261: 589.

Renou F. Histoire de la pharmacie des Carmes à Bordeaux. De sa création à la disparition de sa préparation la plus célèbre: L'eau de Mélisse des Carmes. Thesis No. 86 Université Bordeaux 2–Victor Segalen. UFR des Sciences Pharmacie. December 2005.

Reynolds TB, Lapin AC, Peters RL and Yamahiro HS. Puzzling jaundice.

Probable relationship to laxative ingestion. *JAMA* 1970; 211: 86–90.

Rich MI, Ritterhoff RJ and Hoffman RJ. A fatal case of aplastic anaemia following chloramphenicol (Chloromycetin) therapy. *Ann Intern Med* 1950; 33; 1459–67.

Richet C. Ancient humorism and modern humorism. *BMJ* 1910; October 1st: 911–916

Richet C. *Presse Méd* 1919.

Riggins HM and Hinshaw HC. The Streptomycin–tuberculosis research project of the American Trudeau Society. *Am Rev Tuberc* 1947; 56:168–73.

Rijhsinghani KS, Abrahams C, Swerdlow MA, Rao KVN and Ghose T. Induction of neoplastic lesions in the livers of C57BL × C3HF1 mice by chloral hydrate. *Cancer Detect Prev* 1986; 9(3–4): 279-288.

Ring ME. The advent of printing as an obstacle to the development of rational medicine. *Bull Med Libr Assoc.* 1972; 60(3): 467–470.

Rios Sanchez et al. Agranulocytosis; analisi de 29 episodios en 19 pacientes. *Rev Invest Clin* 1971; 23, 29.

Rives HF, Ward BB and Hicks ML. A fatal reaction to methapyrilene (Thenylene). *JAMA* 1949; July 24th, 1022–4.

Robertson AR and Fleming AG. Mercury poisoning with anaphylactic phenomena and fatal issue fifty-two days later. *Can Med Assoc J* 1918; 8(4): 342–351.

Robinson Nicholas. A new treatise of the venereal disease. In three parts... to which is added a particular dissertation upon the nature and properties of mercury. 1736

Roblot F, Montaz L, Delcoustal M, Robert R, Chavagnat J J, Morichaud G, Scepi M, Roblot P, Gaboriau E and Patte D. Unite d'accueil des urgences, Hopital Jean Bernard, Poitiers. Datura: an easily accessible hallucinogen, a poisoning to be evoked. Apropos of 10 cases. *Rev Med Interne*. 1993; 14(10): 956.

Roche. Personal communication 18th November 2009.

Rodin FH. Cataracts following the use of dinitrophenol: a summary of thirty-two cases. *Calif West Med* April 1936; 44(4): 276–279.

Rogers GA. Addiction to glutethimide (Doriden). *Am J Psychiatry* Dec 1958; 115(6): 551–2.

Rose G. Bias. *Br J Clin Pharmacol* 1982; 13:157–162.

Rosenberg Z. Treating the undesirable effects of radiation and chemotherapy with Chinese medicine, from 'Journal of Chinese Medicine 1997; 55: 29-30 http://www.consumerhealthreviews.com/Articles/ChineseHerbs/TreatingChemoandRadiation.htm. Accessed 25th February 2008.Accessed 25th February 2008.

Rosenthal RL and Blackman A. Bone marrow hypoplasia following the use of chloramphenicol eye drops. *JAMA* 1965; 191: 36–7.

Ross JJ. Shakespeare's chancre: Did the bard Have syphilis? *Clin Infect Dis* 2005; 40: 399–404.

Royal Medical and Chirurgical Society. Report of the Scientific Committee on the uses and the physiological, therapeutical and toxical effects of chloroform, as well as into the best mode of administering it, and of obviating any ill consequences resulting from its administration'. *Medico-Chirurgical Transactions* 1864; 47: 323–442.

Ruef C, Blaser J, Maurer P, Keller H, Follath F. Miscellaneous antibiotics. In: Dukes MNG, editor. *Meyler's side effects of drugs.* 14th ed. Amsterdam: Elsevier; 2000. pp. 848.

Rutstein DD, Stebbins RB, Cathacart RT and Harvey RM. The absorption and excretion of streptomycin in human chronic typhoid carriers. *J Clin Invest* 1945; 24(6): 898–909.

Saad B, Azaizeh H, Abu-Hijleh G and Said O. Safety of traditional Arab herbal medicine. *Evid Based Complement Alternat Med.* 2006; 3(4): 433–439.

Salter J. On the treatment of asthma by sedatives. *BMJ* 1859; s1-4:794

Salvarsen Commitee. Toxic effects of arsenbenzol preparations. *BMJ* 1922; 2(3213): 184.

Samorini G. New data on the ethnomycology of psychoactive mushrooms. *Int J Medicinal Mushrooms* 2001; 3: 257–278.

Sandler DP, Smith JC, Weinberg CR, Buckalew VM, Dennis VW, Blythe WB and Burgess WP. Analgesic use and chronic renal disease. *N Engl J Med* 1989; 320: 1238–43.

Saper RB, Kales SN, Paquin J, et al. Heavy metal content of Ayurvedic herbal medicine products. *JAMA* 2004; 292: 2868–73.

Sarker SK, Forohit SA, Sharma JN, Chawla MP and Gupta DN. Stevens-Johnson syndrome caused by

413

Streptomycin. *Tubercle* 1982; 63: 137.

Savage DC. Neurotoxic effects of piperazine. *BMJ* June 24 1967; 2(5555): 840–1.

Scarborough J. Drugs and narcotics in history. Ed. Roy Porter and Mekuláš, Cambridge University Press. 1945.

Schabez. Thesis, Tübergen 1817. Horn's Archives. *Archiv Für Mediz.* Erfahring, 1825.

Schadelijke invloeden van tetracycline op de vorming van melkgebit en blijvend gebit [Harmful influences of tetracycline on the formation of milk teeth and adult teeth]. Nederlands tijdschrift voor geneeskunde, Ned-Tijdschr-Geneeskd, 9 Oct 1965; 109(41): 1909–10, ISSN: 0028–2162.

Schatz A, Bugie E and Wakeman SA. Streptomycin, a substance exhibiting antibiotic activity against gram positive and gram negative bacteria, *Proc Soc Expl Biol* 1944; 55: 66–69.

Schindel L. Placebo-induced side effects. Drug Induced Disease, Volume 3, 1968 Eds. Meyler L & Peck HM, Ex. Med. Am. p323–330.

Schmiedeberg. *Practitioner* 1885; vol xxxv.

Schreiner GE. Nephrotoxicity and diagnostic agents. *JAMA* 1966; 196: 413.

Schultz W. Über eigenartige Halserkrankungen [On unusual ailments of the throat]. *Dtsch Med Wschr* 1922; 48: 1495.

Schwank R and Friedlanderova B. Severe drug reaction of Stevens-Johnson syndrome type with transition to Lyelle's syndrome following sulphamethoxydiazine therapy of a child. *Cesk Dermatol* June 1977; 52(3):187–92.

Schweiz Med Wschr 1956; 86: 946.

Scott AJ. Drug Anaphylaxis: An illustrative case. *Cal State J Medicine* 1915; 8(5): 189–190.

Scott DF. Pepys and blood transfusion? *BMJ* 2004; 328: 334.

Scrip No. 1128, August 13th 1986, 22.

Scrip. Consumerists draw up own 'blacklist.' *Scrip* September 1982; 831.

Seifert O. Die Nebenwirkungen der Modernen Arzneimittel. Würzburg kabitzsch 1915.

Selbie FR. Experimental production of sarcoma with Thorotrast. *Lancet* 1936; 2: 847.

Selbie FR. Tumours in rats and mice following Thorotrast. *Br J Expertl Path* 1938; 19: 100–107.

Severinus Petrus. Idea Medicinae Philosophicae . Bâle, 1571.

Shapiro S and Lehman L. A case of agranulocytosis following ingestion of cincophen. *Am J Med Sc,* November 1936; 192: 705–709.

Shelton JD. The Harm of 'First, Do No Harm' Washington, DC. *JAMA* 2000; 284: 2687–2688.

Sherratt A. Sacred and Profane Substances: the Ritual Use of Narcotics in Later Neolithic Europe in Sacred and Profane. Eds. P Garwood, R Jennings, J Skeates and D Toms. Oxford: Oxford Committee for Archaeology. Sacred and Profane Conference Proceedings. 1991.

Sherratt A. Alcohol and its Alternatives: Symbol and Substance in Pre-Industrial Cultures. In Consuming Habits: Drugs in History and Anthropology (Goodman J, Lovejoy PE and Sherratt A, Eds.). London, Routledge. 1995.

Shervette RE et al. Jimson 'loco' weed abuse in adolescents. *Pediatrics* 1979; 63: 520–3.

Shryock RH. Citation of verses in the Richmond Enquirer, March 5, 1825. The Development of Modern Medicine. New York: Alfred A. Knopf; 1947.

Sibson LMG. Death from the vapour of chloroform, *London Medical Gazette* 1848; xlii: 109.

Silver S. A new drug in dinitrophenol therapy. *JAMA* 1936; 106: 1085–1096.

Silvestri F. Policlinico Rome. *JAMA* 1914; 177: 1209

Simon MA and Kaufman M. Death following sufathiazole therapy. *Can Med Assoc J* 1943; 48: 23–27.

Sims J. Comunications relative to the datura strammonium, or thorn-apple a cure or relief of asthma. *Edin Med Surg J* 1812; 8: 364.

Singer PN. Galen: selected works. Translated ith noteds written by PN Singer.(Oxford World Classics) 1997. 2002

Singh C. Adverse effects of aspirin: guidebook for medicine, reference, and research.

Sjöstrom H and Nilsson R. Thalidomide and the Power of the Drug Companies. Penguin, 1972 page 192.

Sloane H. An account of symptoms arising from eating the seeds of henbane, with their care, etc. and some occasioned remarks. *Phil. Trans* 2, 1745.

Smalley W. Drug Safety: can simple interventions be effective in a complex world? *Pharmacoepidemiol Drug Saf* 2001; 10: 209–210.

Smick KM, Condit PK, Proctor RL and Sutcher V. Fatal aplastic anemia: an epidemiological study of its relationship to the drug chloramphenicol. *J Chronic Dis* 1964; 17: 859–914.

Smith CM. 'Origin and Uses of Primum Non Nocere—Above All, Do No Harm'. *J Clin Pharmacol* 2005; 45: 371–377.

Smith OC and O'Donnell J. The process of new drug discovery and development. Informa Health Care, 2006.

Smith RG. Assuring the safety of new drugs. *Public Health Rep* 1956; 71(6): 590–3.

Smyth MJ. Carcinogenic effects of thorium. *BMJ* March 23 1940; 1(4133): 504–505.

Sneader W. Drug Discovery. A History. John Wiley & Sons Ltd. 2005.

Snow J. On chloroform and other anaesthetics: their action and administration. The Classics of Medicine series. 1989.

Solecki RS. Shanidar IV, a Neanderthal flower burial in northern Iraq. *Science* 1975; 190 (28): 880.

Sommer JD. 'The Shanidar IV 'Flower Burial': A Re-evaluation of Neanderthal Burial Ritual. *Cambridge Archæological Journal* 1999; 9: 127–129.

Spencer WG. Blood-letting – its past and present use. *Proc R Soc Med* 1927 April 7th; 1547–1574.

Spier J, Cluff LE and Urry WD. Aplastic anaemia following administration of Thorotrast. *J Lab Clin Med* 1947; 321: 147–153.

Spillane JF. Discovering cocaine: an historical perspective on drug development and regulation. *Drug Inf J* 1995; 29: 1519S–1528S.

Spriet-Pourra C and Auriche M. Drug withdrawal from sale. 2nd edition, Richmond – PJB publications 1994.

Spühler O and Zollinger HU. Die chronische-interstitielle Nephritis [chronic interstitial nephritis]. *Zeitsche Klin Med* 1953; 151: 1–50.

Sramek JJ and Khajawall A. Glutethimide abuse. *Am J Psychiatry* 1982; 139(2): 257.

Stang Can J Clin Pharmacol 1998; 4: 53.

Stathakou NP, Stathakou GP, Damianaki SG, Ioannou ET, and Stavarianeas NG. Empedocles' bio-medical comments: A precursor to modern science. www.priory.com/homol/empedocles.htm. Accessed 22nd January 2009.

Stearn WT. Milano: Il Polifilo, 1979.

Steinberg D, Avigan J and Feigelson EB. Effects of triparanol (MER-29) on cholesterol biosynthesis and on blood sterol levels in man. J Clin Invest 1961; 40(5): 884-893.

Stephens MDB. in Chapter 1 of 'Stephens' Detection of New Adverse Drug Reactions'. Eds J. Talbot and P. Waller, 2004.

Stephens MDB. MD thesis. The detection of new adverse drug reactions. London 1985.

Stephens MDB. Pharmaceutical company viewpoint. In Monitoring for adverse drug reactions. Ed.Walker SR and Goldberg A. MTP Press Ltd. 1984. 119 127.

Stephens MDB. Deliberate drug rechallenge. Hum Toxicol 1983;2: 573–577.

Stern R. Indexed surgical procedures. Ann Surg 1891; 13(1): 72.

Sternlieb P and Eisman SH. Toxic hepatitis and agranulocytosis due to cincophen. Ann Int Med 1957; 47: 826.

Stewart DD. Therapeutic Gazette 15th February 1894.

Stolberg M. Inventing the randomized double-blind trial: the Nuremberg salt test of 1835. J R Soc Med 2006; 99: 642–643.

Stolley PD. The risks of phenacetin use. N Engl J Med 1991; 324 (3): 191–193.

Stone E. An account of the success of the bark of the willow in the cure of agues. Phil Trans R Soc 1763; 53: 195–200.

Stone J and Matthews J. Complementary Medicine and the Law. Oxford University Press. 1996.

Stoner HB, Barnes JM and Duff JI. Studies on the toxicity of tin compounds. Br J Pharmacol Chemotheray 1955; 10: 16–25.

Störck A. An essay on the internal use of thorn-apple, henbane and monkshood, which are shown to be safe and efficacious remedies. 1763.

Stormont RT. New program of operation for evaluation of drugs. JAMA 1955; 158(13): 1170–3.

Stratman-Thomas WK. The lure of medical history: Girolamo Fracastoro (1478-1553) – and syphilis. Californian and Western Medicine 1930 October; 739-742.

Stricker. Ueber die Resultate der Behandlung der Polyarthritis mit Salicyläure [On the results of treating polyarthritis with salicylic acid]. Berl. Klin. Wchsr. 1876; 1: 15, 99.

Strom B. What is Pharmacoepidemiology? In Pharmacoepidemiology. 3rd Edition, 2000.

Sughoff K. The earliest printed literature on syphilis being ten tractates from the years 1495-1498. R Lier & Co. (Florence) 1925. http://openlibrary.org/b/OL14733832M. Accessed 5th January 2009.

Sukh Dev. Prime Ayurvedic Plant Drugs. Anamaya, 2006.

Sutrisno R. The SEES theory. Herbal Review 1978 February; 17–8.

Suzuki H. The history of iatrogenic diseases in Japan. In: Ed. Soda T. Drug Induced Suffering. Excerpta Medica. 1980, 35-43.

Swainson Isaac. Mercury stark naked. A series of letters, addressed to Dr. Beddoes; stripping that poisonous mineral of its medical pretensions; ... By Isaac Swainson, ... London, 1797. Based on information from English Short Title Catalogue. Eighteenth Century Collections Online. Gale Group. http://0-galenet.galegroup.com.libsys.wellcome.ac.uk/servlet/ECCO

Swediauer F. (Franz). Practical observations on the more obstinate and inveterate venereal complaints By J. Schwediauer, M.D. London, 1784. Based on information from English Short Title Catalogue. Eighteenth Century Collections Online. Gale Group. http://0-galenet.galegroup.com.libsys.wellcome.ac.uk/servlet/ECCO

Sydenham Thomas. The whole works of that excellent practical physician Dr. Thomas Sydenham wherein not only the history and cures of acute diseases are treated of, after a new and accurate method: but also the shortest and safest way of curing most chronical diseases/translated from the Latin by John Pechy, London 1696

Tainter ML, Cutting WC and Stockton AB. Use of dinitrophenol in nutritional disorders: A critical survey of clinical results. Am J Public Health Nations Health 1934 October; 24(10): 1045–1053.

Talbot CH. Some notes on Anglo-Saxon medicine. Med Hist 1965; 992);156–169

Taylor JM. Early botanists and the introduction of drug specifics. Bull NY Acad Med 1979; 55(7): 684-699.

Temple RJ. The clinical pharmacologist in drug regulation: the US perspective. Br J Clin Pharmacol 1996: 42: 73–79.

The History of Taxonomy 1583–1690 http://www.bihrmann.com/caudiciforms/DIV/ Accessed 25th February 2008.

The James Lind Library, which was created by The Library and Information Services Department of the Royal College of Physicians of Edinburgh.

The Project Gutenberg eBook, The Oldest Code of Laws in the World, by Hammurabi, King of Babylon, Translated by CHW Johns.

The Southwest School of Botanical Medicine http://www.swsbm.com/homepage/. Accessed 25th February 2008.

Thiselton-Dyer TF. The Folklore of Plants, Llanerch Publishers, Lampeter 1994; p315.

Thompson CJS. Mystery and Art of the Apothecary. Kessinger Publishing, 2003.

Thomson S, Steele JC and Reid G. A Dictionary of Domestic Medicine and Household Surgery. Charles Griffin & company. 1896.

Tibi Selma. The Medicinal Use of opium in Ninth-Century Baghdad. 2006.

Tibi Selma. Al-Razi and Islamic medicine in the 9th century. J R Soc Med 2006; 99: 206–7.

Tognoni G, Begher C, Colombo F, Inzalaco M, Mancia M and Masera G. Present limitations and future possibilities of drug surveillance in Italy. In Drug Induced Suffering. Excerpta Medica. Ed. T Soda. 1980.

Tomatis L. Experimental chemical carcinogenesis: Fundamental and predictive role in protecting health in the 1930s–1970s. Eur J Oncol 2006; 11(1): 5–1.

Tsubaki T, Toyokura Y and Tsukagoshi H. Subacute myelo-optic-neuropathy following abdominal symptoms. Jpn J Med 1965; 4(3): 181–4.

Tyson TL. Agranulocytosis following pyrithyldione (Presidon) therapy. JAMA September 10th 1949;141(2):128.

Unschuld P. Medicine in China, a history of pharmaceutics. University of California Press, 1986.

415

Unschuld P. Chinese medicine. Paradigm Publications, Massachusetts, 1998.

Unschuld P. Forgotten tradition of ancient Chinese medicine; a Chinese view from the 18th century. The I-hsüeh Yüan Liu Lun of 1757 by Hsü Ta-Ch'un. Paradigm Publications 1998.

Van Swearingen P. Placidyl and pulmonary odema. Ann Inter Med 1976; 84: 614–15.

Van-der-Linden-F-P. Detrimental effects of tetracycline on the formation of the deciduous and permanent teeth. Ned Tijdschr Geneeskd. 1965 Oct 9; 109(41): 1909–10.

Vane JR, Botting RM. Aspirin and other salicylates. London: Chapman and Hall Medical Publishers; 1992.

Vanherweghem J-L and Even-Adin D. Epidemiology of analgesic nephropathy in Belgium. Clin Nephrology 1982; 17(3): 129–133.

Venning G. Identification of adverse reactions to new drugs. I: What have been the important adverse reactions since thalidomide. BMJ 1983:286: 199–202.

Venning G. Identification of adverse reactions to new drugs. II (continued): How were the important adverse reactions to new drugs discovered and with what delays? BMJ 1983 286; 365–368.

Venning G. Identification of adverse reactions to new drugs. III: Alerting processes and early warning systems. BMJ 1983; 286: 458–460.

Venning G. Identification of adverse reactions to new drugs. IV: Verification of suspected adverse reactions. BMJ 1983; 286: 544–547.

Venning G. Aplastic anaemia due to phenylbutazone. BMJ 1957; 2(5037): 146.

Vépan. Gaz Medic. De Strassb. 1865.

Veterans Administration. The effects of streptomycin on tuberculosis in man (Preliminary Statement) JAMA 1947; 135(10): 634–641.

Violini IF, Schwartz SO, Greenspan I, Ehrlich L, Gonner JA and Felsenfeld O. Hemopoietic changes during Chloromycetin administration. Proc Central Soc Clin Research 1949; 22: 74–75.

Virchow R. Krankheitswesen und Krankheitsurmache [The Nature and Causes of Disease]. Arch für Pathol Anat und Physiol und klinische Med. 1880; 79; Bd. H.1, p10.

Vogl A. The discovery of the organic mercurial diuretics. Amer Heart J 1950; 39:881.

Volmink J. The willow as a Hottentot remedy for rheumatic fever. In: The James Lind Library. http://www.jameslindlibrary.org/trial_records/19th_Century/maclagan/maclagan-commentary.html Accessed 25th February 2008.

Wade OL. Adverse Reactions to Drugs. William Heineman Medical Books, 1970.

Waite AE. Alchemists through the ages. Rudolf Steiner Publications, 1970.

Walch A. An In-Depth Look at The Import Drugs Act of 1848. Harvard Law School, Class of 2002.

Waldman RJ, Hall WN and McGee H. Aspirin as a risk factor in Reye's syndrome. JAMA 1972; 247(22): 3089–94.

Walker GF. Blindness during streptomycin and chloramphenicol therapy. Brit J Ophthalmol 1951; 45: 555–559.

Walker RS and Lintom AL. Phenethyl diguanide: A dangerous side effect. BMJ 1959; 2: 1958–9.

Walker RS, Linton AL and Thomson WS. Mode of action and side-effects of phenformin hydrochloride. BMJ 1960; Nov 26; 2(5212): 1567–1569.

Waller P and Suvarna R. Is aspirin a cause of Reye's syndrome? Drug Saf 2005; 27(1): 71–74.

Waller PC, Wood SM, Langman MJS and Breckenridge AM et al. Review of company postmarketing surveillance studies. BMJ 1992; 304: 1470–1472.

Wallerstein RO, Condit PK, Kasper CK, Brown JW and Morrison FR. Statewide study of chloramphenicol therapy and fatal aplastic anaemia. JAMA 1969; 208(11): 2045–2050.

Walsh JJ. The earliest modern law for the regulation of the practice of medicine. JAMA 1908; 1: 388-9.

Wang JX. The earliest published pharmacopoeia in the world. J. Traditional Chinese Medicine 1987; 7(2): 155-156.

Warkany J and Hubbard M. Mercure dans l'urine des enfants atteints d'acrodynia. Lancet 29th May 1948; 829.

Warkany J. Adverse mercurial reactions in the form of acrodynia and related conditions. Am J Dis Child 1951; 81: 335.

Warner JH. From specificity to universalism in medical therapeutics. In History of Therapy: Proceedings of the 10th International Symposium on the Comparative History of Medicine—East and West. Ed. Yosio Kawakth, Shizo Sakai and Yasuo Cirtsuka. September 8th–15th 1985.

Waugh MA. Role played by Italy in the history of syphilis. Br J Vener Dis 1982; 58(2): 92–95.

Waxman HA. A history of adverse drug experiences: Congress had ample evidence to support restrictions on the promotion of prescription drugs. Food and Drug Law Journal 2003; 58(3):

Weatherall M. Drug treatment and the rise of pharmacology. In The Cambridge Illustrated History of Medicine ED. Roy Porter, Cambridge University Press, 1996.

Welge-Lussen A and Wolfensberaed M. Reversible anosmia after amikacin therapy. Arch Otolaryngology. Head and neck surgery 2003; 129: 1331–5.

West Midlands Centre for Adverse Drug reactions. The Pharmacovigilance Timeline.. http://adr.org.uk/?page_id=94. Accessed 25th February 2008.

Westerhom B. The balance between benefit and risk: The dilemma of the drug legislator. In: Soda T Ed. Drug-Induced Sufferings, Excerpta Medica. 1980, 249–258.

Wetzels JFM. Thorotrast toxicity: the safety of gadolinium compounds. Neth J Med 2007; 65(8): 276-278.

White RHR and Standen OD. Piperazine in the treatment of threadworms. BMJ 1953; 2: 1272.

White William, M.R.C.S. Observations and experiments on the broad-leaved willow bark, illustrated with cases. By W. White, ... Bath, 1798. Based on information from English Short Title Catalogue. Eighteenth Century Collections Online. Gale Group. http://0-galenet.galegroup.com.libsys.wellcome.ac.uk/servlet/ECCO

Willcox W. Toxic jaundice. BMJ 1931; 4th April: 595–7.

Willcox W. Toxicology in relation to medical practice. BMJ 1928; 24th march: 504–5.

Withering William. An account of the foxglove, and some of its medical uses: with practical remarks on dropsy, and other diseases. By William Withering, M.D. ... Birmingham, 1785. Based on information from English Short Title Catalogue. Eighteenth Century Collections Online. Gale Group. http://0-galenet.galegroup.com.libsys. wellcome.ac.uk/servlet/ECCO

Whittet TD. Pepperers, Spicers and Grocers–Forerunners of the apothecaries. *Pro Roy Soc Med.*1968; 61: 801-806.

WHO Drug Information 1997; 11: 4.

WHO Pharmaceutical Newsletter. Thiomersal 2003; 2: 8.

WHO Pharmaceuticals Newsletter No1, 2002.

WHO. The importance of Pharmacovigilance. Safety monitoring of medicinal products. 2002.

WHO, 1969. Pharmacovigilance international: role de l'hôpital, rapport d'une reunion de l'OMS [tenue á Genéva du 18 auguste à 23 novembre 1968].

Wiholm B-E, Kelly JP, Kaufman D, Issaragrisil S, Levy M, Anderson T and Shapiro S. Relation of aplastic anaemia to use of chloramphenicol eye drops in two international case-control studies. *BMJ* 1998; 316: 666.

Willcox W. The uses and dangers of hypnotic drugs other than alkaloids. *BMJ* 1934; 1: 415–418.

Willcox WH and Webster J. The toxicology of Salvarsan. *BMJ* April 1st 1916.

Williams KJ. The introduction of chemotherapy with arsphenamine – the first magic bullet. The James Lind Library (www.jameslindlibrary.org). Accessed Monday 2nd February 2009© Keith Williams, 2009.

Williams, Guy R. The Age of Miracles: Medicine and Surgery in the Nineteenth Century (Academy Chicago Publishers 1981).

Winek CL, Fochtman FW, Trogus WJ Jr, Fusia EP and Shanor SP. Methapyrilene toxicity. *Clin Toxicol* 1977; 11(3): 287–94.

Withington ET. Roger Bacon 'On the errors of physicians' Introduced and translated by ET Withington. In Essays on the history of medicine presented to Karl Sudhoff on the occasion of his seventieth birthday November 26th 1923 London. Oxford University Press.

Witt de. *Medical and Physical Journal* 1799; 1 (1): 84.

Witthauer. Aspirin. *Die Heilkunde*, April 1899 and *BMJ* 68, October 21st 1899.

Wohlgemuth J. Üeber Aspirin (Acetylsalicylsäure) [On aspirin (acetylsalicylic acid)]. *Therap. Monatshefte* 1899; 3: 276–8.

Wohlgemuth, *BMJ*, July 1, 1899, p.34c.

Wong A. A reappraisal of antipyretic and analgesic drugs. *WHO Pharmaceuticals Newsletter* 2002; 1: 15.

Wood A. A new method for treating neuralgia by the direct application of opiates to painful points. Edinburgh *Medical and Surgical Journal*. 1855.

Woodall J. The Surgeon's Mate or Military & Domestic Surgery, London, 1639, 256

Woodville William. Medical botany, containing systematic and general descriptions, with plates, of all the medicinal plants, indigenous and exotic, comprehended in the catalogues of the Materia Medica, as published by the Royal Colleges of Physicians of London and Edinburgh: accompanied with a circumstantial detail of their medicinal effects, and of the diseases in which they have been most successfully employed. By William Woodville, ... In three volumes. ... Vol. 1. London, 1790-93. 3 vols. Based on information from English Short Title Catalogue. Eighteenth Century Collections Online. Gale Group. http://0-galenet.galegroup.com. libsys.wellcome.ac.uk/servlet/ECCO

Worster-Drought C. Atophan poisoning. *BMJ* 1923; 1:148–149.

Wulff HR. The language of medicine. *BMJ* 2004; 97: 187–188.

Wysowski DK and Swartz L. Adverse drug event surveillance and drug withdrawals in the United States, 1969-2002. *Arch Intern Med* 27th June 2005; 165: 13611-369.

Yamagiwa, K. & Ichikawa, K. Experimentelle Studie über die Pathogenese der Epithelialgeschwülste. *Mitt. Med. Fak. Kaiserl. Univ. Tokio* 15, 295-344 (1915).

Yohai D and Barnett SH. Absence and atonic seizures induced by piperazine. *Pediatr Neurol* 1989; 5(6); 393–394.

Young NS. Introduction. *Eur J Haematol. Supplement.* 1996; 60(57): 6–8.

Zhu You-Ping, Toxicity of the Chinese herb Mu Tong {Aristichia manshuriensis} (What history tells us), *Adv Drug React Toxicol Rev* 2002; 21(4): 171–177.

Zintel HA, Flippen HF, Nichols AC, Wiley MM and Rhoads JE. Studies on streptomycin in man 1. Absorption, distribution, excretion and toxicity. *Am.*

J. Med Sci 1945; 210: 421–430.

Ziporin T. The Food and Drug Administration: how 'those regulations' came to be. *JAMA* 1985; 254(15): 2037–2046.

Ziporin T. AMA's Bureau of Investigation exposed fraud. *JAMA* 1985; 254(15): 2043

Zolov B. Agranulocytosis resulting from sandostene *J Maine Med Ass* 1958; 49: 335.

Index

426

Extra Reference Section

I apologise to the reader for the necessity of adding a second reference section. Numerous references in the text are not matched in the reference section due to my inept proofreading.

Aspirin references will be found on pages 283 – 292.

Abramowitz EW. Erythema multiforme associated with cutaneous pigmentation (Melanin) *J Cutan Dis* 1918; 36: 11.

Aery L. The symptoms, nature, causes and cure of the essera, or nettle-rash: To which are added some general observations on the cure of cutaneous diseases. Whitehaven : J. Ware, 1774.

Akabane T. Mercury. In: Behrman RE, Vanaughan VC (ed) Nelson Textbook of Pediatrics. WB Saunders Company 1983.

Albahary C. Maladies médicamenteuses d'ordre thérapeutique et accidental. Masson 1953.

Alexander HL. Reactions with drug therapy. WB Saunders Company 1955.

Almkvist J. Ueber merkurielle Dermatosen; klinische, histologische und experimentelle Studien, *Arch. f. Derm. u. Syph.*, 1922, 141:342; also, Quecksilberschiidigungen, Handbuch der Haut und Geschlechtskrankheiten, Berlin, 1928, v. 18, p. 178; also, Aus der Geschichte der Quecksilbersehadigung, Dorm. Wchnschr., 1932, 95:1720.

Amelung W and Püntamann E. Clinical aspects and therapy of the so-called Contergan-polyneuropathy. *Der Nervenarzt,* 1966; . 37 (5): 189-99.

Ballet F. Hepatotoxicity in drug development: detection, significance and solutions, *J Hepatol* 1997; 26 (Suppl. 2): 26–36.

Baral J. Aspirin and the Reye syndrome. *Pediatrics* 1988; 82(1); 135.

Basch von S. Über die Messung des Blutdrucks am Menschen, *Zt. Klin. Med.,* 1880, 2:78-96.

Basilius Valentinus. The Triumphal Chariot of Antimony, 1685.

Baxby D. The genesis of Edward Jenner's Inquiry of 1798: a comparison of the two unpublished manuscripts and the published works. *Med Hist* 1985; 29(2): 193-199.

Bell B. A treatise on gonorrhoea virulenta and lues venere. Edinburgh, 1793.vol 2, 288.

Bergman et al., Epidemiology of adverse drug reactions to phenformin and metformin. *BMJ* 1978; 2 (6135):464-6.

Bignall JR, Crofton JW and Thomas JAB. Effect of Streptomycin on vestibular function. *BMJ* 1951; 1: 534-59.

Bilderback JB. Group of cases of unknown etiology and diagnosis *Northwest Med* 1989; 19:263.

Black J. The puzzle of pink disease. *JRSM* 1999; 92: 478-481.

BMJ 1959. Walker RS, Linton AL and Thomson WST. Mode of action and side-effects of phenformin hydrochloride. *BMJ* 1960; Nov: 1567.

Bonah C. L'affaire du Stalinon : et ses conséquences réglementaires, 1954-1959 «Sécurité sanitaire» et innovation thérapeutique en France il y a 50 ans *Rev Prat* 2007,Sep,15;57(13):1501-5;

Broadbent WH. The relation of pathology and therapeutics to clinical medicine. *BMJ* 1887 Feb 5th; 253.

Brock AJ. On the natural faculties / Galen; with an English translation by Arthur John Brock Cambridge, Mass. : Harvard University Press ; London : W. Heinemann, 1991.

Brunton TL. An address on the experiments on anaesthetics. *BMJ* 1890; Feb 15th : 347-360.

Burley DM. The rise and fall of Thalidomide. *Pharmaceut Med* 1988; 3: 231-237.

Burns R, Thomas DW and Barron VJ. Reversible encephalopathy possibly associated with Bismuth subgallate ingestion. *BMJ* 1974; 1:220-223.

Castle W et al., Serevent nationwide surveillance study: comparison of salmeterol with salbutamol in asthmatic patients who require regular bronchodilator treatment. *BMJ* 1993; 306:1034-7.

Cavers DF, The Food, Drug, and Cosmetic Act of 1938: Its Legislative History and Its Substantive Provisions, 6 Law & Cont. Probs. 2 (1939).

Chalmers I and Tröhler U. Helping physicians to keep abreast of the medical literature: Medical and Philosophical Commentaries, 1773-1795. *Annals Intern Med*, 2000; 133(3): 238-43.

Choulis NH and Dukes MNG. In *Meyler's Side-Effects of Drugs* 14th edition, Elsevier Science 2000: 686.

Cobert BL and Biron P. Pharmacovigilance from A to B. Blackwell Science 2002.

Committee of Principal Investigators. A cooperative trial in the primary prevention of ischaemic heart disease using clofibrate. *Br Heart J* 1978; 40(10): 1069-1118.

Cunningham ML. NTP Technical Report on the Hepatotoxicity Studies of the Liver Carcinogen Methapyrilene Hydrochloride National Toxicology Program Toxicity Report Series Number 46. 2000.

Dawson WR. A leechbook or collection of medical recipes of the fifteenth century. 1934.

Debré R Thieffry St, Brissand ED and H Noufflard Streptomycin and tuberculosis in children *BMJ* 1947; 2: 897.

Delay J and Pichol P. Medizinische Psychologie Thieme:Stuttgart.

Demaitre L. The Fasciculus Medicinae, translated by Luke Demaitre, Birmingham, The Classics of Medicine Library, 1988.

Dharmananda S. Kampo medicine. The Practice of Chinese Herbal Medicine in Japan http://www.schmerzinstitut-duesseldorf. de/uploads/media/Kampo_MFZD.pdf

Duchesney G. Le risque thérapeutique, prevention et traitement des accidents. Doing et Cire, 1954

Ellis H. Penicillin: the early days. *Int J Pharm Med* 1997; 11: 275-279.

Ewing Hunter J. Acute poisoning after one dose of Exalgin and Antipyrin combined. *BMJ* 1908; October 3rd: 1052

Fanconi, Botsztejn and Shenker. Réaction d'hypersensibilité à la medication mercurielle dans l'enfance avec une consideration particulière de la maladie du calomel. Clinique Infantile de Zurich. *Helv Paed Acta* 1947; Suppl. 2.

FDA. 2006 http://www.fda.gov/AboutFDA/WhatWeDo/History/ CentennialofFDA/TheLongStrugglefortheLaw/default.htm

Feer E. Eine eigenartige Neurose des vegetative Systems bei Kleinkinde. *Ergeb Inn Med Kinderheilkd* 1923;24:100-2.

Floyer J. The physician's pulse-watch or, an essay to explain the old art of feeling the pulse, and to improve it by the help of a pulse-watch. Printed for Sam. Smith and Benj. Walford at the Prince's Arms in St Paul's Churchyard 1707.

Freudenberg F. Über ein neues Arzneixanthem. *Berliner Klinische Wochenschrift* 1878: 630.

Fühner von H. Medizinische Toxikologie: Lehrbuch für Ärzte, Apotheker und Chemiker. Stuttgart: Georg Thieme

Gordon L. Green magic: flowers, plants, & herbs in lore & legend. Viking Press, 1977

Hanif M et al., Fatal renal failure caused by diethylene glycol in paracetamol elixir: the Bangladesh epidemic. *BMJ* 1993; 311: 88-91.

Hecht A and Janssen W. Diet drug danger déja vu. *FDA Consumer* 1987; 21(1):22-27.

Hess W, Eberlein HJ and Pöthe H. Fleher und gefahren: Zyanose durch eine medikamentös induzierte methemoglobinaemie *Anaesthetist* 1983; 32:124.

Hitch JM and Raleigh N. Neurotoxic symptoms following use of Asterol dihydrochloride. *JAMA* 1952; 150: 1004.

Horner WD, Jones RB and Boardman WW. Cataracts, Following the use of Dinitrophenol. *JAMA* 1935; 105: 108-110.

Hoyne AL and Larrimore GW. Sulfathiazole as a cause of death: report of patient with acute agranulocytosis. *JAMA* 1941; 117(16): 1353-1354

Jacob FH. Reviews. *BMJ* 1909; April 17th : 955

JAMA 1962. Laughlin RC and Carey TF. Cataracts in patients treated with triparanol *JAMA* 1962; 181: 339-40.

James A. Pfister JA. Behavioral Strategies for Coping with Poisonous Plants. Presented in "Grazing Behavior of Livestock and Wildlife." 1999. Idaho Forest, Wildlife & Range Exp. Sta. Bull. #70, Univ. of Idaho, Moscow, ID. Editors: K.L. Launchbaugh, K.D. Sanders, J.C. Mosley.

Jellinek EH. Chronic alpha-irradition of the nervous system from thorium dioxide. *JRSM* 2004; 97:345-349.

Juhlin L. The history of urticaria and angioedema. ESHDV Special annual lecture Geneva Oct 11th 2000 www. Bium.univ-paris5.fr/ sfhd/ecrits/urtic.htm

Kaddu AMM. *Meyler's Side Effects of Drugs Annual*; 2000; volume 12: 267.

Kline NS. Clinical experience with Iproniazid *J clin exp Psychopath.* 1958;19, Suppl 1:72.

Knopp J et al., Thalidomide in the treatment of sixty cases of chronic discoid lupus erythematosus. *Br J Dermatol* 1983; 108: 461-466.

Lagier G. Encephalopathies bismuthiques: situation dans les pays autres que la France. *Thérapie* 1980; 35(3): 315-317.

Lamotte E. Le Traité de la grande vertu de sagesse de Nāgārjuna. Leuvain,1966

Lasagna 1990. Brent RL. The prediction of human diseases from laboratory and animal tests for teratogenicity, carcinogenicity and mutagenicity. In: Lasagna L ed. *Controversies in Therapeutics.*. Philadelphia, PA: WB Saunders; 1980:134-150.

Le Quesne PM. Toxic substances and the nervous system: the role of clinical observation. *J Neurol Neurosurger Psychiatry* 1981; 44:1-8.

Leader 1976. D A Isenberg. General practitioners and barbiturates. BMJ Oct 1976; 2: 939 – 940.

Leader. The dangers of Amidopyrine. *BMJ* 1952; June 14th : 1292.

Lederer M and Rosenblatt P. Death during Sulfathiazole Therapy *JAMA* 1942; 119: 8-18.

Leube. In 'Untoward effects of drugs'. Lewin L. 1881, Geo. S Davis Published, Detroit. Page 45.

Lind J (1753). A treatise of the scurvy. In three parts. Containing an inquiry into the nature, causes and cure, of that disease. Together with a critical and chronological view of what has been published on the subject. Edinburgh: Printed by Sands, Murray and Cochran for A Kincaid and A Donaldson.

Lindsay DG et al., Cutaneous reaction to sulfamethoxypyrazine *Arch Derm (Chicago)* 1958; 78:299.

Magendie F. De l'influence de l'émétique sur l'homme et les animaux. Paris Crochard, 1813.

Martin–Bouyer G. Epidemiological study of encephalopathies myocloniques iatrogènes aux sels de bismuth *j Neurol Sci* 1976; 27: 133-143.

McKendrick JG. Report on the action of anaesthetics *BMJ* 1880; Dec 18th : 957-971.

McKeown T. Medical issues in historical demography. In: Clarke E (ed.). *Modern Methods in the History of Medicine.* London: Athlone Press, 1971, pp. 57–74. (Reprinted *Int J Epidemiol* 2005;34:515–20.)

Melvin KE and Howie RN. Fatal case of Stevens-Johnson syndrome after sulphamethoxypyridazine treatment. *BMJ* 1961; 2(5256): 869-70.

Midy. Les médications anti-goutteuses, à travers les âges. Broché Paris la piperazine midy 1910 sans auteur précisé . Edité par la piperazine midy à Paris en 1910

Morgan G. Reye's Syndrome: the beginning. *Journal of the National Reye's Syndrome Foundation* 1985; 5: 2-8.

Nelson CW. Early efforts at Mayo on the safety of therapeutic agents. *Mayo Clin Proc* 1997; 72: 798.

Ohler RI, Houghton JD and Moloney WC. Urethane toxicity. *N Eng J Med* 1950; Dec 21. 984-988.

Palfi G et al., Pre-Columbian Congenital Syphilis from the Late Antiquity in France. *International Journal of Osteoarchaeology* 1992; 2, 3: 245-261.

Patel PM et al. Anthraquinone laxatives and human cancer: an association in one case. *Postgrad Med J* 1989; 65: 216–17.

Piria R. Sur des nouveaux produits extraits de la salicin. *C R Acad Sci Paris.* 1838;6:620-624.

Piria R. Sur la salicine et les produits de sa decomposition. Mémoire lu l'Academie des Sciences de l'Institut de France le26 nov. 1838 Paris, Crochard Ed.

Pliny Gaius Secundia. Historia Naturalis. AD 77.

Rawlins MD and Thompson JW. Pathogenesis of adverse drug reactions. In Textbook of Adverse Reactions (Davies DM (ed.) Oxford University Press. 44.

Repertoire du Registre CC. *Maladies Vénériennes, et la Chambre Noble.* Arch Hosp Aa 104. Geneva: Archives d'Etat de Genève; 1761. p. 53 (18 January), 135–6 (6 December).

Report 1935. Special report of the Council. Council on Pharmacy and Chemistry. On July 6, 1935, the AMA's Council on Pharmacy and Chemistry reported dinitrophenol would not be included in its quasi-official list of acceptable remedies.

Reye RDK, Morgan G and Baral J, Encephalopathy and fatty degeneration of the viscera. A disease entity in childhood. *Lancet*, 1963;11:749-53.

Roberts R. Studies in Paediatrics: special issues. In *DIA Conference*, *15-16 April 1996 Assessing Safety of Investigational Drugs.*

Ross. Chemin E. Ross defends Haffkine: the aftermath of the vaccine-associated Mulkowal Disaster of 1902. *J History Med* 1991; 46: 201-218

Russell JC. British Medieval Population. Albuquerque 1948

Scott, J.M. The White Poppy. New York: Funk & Wagnells, 1969; 5, 46-82, 109-125.)

Selter P. Über Trophdermatoneurose. *Verh ges kinderheilkd 20* Versammiung. 1903; 45-50.

Shah RR. Thalidomide, drug safety and early drug regulation in the UK. *Adv Drug React Toxicol* 2001; 20(4): 188-255.

Shimoto and Aoki. Kushimoto H and Aoki T. Toxic erythema with generalized follicular pustules caused by streptomycin. *Arch Dermatol* 1981;117(7):444.

Silver S. A new danger in dinitrophenol therapy *JAMA* 1934; 103: 1058.

Singer C and Underwood EA. *A Short History of Medicine*, New York and Oxford: Oxford University Press, Library of Congress ID: 62-21080. (1962)

Smadel JE. Chloramphenicol (Chloromycetin) in the treatment of infectious diseases. *Am J Med.* 1949; 7: 671-685.

Smith S and Hollman A. Digoxin comes from digitalis lanata. *BMJ* 1996; 312:912 (6 April).

Standen and White. White HR and Standen OD Piperazine for Threadworms *BMJ* 1953; 2: 1272.

Staudt N and Rudert H. Das Stevens-Johnson-Syndrom nach Sulfamethoxydiazin-Behandlung.*HNO*, 1968; Aug 16(8): 242-3.

Stearn WT. Herbarium Apulei. *Il Polifilo,*Milano 1979.

Stephens CAL et al., Benefits and toxicity of phenylbutazone in rheumatoid arthritis. *JAMA* 1952; 150: 1084-1086.

Sterpellone L and Elsheikl MS. L'arte medica nei Califfati d'oriente e d'occidente. Saranno, Ciba Editzione, 1995: 45.

Swift H. Erythodema. In: *Australian Medical Congress Transactions.* 10th session New Zealand 1914; 575.

The Poh, 1985. Citizen Action Group Chapter 7. The politics of health 2nd January 2004 http://www.nader.org/history/bollier_chapter_7.html

Thiele H, Warkany J and Hubbard DM. *Journal of Pediatrics*, 1958; 42: 239.

Thomas KB. Chloroform: commissions and omissions. *Proc R Soc Med* 1974; 67(8): 723-730.

Thorwald J. Science and secrets of early medicine. Thames and Hudson, London 1965; 65.

Tilles G and Wallach D. Le traitement de la syphilis par le mercure: une histoire thérapeutique exemplaire. *Hist Sci Med* 1996; 30(4); 501-510.

Tschanz DW, The Arab Roots of European Medicine, in *Aramco World*, May/June 1997, pp. 31.

Turner M. An Account of the Extraordinary Medicinal Fluid, called Aether. (1761) Project Gutenberg Ebook. 12522

Venice. Nicholas Salernitana. Antidotarium. 1471.

Walford.L Retrospective Address of the Reading Pathological Society. *Prov Med Surg J* Sep 1845; s1-9: 589 – 591.

Waller AD. A demonstration on man of electromotive changes accompanying the heart's beat. *J Physiol* 1887; 8: 229-34.

Wax PM. Elixirs, diluents, and the passage of the 1938 Federal Food, Drug and Cosmetic Act. *Ann Intern Med* 1995; 122(6):456-61.

Webster C. Medicinae praxeos systema, ex Academiae Edinburgenae disputationibus inauguralibus praecipue depromptum, et secundum naturae ordinem digestum. 1780. 465 pp. Edinburgh.

Wechselmann W. Über die behandlung der Syphilis mit Dioxydiamido-arseno-benzol. *Berlin Klinische Wochenschrift* 1910; 47:1261-1264.

Weisburger JH. Carcinogenicity and mutagenicity testing, then and now. *Mutation Research. Reviews in mutation research* 1999: 437(2): 105-112.

Willcox W. The uses and dangers of hypnotic drugs other than alkaloids. *BMJ* 1934; 1: 415-418.

Wilson A and Shild HO. (1952). *Clark's Applied Pharmacology.* J & A Churchill Ltd.

Wright DJM. & Csonka GW. 1996 Syphilis. In *Oxford textbook of medicine*, 3rd edn (ed. D. J. Weatherall, J. G. G. Ledingham & Warrell DA, pp. 706–719. Oxford University Press.

Errata

p.14, line 16: 'Nipper' should be 'Nippur'

p.18, line 12: 'Caraka' should be 'Charaka'

p.51, line 13: Swap 'emetics' and 'purges'

p.78, line 23: 1741 should read 1775

p.113, line 26: 1656 should read 1546

p.133, line 16: For the first '$\mathfrak{z}$i' read '$\mathfrak{z}$ss'

p.219, line 10: (Marker drugs) should read (Part3)

p.222, line 12: 1838 should be 1938

p.265, The table entry 'Acrodynia' should show a cross for SED of Drugs 1952

p.278, line 22: for 'BP☐' read 'BP⇧'

p.278, line 23: for 'BP☐' read 'BP⇩'

p.283, References numbers after No.20 should be one less than stated in the tables

p.343, line 2: 'Hörein' should be 'Hörlein'

p.366, line 20: '0.5% of the cases' should be '5 cases'

p.378, line 1: '49' should be '50'

p.333, line 29: 'Lifespan' should be 78 years

p.346, line 28: 'Lifespan' should be 73 years

p.346, line 29: 'Delay in recognition' should be 88 years

p.345, line 23: 'Delay in recognition' should be 14 years

p.345, line 24: 'Delay in regulatory action' should be 28 years